Telemedicine in Dermatology

Hans Peter Soyer • Michael Binder
Anthony C. Smith • Elisabeth M.T. Wurm
Editors

Telemedicine in Dermatology

Springer

Editors
Hans Peter Soyer, M.D., F.A.C.D.
Dermatology Research Centre
The University of Queensland
School of Medicine
Princess Alexandra Hospital
Brisbane
Australia

Michael Binder, M.D.
Department of Dermatology
Medical University Vienna
Vienna
Austria

Anthony C. Smith, Ph.D., M.Ed., B.Nurs., RN
Centre for Online Health
School of Medicine
The University of Queensland

Queensland Children's Medical Research Institute
The University of Queensland
Royal Children's Hospital
Brisbane
Australia

Elisabeth M.T. Wurm, M.D.
Dermatology Research Centre
The University of Queensland
School of Medicine
Princess Alexandra Hospital
Brisbane
Australia

ISBN 978-3-642-44166-0 ISBN 978-3-642-20801-0 (eBook)
DOI 10.1007/978-3-642-20801-0
Springer Heidelberg Dordrecht London New York

Printed on acid-free paper

Springer is part of Springer Science+Business Media (www.springer.com)

Contents

Introduction to Teledermatology

1

Elisabeth M.T. Wurm, H. Peter Soyer,
and Anthony C. Smith

Core Messages

- Telemedicine is the use of telecommunication technologies for the exchange of medical information over a distance.
- Teledermatology is a subcategory within telemedicine providing specialist service by a dermatologist over a distance.
- Two modes of image and data transmission are commonly applied in teledermatology: store-and-forward systems (SAF) and real-time applications (RT).
- Store and forward is a technique in which information is sent to a data storage unit to be retrieved anytime.
- In real-time/live interactive telemedicine, information is delivered simultaneously with little or no delay.

E.M.T. Wurm (✉) • H.P. Soyer
Dermatology Research Centre, The University of Queensland, School of Medicine, Princess Alexandra Hospital, Brisbane, QLD, Australia
e-mail: e.wurm@uq.edu.au, lissy.wurm@gmail.com; p.soyer@uq.edu.au

A.C. Smith
Centre for Online Health, School of Medicine, The University of Queensland,

Queensland Children's Medical Research Institute
The University of Queensland
Royal Children's Hospital
Brisbane, Australia
e-mail: asmith@uq.edu.au

Definition

Telemedicine is an emerging field of medicine, providing access to medical knowledge that would otherwise not be available at a particular location. It is commonly defined as the use of telecommunication technologies for the exchange of medical information over a distance for the purpose of patient management (including triage, diagnosis, therapeutic suggestions, as well as follow-up) and medical education [1]. There is no consistent terminology, however. What is called telemedicine in this book might be called e-health, telehealth, online health, or simply "medicine at a distance" elsewhere. Teledermatology is a subcategory within telemedicine providing specialist service by a dermatologist to another health professional or directly to a subject with a skin disorder. Due to the visual oriented nature and the gaining importance of digital imaging in this speciality, dermatology is well suited for application in telemedicine, especially in dermoscopy, dermatopathology, and reflectance confocal microscopy [2]. A study performed in Norway listed teledermatology among priority telemedicine specialities for large-scale implementation [3] underlining the growing interest in this field.

Historic Review of Telemedicine and Teledermatology

The history of telemedicine is closely linked to the evolution of telecommunication and information technology. The term telemedicine itself was first used in

H.P. Soyer et al. (eds.), *Telemedicine in Dermatology*,
DOI 10.1007/978-3-642-20801-0_1, © Springer-Verlag Berlin Heidelberg 2012

1970, although the concept of transferring medical information over a distance itself is much older. In fact, distance communication has been used for centuries to convey messages comprising medical information by means of bonfires, telegraphs, and the telephone, for example [4]. However, it has been the ongoing technical evolution of the last two centuries that has led to a boom in telemedicine.

One of the first reported telemedicine projects was the "telecardiogram" in 1906, which transmitted electrocardiograms via a telephone network, created by Wilhelm Einthoven, the inventor of the electrocardiograph [5]. Between the 1950s and 1970s, a variety of telemedicine projects were performed. The Nebraska Project in the 1950s included interviews with psychiatric patients performed by doctors in another hospital 150 km away via a closed-circuit TV network. The NASA employed various other telemedicine projects in manned space flight, such as the remote monitoring of cardiovascular and other physiological parameters of astronauts in space crafts. Furthermore, NASA launched some terrestrial projects such as the STARPAHC (*Space Technology Applied to Rural Papago Health Care*) program for Papago Indians in Alaska [4].

The majority of these early telemedicine projects, however, did not stand the test of time due to their poor cost-effectiveness. It was not until the early 1990s that telemedicine experienced a revival, fuelled by rapid advancements and reduction of price in information and communication technology as well as digital imaging. Whereas such a Pubmed literature search 15 years ago, using the search phrase "telemedicine" in 1994, would have produced about 300 publications in total, by May 2011, there were nearly 13,000 entries under the search term "telemedicine" in Pubmed, and more than 300 using the search terms "teledermatology" as well as "telemedicine" and "dermatology."

The probably first reported use of telemedicine in dermatology dates back to 1972, when skin lesions of patients of the Logan International Airport Medical Station were assessed by dermatologists at the Massachusetts General Hospital telemedicine center on a television screen [6]. The term teledermatology itself was coined in a publication by Perednia and Brown in 1995 [7] that described the benefits of a teledermatologic application in rural Oregon, USA, in a region that was underserved by dermatologists. Various scientific publications have assessed the diagnostic accuracy of teledermatology. Store-and-forward teledermatology, compared to direct physical examination, has reportedly a total agreement rate of 41–94%, and partial agreement in 50–100% [8].

The most recent development are mobile telemedicine solutions that do not depend on stationary systems, but utilize mobile satellite and cellular telecommunication networks for the delivery of health care [9–13].

Stimuli to Implement Teledermatology

The stimulus to implement telemedicine derives from the need to address several problems such as inequity in access of (specialist) medical care as well as rising costs of medical care. Teledermatology is a unique tool to provide dermatologic care, its application comprise the entire field of dermatology ranging from primary diagnosis and treatment management to homecare, specialist consultations, and research and teaching purposes. It can be applied in remote locations, including underserved rural areas as well as developing countries with a shortage of trained dermatologists without inconvenience, time expenditure, and involved costs of patient travel. Furthermore, in urban areas, teledermatology has valuable applications in patient management and medical education and opens the door for telework options with flexible hours for dermatologists.

Approaches to Teledermatology Communication

The most common application of teledermatology is specialist referral. This involves telecommunication between a medical professional and a remote specialist/specialized center in order to get a second opinion on diagnosis and/or treatment advice in an equivocal case, thereby avoiding moving the patient to another location. A study conducted by Lozzi and colleagues showed that diagnostic accuracy in equivocal inflammatory and neoplastic skin conditions can be increased by up to 30% with the aid of teledermatology [14]. Dermoscopy is specially suited for this, because images can be easily obtained by a health care worker and interpreted in a store-and-forward application by a specialist.

Digital dermoscopic imaging enables to forward dermoscopic images (together with clinical information and macroscopic images) to specialists using a store-and-forward approach [15]. This is called teledermoscopy [1]. As dermoscopy itself is based on evaluation of a two-dimensional image, it is ideally suited for telemedicine purposes. Various studies to assess the power of teledermoscopy have been performed during the last years. A good correlation between face-to-face (FTF) diagnosis and teledermoscopy has been shown, and, more importantly, a good correlation between teledermoscopy and histopathology (the diagnostic gold standard for diagnosis of skin lesions). Interestingly, some studies even indicated that teledermoscopic diagnosis is superior to FTF diagnosis, especially when performed by experts [16–18]. However, there is concern that solely remote diagnosis could lead to mismanagement of melanoma patients [19] Therefore, teledermoscopy has been suggested as a triage tool to filter out clearly benign lesions, allowing obvious malignancy and equivocal lesions to be appropriately managed in specialized facilities.

A study by Moreno-Ramirez et al. showed that 51% of (benign) skin lesions could be filtered by a teledermatologic triage system, with excellent interobserver agreement for management decisions between FTF and teledermoscopy [20]. A recent study by Tan and coworkers [16] assessed the potential of teledermoscopy as a triage tool for 200 patients with 491 lesions referred to a skin lesions clinic in New Zealand. Patients were seen FTF by two of three dermatologists respectively; two telediagnoses were acquired. The diagnoses were compared to histopathology for those lesions excised. The exact concordance between FTF and teledermatology was 74% with predominately minor discrepancies in diagnoses. The concordance between FTF diagnoses ranged between 75.5% and 82.2%. However, for those lesions excised, teledermoscopy was superior to FTF when compared to histopathology.

Teledermoscopy is, of course limited as it relies on images of acceptable quality (which, with recent advances in imaging technology is becoming a minor problem) and, more importantly the risk of missing other clinically important lesions. However, it has great potential as a supportive complement to current FTF management plans which leave gaps in between routine FTF examinations and a tool to decrease the personal barrier to approach a specialist, thus enabling timely and appropriate treatment of melanoma.

Until recently, digital dermoscopic imaging (with acceptable quality) required possession of costly imaging devices for videodermoscopy or the quite time-consuming use of digital cameras with special attachments for dermoscopy. With a specially designed dermoscopic attachment with corresponding application software for commercially available Smartphones, for taking of dermoscopic images a relatively affordable device is now available for use of wider populations [21].

Teledermatology also enables international exchange of expert opinions. Online forums for teleconsultation provide discussion views enabling presentation of interesting cases. This exchange of knowledge and discussion of medicine-related topics between health care providers, especially between a physician and a specialist, has a valuable educational benefit for all participants and enhances quality assurance in dermatology. An example for this is the website http://www.telederm.org launched by the Department of Dermatology, Medical University of Graz, Austria, aiming to provide a user-friendly teledermatology consultation service connecting physicians and dermatologists worldwide.

Telehomecare is another evolving telemedicine application. It describes remote follow-up and monitoring of an individual with a chronic condition "at home" or outside the hospital. An emerging field of interest of telehomecare in dermatology is the follow-up treatment of crural ulcers.

The most simple, but at the same time most complex form of teledermatology interaction, direct teleconsultation involves direct telecommunication between an individual with a dermatologic disorder and an expert in the absence of guidance of other trained medical personnel in a face-to-face visit. It is most complex, since it deeply affects existing structures in medicine. It requires active participation of the patient in order to avoid improper management. For primary diagnosis, a visit to trained medical personnel might be indispensable; teledermatology might be very valuable as a tool for triage and aftercare, however. Mobile applications might be considered especially useful for these applications [15].

Medical Education

Internet and e-mail based teleeducation services, better known as e-learning, are becoming increasingly ubiquitous as a means of providing (continuous) medical education. E-learning avoids limitations of time and location imposed by attendance of lectures, seminars, or conferences in person. Online atlases provide a steadily expanding collection of dermatologic images. Various online courses, computer-based training, and web applications in dermatology principally aim at medical students, physicists, and dermatologists. They provide connection of text, images, video and audio files, and thus go far beyond merely displaying the context of a textbook on a computer monitor. Revisions can be individually adapted which can increase learning efficacy considerably. E-learning itself needs to be trained by individuals used to learn with textbooks or lectures, however.

Another teledermatology development are websites that offer general information about skin conditions for affected individuals and their relatives. A recent survey conducted in seven European countries revealed that 44% of citizens have reportedly used the Internet for health purposes [22]. Peer support groups of individuals affected by the same skin condition are valuable to reduce the burden of the disease. Specialist training courses via Internet are available particularly in dermoscopy as well as reflectance confocal microscopy. [15]

Obstacles to Implement Teledermatology

There are numerous advantages of teledermatology but there are some obstacles to implementation of such a system. There is a constant technical development that facilitates practical applicability, but there are still restraints arising from questions of data security, medical liability, reimbursement, and sociocultural barriers to acceptance of the method. These issues will be addressed with greater detail in determined chapters of this book. Legal issues with regard to responsibility and liability are complicated by teleconsultations performed between two or more countries, with differing legal systems. However, when teleconsultation is used to obtain a second opinion, the responsibility always remains with the primary care physician. Confidence about the security of personal data is critical for the practical implementation of a telemedicine network but is part of a wider problematic issue arising with the use of telecommunication in general. There also is the fear of a continuing deterioration of the relationship between physician and patient by loss of personal human contact in medicine. Whereas these issues must be addressed, to overcome resistance to implement telemedicine, they should be seen in the context of wider social phenomenon in the wake of persistent development and integration of new technology in all areas of medicine and modern life.

Standard Workflow

There is a vast variety of communication technologies that can be used for telemedicine. In general, however, two modes of image and data transmission, which sometimes overlap, are commonly applied: store-and-forward systems (SAF) and real-time (live-interactive) applications, also referred to as "asynchronous" and "synchronous" teledermatology.

Store and forward is a technique in which information (primarily still images and sometimes video clips with accompanying data) is sent to a data storage unit to be retrieved anytime. E-mail conversation and specially designed telemedicine web applications are examples for this modality. The sender can enter data at his or her convenience, and the recipient can later retrieve and analyze it. Communication is thus facilitated independent of the availability of the participants and independent of time zones. This asynchronous system facilitates international cooperation. The SAF method also allows a relatively large number of consultations to be managed in a brief period of time [23]. Communication is not interactive, however. Participants are not able to ask questions directly. In addition, the recipient only obtains information preselected by the sender. Despite rapid technical advance and market price change, the equipment for store and forward is still comparatively more affordable. In teledermatology, the SAF method has a wider use. A review by Levin et al. published in 2009 [8] showed a variation of partial diagnostic agreement of teledermatologist and clinical dermatologist ranging from 50% to 100%, and total agreement of 41–94% in studies applying SAF teledermatology. In comparison, total diagnostic agreement between clinic dermatologists ranged between 54% and 95%, and partial agreement was reported in 90–100%.

A "classic" example for a SAF consultation is as follows: An individual with an unusual skin lesion seeks advice at an outpatient service/teledermatologic service. Macroscopic and, if necessary, also dermoscopic digital images are taken. Via a secure web application/a standard e-mail program, these pictures are sent together with anonymous patient data (age and sex of patient, side of the lesion, current growth, etc.) to one/numerous experts for consultation. The consulted expert retrieves the data at a later time. The expert then sends back a report to the referring sites, including a diagnosis, a treatment advice, or a triage plan (advice for further referral).

In *real-time/live interactive* telemedicine, information is delivered simultaneously without any latency. It is most commonly performed in the form of a patient interview via a videoconference. Sender and recipient communicate over a distance but interact directly. The consulted teleexpert can ask direct questions about case history, and give instructions about the body sites he/she wants to view. Besides impossibility to touch the skin directly, a conventional face-to-face consultation is mimicked. Presence of all participants at the same predetermined time is required, however. Individual sessions generally last as long as, or even longer than, traditional face-to-face consultation. Furthermore, the equipment for real-time technology can be comparatively more costly as higher bandwidth is required. This modality also encompasses telesurgical procedures as well as robotic microscopy over a distance. A review performed by Whited et al. in 2007 reported partial agreement of 80–99% and total agreement 54–89% in studies performed with RT teledermatology systems [24].

A "classic" example for a real-time consultation is as follows: A subject with a skin condition living in a remote area seeks advice at a nearby teledermatologic center. In a videoconference, he is interviewed by a remote teledoctor, who asks anamnestic questions and tells the personnel on the referring site which body area he/she wants to view. The patient can ask relevant questions too. The interview ends with a diagnosis and management advice or advice for further referral.

Both systems can be merged; these systems are usually called combined or *hybrid teledermatology*. An example for this would be the discussion of patient information that has been sent beforehand in videoconference, or vice versa, sending further data via store-and-forward mode concerning a previous real-time patient interview. The benefit of this model is that it combines advantages of both methods. It has been reported to increase diagnostic accuracy of diagnosis when compared to SAF teledermatology alone [25].

In a clinical setting, this could work as follows: Trained personnel (e.g., a specially trained nurse) on the referring site completes a patient anamnesis form and obtains digital images of relevant skin lesions. This information is sent to the consulted expert via e-mail. During the following videoconference, the teleexpert can ask the patient for more information and ask the trained personnel for further images, which are forwarded during the live interactive consultation.

Aim of This Book

The aim of this book is to provide practical guidance for dermatologists who are interested in implementing a teledermatology program or are simply interested in the topic. Presumably, every dermatologist will be directly or indirectly confronted with telemedicine procedures. Teledermatology has proliferated in countries all over the world, as distinctive as Pakistan, Australia, and developing countries. Medical systems and geographical and demographic features with consequent arising problems in access to dermatologic care that stimulated implementation of teledermatology vary from country to country. The knowledge and practical experiences of experts all over the world involved in teledermatology projects will be presented in this book. We do believe that teledermatology is a promising technique to equalize access to dermatologic specialist knowledge, offering management and treatment benefits for dermatologic patients as well as educational benefits for primary care providers.

References

1. Wurm EM, Hofmann-Wellenhof R, Wurm R, Soyer HP (2008) Telemedicine and teledermatology: past, present and future. J Dtsch Dermatol Ges 6:106–112
2. Hofmann-Wellenhof R, Wurm EM, Ahlgrimm-Siess V, Richtig E, Koller S, Smolle J et al (2009) Reflectance confocal microscopy – state-of-art and research overview. Semin Cutan Med Surg 28:172–179
3. Norum J, Pedersen S, Stormer J, Rumpsfeld M, Stormo A, Jamissen N et al (2007) Prioritisation of telemedicine services for large scale implementation in Norway. J Telemed Telecare 13:185–192
4. Zundel KM (1996) Telemedicine: history, applications, and impact on librarianship. Bull Med Libr Assoc 84:71–79
5. Stanberry B (2000) Telemedicine: barriers and opportunities in the 21st century. J Intern Med 247:615–628
6. Murphy RL Jr, Fitzpatrick TB, Haynes HA, Bird KT, Sheridan TB (1972) Accuracy of dermatologic diagnosis by television. Arch Dermatol 105:833–835
7. Perednia DA, Brown NA (1995) Teledermatology: one application of telemedicine. Bull Med Libr Assoc 83:42–47
8. Levin YS, Warshaw EM (2009) Teledermatology: a review of reliability and accuracy of diagnosis and management. Dermatol Clin 27:163–176, vii

9. Ebner C, Wurm EM, Binder B, Kittler H, Lozzi GP, Massone C et al (2008) Mobile teledermatology: a feasibility study of 58 subjects using mobile phones. J Telemed Telecare 14:2–7
10. Massone C, Lozzi GP, Wurm E, Hofmann-Wellenhof R, Schoellnast R, Zalaudek I et al (2006) Personal digital assistants in teledermatology. Br J Dermatol 154:801–802
11. Massone C, Lozzi GP, Wurm E, Hofmann-Wellenhof R, Schoellnast R, Zalaudek I et al (2005) Cellular phones in clinical teledermatology. Arch Dermatol 141:1319–1320
12. Tran K, Ayad M, Weinberg J, Cherng A, Chowdhury M, Monir S et al (2011) Mobile teledermatology in the developing world: implications of a feasibility study on 30 Egyptian patients with common skin diseases. J Am Acad Dermatol 64(2):302–309
13. Massone C, Brunasso AM, Campbell TM, Soyer HP (2009) Mobile teledermoscopy – melanoma diagnosis by one click? Semin Cutan Med Surg 28:203–205
14. Lozzi GP, Soyer HP, Massone C, Micantonio T, Kraenke B, Fargnoli MC et al (2007) The additive value of second opinion teleconsulting in the management of patients with challenging inflammatory, neoplastic skin diseases: a best practice model in dermatology? J Eur Acad Dermatol Venereol 21:30–34
15. Wurm EM, Campbell TM, Soyer HP (2008) Teledermatology: how to start a new teaching and diagnostic era in medicine. Dermatol Clin 26:295–300, vii
16. Tan E, Yung A, Jameson M, Oakley A, Rademaker M (2010) Successful triage of patients referred to a skin lesion clinic using teledermoscopy (IMAGE IT trial). Br J Dermatol 162:803–811
17. Braun RP, Meier M, Pelloni F, Ramelet AA, Schilling M, Tapernoux B et al (2000) Teledermatoscopy in Switzerland: a preliminary evaluation. J Am Acad Dermatol 42:770–775
18. Piccolo D, Smolle J, Argenziano G, Wolf IH, Braun R, Cerroni L et al (2000) Teledermoscopy – results of a multicentre study on 43 pigmented skin lesions. J Telemed Telecare 6:132–137
19. Halpern SM (2010) Does teledermoscopy validate teledermatology for triage of skin lesions? Br J Dermatol 162:709–710
20. Moreno-Ramirez D, Ferrandiz L, Galdeano R, Camacho FM (2006) Teledermatoscopy as a triage system for pigmented lesions: a pilot study. Clin Exp Dermatol 31:13–18
21. GmbH FS (2010) Fotofinder Handyscope. (cited 21 Dec 2010). Available from: http://www.prlog.org/10968569-fotofinder-presents-handyscope-mobile-skin-cancer-screening-with-iphone.html
22. Andreassen HK, Bujnowska-Fedak MM, Chronaki CE, Dumitru RC, Pudule I, Santana S et al (2007) European citizens' use of E-health services: a study of seven countries. BMC Public Health 7:53
23. Wooton R, Krupinski E, Hailey D, Patterson V, Scott R, Whited J et al (2008) Memorable telemedicine experiences. J Telemed Telecare 14:50–54
24. Whited JD (2006) Teledermatology research review. Int J Dermatol 45:220–229
25. Baba M, Seckin D, Kapdagli S (2005) A comparison of teledermatology using store-and-forward methodology alone, and in combination with Web camera videoconferencing. J Telemed Telecare 11:354–360

Part I

International Experience

2 Teledermatology: The Atlantic Experience

Lars Erik Bryld, Michael Heidenheim, Tomas N. Dam, Deirdre Nathalie Dufour, Edith Vang, Tummas í. Garði, and Gregor B.E. Jemec

Core Messages

- It is beneficial if teledermatology is integrated in an existing structure for optimum utilisation of resources.
- Teledermatology has been used to redistribute the workload of specialists.
- Teledermatology provides continuous access to specialist assessment of patients in collaboration with local physicians.
- Simple store-and-forward teledermatology is well suited for follow-up of patients initially seen by a specialist.
- Milder cases of some clinically characteristic diseases such as acne are well suited to management through teledermatology.
- Teledermatology offers the possibility of case-based continued medical education of non-specialists.
- Teledermatology generally follows the life curve of other successful new organisational models and does not affect demand for health services.

Introduction

Ideally all patients should be seen in person by physicians, as this not only allows the optimal setting for clinical diagnosis and treatment, but also provides the human interaction which is an indispensable element of the patient–doctor relationship. Nevertheless, geography and scarcity of resources (both human and financial) have created the need for alternative solutions in many areas of the world. Telemedicine has proven to be an important alternative, which may help overcome a physical distance between patient and specialist.

Strongly visual specialities such as radiology, histopathology and dermatology are naturally well suited for telemedical applications, just as strongly sound-oriented specialities, e.g., psychiatry. Specialities relying on other senses derive less benefit from telemedicine. Although all clinical specialities require substantial direct interaction with patients for a successful outcome, medical specialities where treatment is not operator-dependent are better suited to telemedicine than specialities based on physical interventions such as surgery [1–5]. Technically complex direct patient–physician interactions via remotely operated robotics have been

L.E. Bryld • M. Heidenheim • T.N. Dam • D.N. Dufour • G.B.E. Jemec (✉)
Department of Dermatology, Health Sciences Faculty, Roskilde Hospital, University of Copenhagen, Roskilde, Denmark
e-mail: lebr@regionsjaelland.dk; mih@regionsjaelland.dk; tnd@regionsjaelland.dk; dndu@regionsjaelland.dk; gbj@regionsjaelland.dk

E. Vang • T.í. Garðí
Landssjúkrahúsið (Main Hospital), Tórshavn, Faroe Islands
e-mail: lsediva@ls.fo; lstumga@ls.fo

H.P. Soyer et al. (eds.), *Telemedicine in Dermatology*,
DOI 10.1007/978-3-642-20801-0_2, © Springer-Verlag Berlin Heidelberg 2012

created to overcome these limitations, whilst at the same time imposing technical and organisational limitations which restrict their use [6,7,8,9,10,11,12,13,14]. Simple use and access are important characteristics of successful technological and organisational interventions.

The Atlantic Setting

The Faroe Islands consist of 18 major islands about 750 km off the coast of Norway and 650 km off the coast of Iceland. The capital Tórshavn (population 12,300) is situated at 62°00′N 06°47′W/62°N 6.783°W/62; –6.783. Located 1,300 km from Copenhagen, the islands have extensive local autonomy as an autonomous province within the Kingdom of Denmark. The islands have a local democratically elected parliament and government. The population of approximately 48,000 persons is serviced by 82 doctors employed either as general practitioners (GPs) or at one of the three hospitals. The combined total number of hospital beds is 245. The main hospital in Tórshavn has approximately 220 beds and provides a broad range of regional medical and surgical services. Specialist services (e.g., rheumatology) are currently provided by visiting consultants. Telemedicine is actively used by the hospital in pathology and radiology, for example. Danish is spoken by all Faroese as the primary foreign language, and accepted as valid for medical records within the Faroese health system.

The Challenge

The aim of the health service is to establish a full service health system that provides both basic and specialist treatment to all inhabitants. This is done by actively attracting specialists, promoting specialist education of Faroese nationals and establishing close ties with collaborating partners abroad.

Dermatology services were previously provided by a single specialist resident in Tórshavn, and when he retired from practice it was maintained through visiting consultants who worked periodically at the hospital in Tórshavn. Over the course of the years, a set of core facilities have been established such as UV-therapy and CO_2 laser therapy, as well as a capacity for hospital admission of patients. These facilities provide a strong organisational background for the establishment of a successful teledermatological service. For the outpatient facility, auxiliary staff was hired, and throughout the preceding period the expectation of the society required that regular dermatological services were available locally.

Alternative solutions could be considered: One alternative solution would be to send patients abroad for treatment, which is an option regularly used for highly specialised therapy but not practically feasible for a high patient volume such as that seen in dermatology. Another alternative solution is to increase the training of the general practitioners to handle a larger share of the dermatological patients. However, whilst this strategy may help to reduce the demand for specialist treatment of simple cases, it cannot provide highly specialised dermatological treatment. Neither of these two solutions would furthermore ensure the full use of the existing facilities.

In addition to the organisational challenge, the proposed solution should be able to handle a high volume of patients with chronic, recurrent diseases in which consultations can be segregated into two types: initial diagnostic or therapeutic consultations, and subsequent follow-up consultations aimed at controlling side effects and monitoring progress and adherence (see Fig. 2.1).

The Solution

The solution has been the use of simple store-and-forward teledermatology integrated in a nurse-led clinic at the main hospital in Tórshavn [15]. This set-up allows daily access to specialist assessment of patients; it allows nurse–patient interaction and the possibility of continuous use of the facilities locally available for maximum operating efficiency. By design, the system has not completely replaced specialist visits, as these are perceived to be necessary not only for the more complex diagnoses, but also for implementing treatment. Conversely, follow-up consultations take the simpler and more structured format of store-and-forward teledermatology, and thereby do not require the physical presence of specialists. The clinic is permanently staffed by a nurse and a secretary, and eight times a year a dermatologist comes in for 4 days. Between physician visits, patients are managed by the nurse, who is supervised through daily use of the telemedicine system. Patients seen by the dermatologist predominantly need physical intervention, e.g., dermatosurgery, more

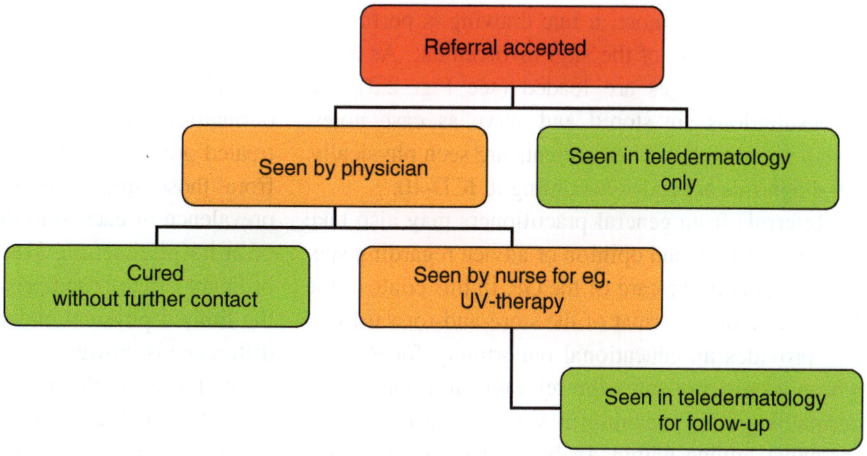

Fig. 2.1 Patient flow

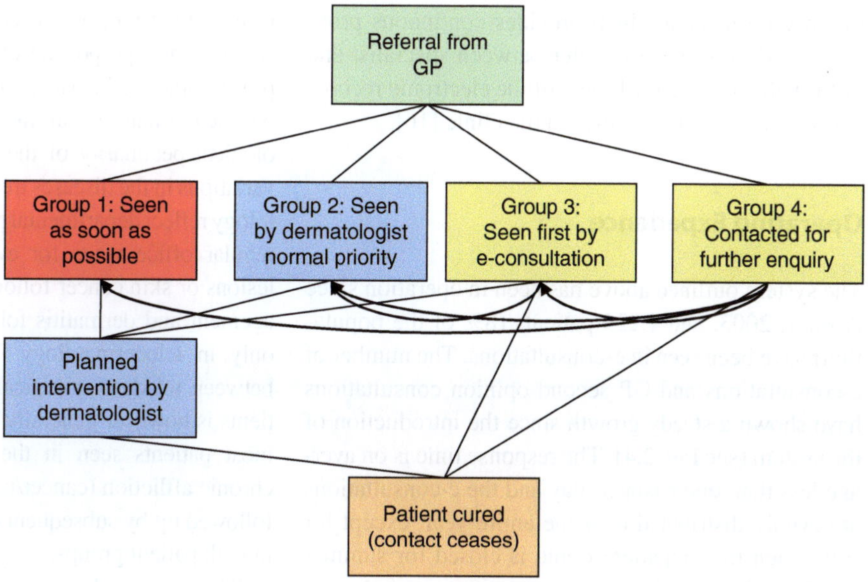

Fig. 2.2 Triage of referrals

complex diagnosis or treatment. Because the time available for direct patient–physician interaction is limited, selected benign or cosmetic conditions are not treated, e.g., benign skin tumours such as seborrheic keratoses.

Referrals are received from general practitioners and the local hospitals. The referrals are made either directly (electronically) into the system or forwarded by paper to the outpatient department. Initial triage sorts the referrals as shown in Fig. 2.2.

Patients seen by the consultant dermatologist are either: (1) treated and cured without need for further contact, (2) returned to the referring physician with suggestions for therapy or (3) scheduled for a follow-up teledermatological consultation (e-consultation). Every e-consultation is stored in a database on the server, and all communication via the Internet is encrypted to the SSL standard.

Primary e-consultations involve the nurse, who provides a structured history entered in a standardised form with specific questions, and supplies this data as well as electronic pictures via a web-based store-and-forward system, via a website for storage of all data (Dansk Telemedicin, Copenhagen, Denmark). The format is highly structured. Patient data including age, sex, date of birth, etc. are entered first. Then the patient history is entered with form fields provided for: (1) clinical problem, (2) case history, (3) duration of disease, (4) presence of itch, (5) known allergies, (6) medication, (7) concomitant diseases, (8) similar diseases in the household and (9) a space for free comments. Furthermore, a line drawing is performed marking the extent of the skin involvement. As a last step, patient images are loaded (see Fig. 2.3). All e-consultations are stored and serve as case notes, which are available when patients are seen physically. All diagnoses are coded according to ICD-10.

Referrals from general practitioners may also take the form of a second opinion or advice regarding specific patients in the care of the GP. In this context, the highly structured format of the store-and-forward system provides an educational opportunity for the GP, who not only structures the relevant information in a dermatologically meaningful way, but also receives specialist advice within 48 h and has an electronic record of event. These electronic records then constitute a vade mecum which provides continuous problem-based knowledge transfer between specialist and GP. Finally, the establishment of the electronic records allows future quality control in the clinic [16].

Operating Experience

The system outlined above has been in operation since April 1, 2003, and 4,225 patients (8% of the population) have been seen in e-consultations. The number of e-consultations and GP second-opinion consultations have shown a steady growth since the introduction of the system (see Fig. 2.4). The response time is on average less than one business day and the e-consultations are evenly distributed over the entire year, except for July when the outpatient clinic is closed for summer holidays (data not shown).

The introduction of second-opinion consultations with GPs provides continuous case-based medical education for the GPs involved and has been greatly appreciated. The structured information transfer to the nurse-led clinic is also helpful to the general organisation, which makes it possible to handle a larger number of minor complaints without taxing the specialist resources, similarly to what happens in more specialised clinics [17].

Furthermore, the spreading of routine consultations allows more continuous access to specialist treatment for the patient, i.e. a case need not only be assessed every sixth week when the specialist is physically present. The overall system thus provides comprehensive dermatological health care. However, the diseases treated predominantly in physical consultations differ from those treated in e-consultations. The relative prevalence of each skin disease while mimicking that of at hospital setting [18,19] differs, somewhat from ordinary office-based private practice [20], because of the limited physical attendance of the physician. The difference is, however, medically rational and pose no health hazard to the population. For example, removal of warts and other benign skin growths are not offered because of resource limitations.

On the other hand, management of dermatitis and investigation for possible contact allergy constitute a relatively larger proportion of office visits compared with private practice in America. This reflects European and Nordic dermatological tradition more than any epidemiological peculiarity of the Faroe Islands. Furthermore, variations in the diseases treated directly or by teledermatology reflect departmental policy to, for example, reserve regular office visits for evaluation of pigmented skin lesions or skin cancer follow-up. Conversely, acne management and dermatitis follow-up are generally treated only in teledermatology. The difference in case-mix between teledermatological patients and regular outpatients is however generally averaged out by the fact that most patients seen in the outpatient clinic for some chronic affliction (cancer/nevi group excepted) are often followed up by subsequent e-consultation, and so appear in both patient groups.

The continued increase in demand for dermatological consultations and advice suggests that the system is functioning well, but also introduces problems known from other systems. In particular, the steady accumulation of patients under care in the telemedical system poses a problem, as it has lead to increasing waiting times and stretching of the nursing resources available. In as far as these problems are seen in all health care systems, it suggests that this model for the introduction of telemedicine bears great resemblance to other organisational innovations.

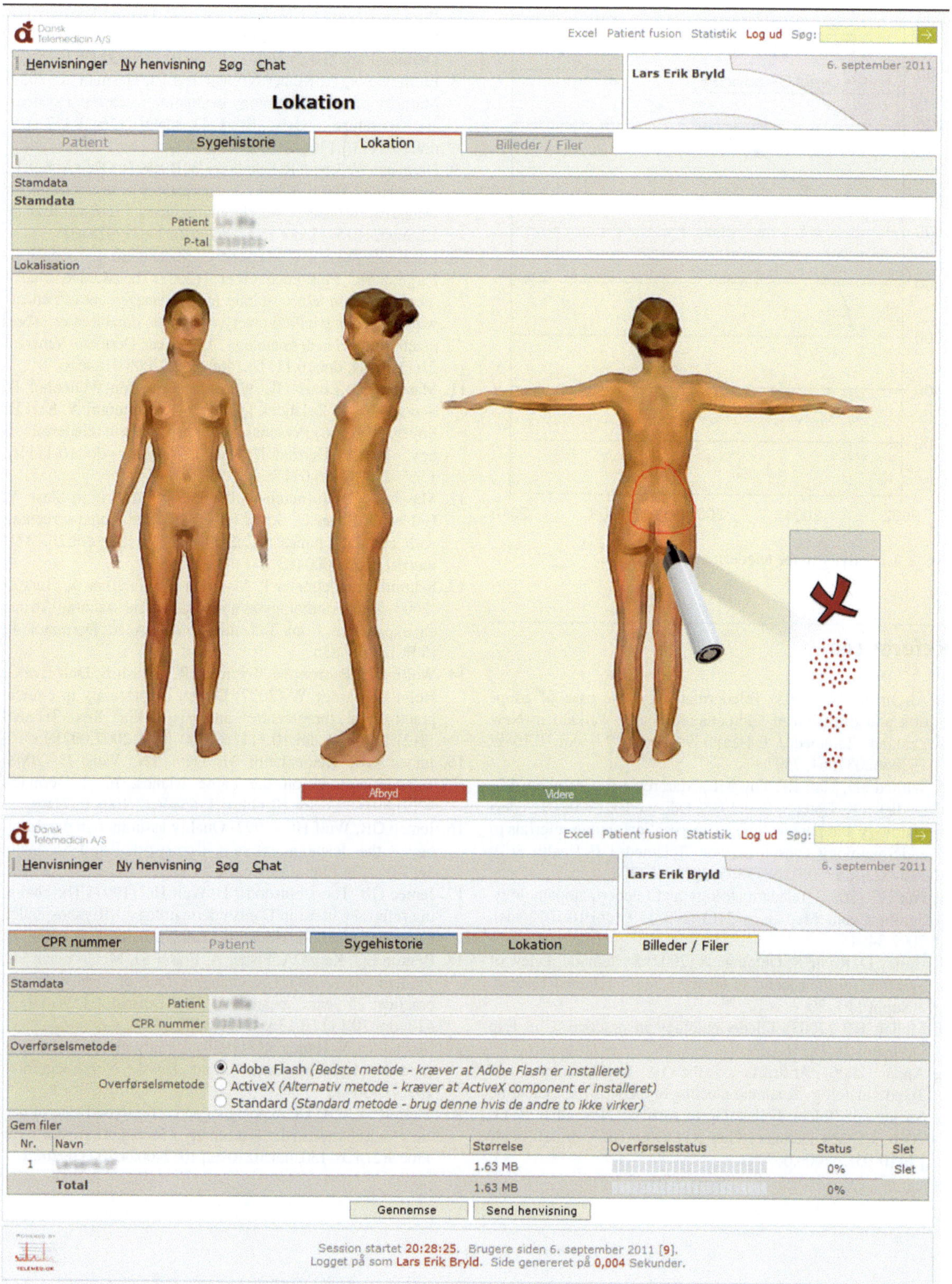

Fig. 2.3 The web-based store-and-forward system

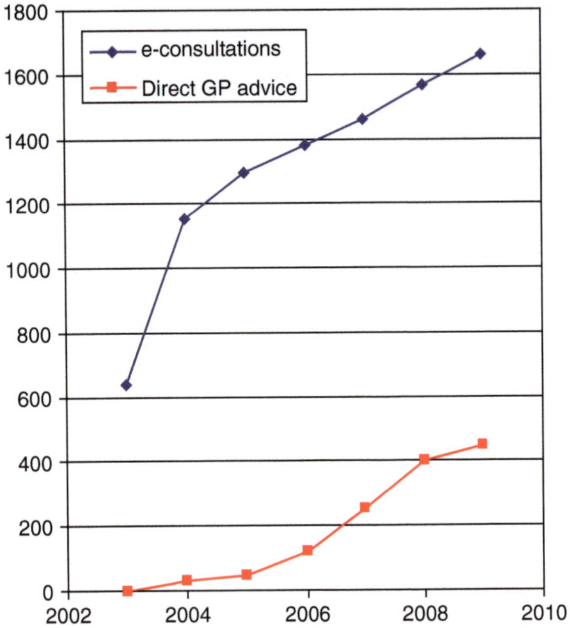

Fig. 2.4 Activity in the teledermatology system

References

1. Al-Qirim NA (2003) Teledermatology: the case of adoption and diffusion of telemedicine health Waikato in New Zealand. Telemed J E-Health 9(2):167–177. doi:10.1089/153056203766437507
2. Whited JD, Hall RP, Foy ME, Marbrey LE, Grambow SC, Dudley TK, Datta S, Simel DL, Oddone EZ (2002) Teledermatology's impact on time to intervention among referrals to a dermatology consult service. Telemed J E Health 8(3): 313–321. doi:10.1089/15305620260353207
3. Pak HS (2002) Teledermatology and teledermatopathology. Semin Cutan Med Surg 21(3):179–189. doi:10.1053/sder.2002.34945
4. Hailey D, Roine R, Ohinmaa A (2002) Systematic review of evidence for the benefits of telemedicine. J Telemed Telecare 8(Suppl 1):1–30
5. Mallett RB (2003) Teledermatology in practice. Clin Exp Dermatol 28(4):356–359
6. Anon (2006) Abstracts of the 1st world congress of Teledermatology & annual meeting of the Austrian Scientific Society of Telemedicine, Graz, Austria, November 9–11, 2006. J Dtsch Dermatol Ges 4(11):999–1017. doi:10.1111/j.1610-0387.2006.06798.x
7. Burg G, Hasse U, Cipolat C, Kropf R, Djamei V, Soyer HP, Chimenti S (2005) Teledermatology: just cool or a real tool? Dermatology 210(2):169–173. doi:10.1159/000082573
8. Eminović N, de Keizer NF, Bindels PJ, Hasman A (2007) Maturity of teledermatology evaluation research: a systematic literature review. Br J Dermatol 156(3):412–419. doi:10.1111/j.1365-2133.2006.07627.x
9. Hofmann-Wellenhof R, Salmhofer W, Binder B, Okcu A, Kerl H, Soyer HP (2006) Feasibility and acceptance of telemedicine for wound care in patients with chronic leg ulcers. J Telemed Telecare 12(Suppl 1):15–17. doi:10.1258/135763306777978407
10. Lozzi GP, Soyer HP, Massone C, Micantonio T, Kraenke B, Fargnoli MC, Fink-Puches R et al (2007) The additive value of second opinion teleconsulting in the management of patients with challenging inflammatory, neoplastic skin diseases: a best practice model in dermatology? J Eur Acad Dermatol Venereol 21(1):30–34. doi:10.1111/j.1468–3083.2006.01846.x
11. Massone C, Lozzi GP, Wurm E, Hofmann-Wellenhof R, Schoellnast R, Zalaudek I, Gabler G, Di Stefani A, Kerl H, Soyer HP (2006) Personal digital assistants in teledermatology. Br J Dermatol 154(4):801–802. doi:10.1111/j.1365–2133.2006.07175.x
12. Massone C, Hofmann-Wellenhof R, Ahlgrimm-Siess V, Gabler G, Ebner C, Soyer HP (2007) Melanoma screening with cellular phones. PLoS One 2(5):e483. doi:10.1371/journal.pone.0000483
13. Schmid-Grendelmeier P, Masenga EJ, Haeffner A, Burg G (2000) Teledermatology as a new tool in sub-saharan Africa: an experience from Tanzania. J Am Acad Dermatol 42 (5 Pt 1):833–835
14. Wollina U, Burroni M, Torricelli R, Gilardi S, Dell'Eva G, Helm C, Bardey W (2007) Digital dermoscopy in clinical practise: a three-centre analysis. Skin Res Technol 13(2):133–142. doi:10.1111/j.1600–0846.2007.00219.x
15. Jemec GB, Heidenheim M, Dam TN, Vang E (2008) Teledermatology on the Faroe Islands. Int J Dermatol 47(9):891–893. doi:10.1111/j.1365–4632.2008.03718.x
16. Jemec GB, Wulf HC (1997) Quality assurance in dermatology – the development of a framework. Int J Dermatol 36(10): 721–726
17. Jemec GB, Thorsteinsdóttir H, Wulf HC (1997) The changing referral pattern in Danish dermatology – Rigshospitalet, Copenhagen, 1986–1995. Int J Dermatol 36(6):453–456
18. Benton EC, Kerr OA, Fisher A, Fraser SJ, McCormack SK, Tidman MJ (2008) The changing face of dermatological practice: 25 years' experience. Br J Dermatol 159(2):413–418. doi:10.1111/j.1365-2133.2008.08701.x
19. McFadden N, Hande KO (1989) A study of new patients at a dermatologic outpatient clinic. Tidsskr Nor Laegeforen 109(4):436–437
20. Stern RS (2004) Dermatologists and office-based care of dermatologic disease in the 21st century. J Investig Dermatol Symp Proc 9(2):126–130. doi:10.1046/j.1087–0024.2003.09108.x

3 Health Management Practice as a Method to Introduce Teledermatology: Experiences from the Netherlands

Leonard Witkamp and Job Paul van der Heijden

Core Messages

- Because of increased demand, healthcare provision will come to a standstill if its efficiency is not changed rigorously.
- Telemedicine is a solution to increase healthcare efficiency.
- The Health Management Practice (HMP) model is a roadmap for developing, investigating and implementing telemedicine tools.
- Teledermatology after selection by the general practitioner has been fully integrated in the Netherlands.
- Teledermatology has led to higher satisfaction and learning effect, 75% reduction of all physical referrals to dermatologists, 20.6% cost savings and better quality of care.
- HMP has enabled KSYOS to perform over 50,000 teledermatology consultations, expand teledermatology to other EU countries, as well as to other areas such as teleophtalmology, telespirometry and telecardiology.

L. Witkamp (✉)
KSYOS TeleMedical Center, Amstelveen, The Netherlands
e-mail: l.witkamp@ksyos.org

J.P. van der Heijden
Department of Dermatology, Academic Medical Centre, University of Amsterdam,
e-mail: j.vanderheijden@ksyos.org

Introduction

Increasing pressure on the healthcare sector makes it necessary to design a new model of how to provide care. Without radical changes in the way care is provided, healthcare costs will increase extensively in the coming decades. With a population pressure of 60% at this moment, in the Netherlands 40% of the population is active to maintain the others, of which one-third are older than 65 and two-thirds are younger than 20 years. In the coming decades, the population pressure will grow to 85% of which half will be over 65 and of those a major part will be 75 plus [1] (Fig. 3.1). This group is bulk consumer in health care. This extensive increase in demand of care will not be followed up by an increase in care providers and care capacity. If the healthcare sector is not going to change, it will probably grind to a standstill. The improved awareness of the need for change in health care has as yet not fully led to a powerful introduction of tools that help to improve (the efficiency of) health care. Developments in the field of integrated care applications are characterised by fragmentation and lack of proficiency and marketing insight. The lack of prospect to reimbursement turns investing for parties into a risk. Promising projects remain therefore often on a relatively small scale invisible or just disappear after subsidies are terminated. Successful initiatives so far are scarce. However, some are successful. Because integrated services bear many aspects such as healthcare delivery by various care providers, development of software, hosting, research, marketing on the medical market, quality control and negotiations with care providers and health insurers, participants with expertise in the

H.P. Soyer et al. (eds.), *Telemedicine in Dermatology*,
DOI 10.1007/978-3-642-20801-0_3, © Springer-Verlag Berlin Heidelberg 2012

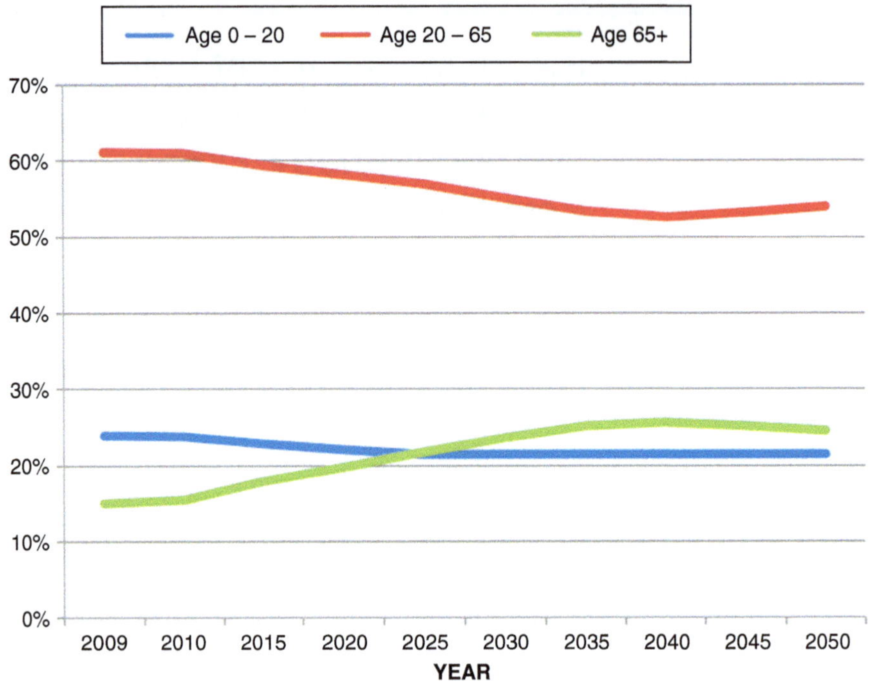

Fig. 3.1 Dutch population prognosis

various fields need to cooperate. Successful initiatives are mainly combinations of public and private parties that have the courage to work together, share their knowledge and invest jointly. A requirement for a responsible introduction of integrated services in regular care has proved to be meeting demands for security, connectivity and user friendliness. The Health Management Practice model addresses all these aspects.

Health Management Practice

With the use of Health Management Practice, private and public parties and independent knowledge institutes jointly develop telemedicine tools, study their effect on efficiency increase of the primary healthcare process and empower their modular and subsequent upscaled introduction in regular care [2]. It enables the step-by-step introduction of new telemedicine tools in day-to-day care not by weakening it but on the contrary by intensifying it.

Telemedicine Development

Partners elaborate a telemedicine tool to an integrated service including security, software, hardware, infrastructure, hosting and management. Telemedicine tools developed meet requirements of safety, connectivity and user friendliness [3]. They adhere to national ICT healthcare infrastructures and on the long term add to the development of the electronic patient record.

Health Management Research

Health Management Research aims to prove that the use of telemedicine services increases efficiency; it brings more satisfaction with users, increased production volume and better quality at equal or lower costs, thus re-routing the dramatic growth in costs in the healthcare sector. It entails usability and efficiency research aiming at professionalising new telemedicine tools in a phased way, obtain support, prove the effect on improvement of efficiency and after that study the user and reimbursement model. Independent scientific parties protocol the various stages of the research and monitor its quality and independence.

Health Management Implementation

All stakeholders – manufacturers, users, policy makers and health insurers – are involved in the design of practice and reimbursement research. Starting point here are significant reductions in costs on a macro level and a healthy business case with surplus reimbursement per use for manufacturers, users and policy makers. The interested parties together establish a price for the use of the telemedicine tool and predefine performance indicators that are conditional for reimbursement. These performance indicators may entail outcomes on health as well as logistic outcomes. In order to guarantee successful up-scaling in regular care, the benefits of the telemedicine instrument for and its synergy with regular care are actively marketed and communicated.

Success of Teledermatology in the Netherlands

Health Management Practice has been successfully applied to develop, investigate and upscale teledermatology in the Netherlands. Teledermatology has proven to enable the general practitioner to provide a dermatologist with digital images and short description through a secure Internet connection. As both general practitioner and dermatologist experienced teledermatology as enrichment of their work, with emphasis on quality improvement and learning effect, teledermatology has been widely accepted now in regular health care. Teledermatology has led to higher volume growth of dermatological care at equal costs in the Netherlands.

Development: KSYOS Teledermatology Consultation System (TDCS®) as an Integrated Service

Health Management Practice has led to the introduction of the KSYOS Teledermatology Consultation System (TDCS®), through which general practitioners perform teledermatology consultations safely with the use of the unique health worker identification passport (UZI-pas), guaranteeing all patient data to remain confidential, integer and available. This digital pass is issued by the Dutch Ministry of Health. The TDCS® does not only include software, but also the provision of hardware (digital camera, docking station, UZI-pas and card reader), quality monitoring, helpdesk, on-site monitoring, billing, administration, education and malpractice insurance. The expansion of this teleconsultation system to other disciplines has added to the accelerated development of the electronic health record (Fig. 3.2).

Research: Performance Indicators

In usability studies, the complete service including the infrastructure of the Teledermatology Consultation System has been tested under intensive monitoring amongst a relatively small group of future users (10–20 medical specialists and family doctors) during a short period (4–8 weeks). In these studies software, hardware, logistics and experience of the user have been investigated.

Health Insurance companies and policy makers have agreed upon the following performance indicators of teledermatology that are conditional for its reimbursement:

- Use of the Dutch national Unique Health Worker Identification pass (UZI-pas)
- Monitoring of the number of prevented physical referrals to the dermatologist
- Monitoring of the response time of the dermatologist

Unique Health Worker Identification Pass

On the 1st of June 2007, in total 1,732 health workers were working with the UZI-pas; 733 of them have been provided by KSYOS for the use of the KSYOS Teledermatology System (43% of all UZI-passes in the Netherlands). This UZI-pas can be used for different other (transmural) services and by other institutions [4]. Teledermatology thus adds significantly to the development of the national health infrastructure and the electronic patient record.

Number of Prevented Physical Referrals to the Dermatologist

KSYOS has monitored the general practitioner's decision points before and after the Teledermatology Consultation. Before the TeleConsultation, the general practitioner answered the standard question: "Would you physically refer this patient to the dermatologist without the availability of teledermatology?" After the

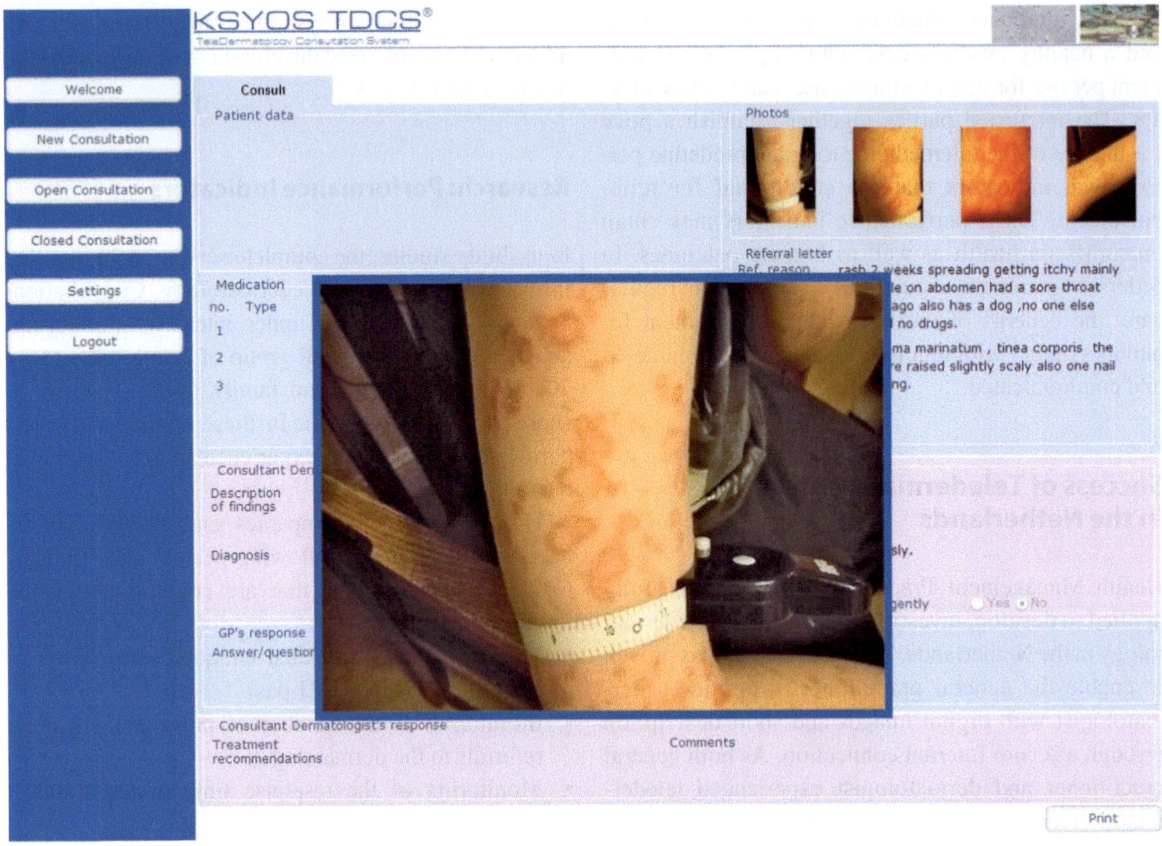

Fig. 3.2 TeleDermatology consultation system

TeleConsult, he answered the following question: "Do you refer the patient physically to the dermatologist?" Of 13,710 TeleConsultations evaluated, 72% of the population selected for a teledermatology consultation by the GP would have been referred to the dermatologist without the availability of teledermatology (Group A). In 28%, this would not have been the case (Group B). In this group, a TeleConsult is performed for general advice in order to improve the quality of the treatment. After the Teledermatology Consultation, of group A (would have been referred without the availability of teledermatology) 25% are referred a 75% reduction. Of group B (would not have been referred without the availability of teledermatology), 15% are physically referred to the dermatologist (4% of the total population). In the whole population, the total number of physical referrals to the dermatologist decreases from 71% to 22%, an overall reduction of 69%. This reduction includes extra referrals due to advice, quality improvement and potential lowering of the referral threshold. This reduction does not include the long-term reduction of referral due to the learning effect of teledermatology, nor to the advices that have been given in Group B.

Cost Reducing Effect of Teledermatology

The reimbursement for a Teledermatology Consult is €67,50. This includes reimbursement for the general practitioner, dermatologist and KSYOS TeleMedical Centre. The reimbursement for KSYOS includes the complete integrate service. The reimbursement of the general practitioner includes the extra work for Teledermatology Consultation (10 min) and all to the TeleConsultation-related visits to general practitioner. The general practitioner is not allowed to also charge these visits to his regular system. The mean costs of a physically referred patient including treatment are €202,18. The size of Group A is 72% of the total population selected for a teledermatology consultation by

Table 3.1 Perceived benefits of teledermatology

	Higher satisfaction	Cost reduction and/or higher production volume at equal or lower costs	Better quality of care
Patient	Answer within 2 days, no waiting list	Accessibility of care in the coming decades, no costs for travelling and absence of work	Quicker and better care, advice in case of non-referral, emergencies
General practitioner	Working satisfaction, service to the patient, learning effect, innovation	Extra budgetary income	Learning effect, advices, emergencies
Dermatologist	Working satisfaction, service to general practitioners, increased adherence	Extra budgetary income	Learning effect, more time for more dermatology suited patients
Hospital	Service to general practitioners, increased adherence	Increased adherence to general practitioners, dosage of waiting lists, marketing instrument, free service (no investment for the hospital)	
Policy maker	Innovation	Accessibility or care in the view of the ageing population	Quicker better care
Health insurance company	Service to clients	Accessibility or care in the view of the ageing population	Quicker better care, better service for clients

the GP; the referral reduction is 75% in this group. The size of Group B is 28% of the total population; the referral increase in this group is 15%. The cost reducing effect in group A is somewhat reduced by the quality increase in group B, still leading to a cost reduction of 20.6%. The breakeven point for teledermatology is €124,25/TeleConsult. However, due to a long-term reduction of physical referral, the cost saving effect of teledermatology will further increase.

Service for the Patient: Response Time of the Dermatologist

The trimmed mean response time of the dermatologist was 4.2 h, the median 2 h. Of all patients, 95% received a response within 2 working days. Most TeleConsultations were sent at the end of the morning or afternoon. This applied also for the response by the dermatologist.

Perceived Benefits of Teledermatology

In interview sessions amongst patients, general practitioners, dermatologists, hospital management, policy makers and account managers of health insurance companies, teledermatology was considered to lead to increased service, more working satisfaction, cost saving and higher production volume at equal costs and better quality of care (see Table 3.1).

More structured independent qualitative research amongst 205 general practitioners that work with KSYOS Teledermatology concluded that general practitioners see teledermatology as enrichment of their work. General practitioners considered teledermatology to have a learning effect, to be important for their work, to add to the efficiency of the care process, to increase work satisfaction and to fit into their regular work activities (Table 3.2).

Implementation of Teledermatology

At this moment, 8,200 general practitioners and 350 dermatologists on a population of 16 million are registered and actively practising in the Netherlands [5]. Eight percent of all general practitioners' consultations concern dermatology. Hereof, 93% are treated by the general practitioner, 7% are referred to the dermatologist, leading to 45 referrals per year per GP. Within the last 1.5 years, KSYOS TeleMedical Centre has connected 1,500 general practitioners and 142 dermatologists. However, 40% of the general practitioners are active in teledermatology, performing 4.0 TeleConsultations per quarter. Overall, all general practitioners perform 0.5 TeleConsultations per month. Despite regular extra budgetary reimbursement for general practitioners and dermatologists, the rapid growth of general practitioners connected is not followed by an equal increase in number of Teledermatology Consultations. In total, over

Table 3.2 Perceived benefits of teledermatology by general practitioners performing teledermatology

	Fairly positive – positive and very positive (%)
Teledermatology has a learning effect	
I can treat more dermatological conditions by myself	78
I learn from teledermatology	83
Teledermatology is important for general practitioners	
Teledermatology is important in my work	79
Teledermatology is useful	84
Teledermatology is efficient	
Teledermatology makes healthcare provision in general more effective	94
Teledermatology prevents live referrals to the dermatologists	79
Teledermatology enables me to service my patients quicker	87
Teledermatology simplifies the treatment process of patients	86
Teledermatology increases satisfaction	
I like to work with teledermatology	88
Teledermatology fits into my routine practice	
Teledermatology adheres to my daily activities	81

70,000 TeleConsultations have been performed through KSYOS in TeleDermatology, TeleOpthalmology, TeleCardiology and TelePulmonolgy. Recent results based on 40.000 TeleDermatology Consultations show TeleDermatology as an fully integrated service in regular healthcare contributing to more efficient and cheaper healthcare. [6]

KSYOS TeleMedical Centre: The First Virtual Hospital in the Netherlands

Safe, prosperous and socioeconomic balanced introduction of teledermatology demands its provision by certified centres that meet minimal quality requirements and that guarantee reasonable reimbursement of general practitioner and dermatologist, additional to regular reimbursement. KSYOS TeleMedical Centre has been officially recognised as a healthcare organisation in December 2005 performing teledermatology consultations. KSYOS contracts health insurance companies that pay for each teleconsultation that is performed. KSYOS in return pays the general practitioners and dermatologists, manages security, software and hardware (digital camera, docking station, UZI-pas and card reader), all logistics and infrastructure with ongoing instruction, quality monitoring and helpdesk function, takes care of invoicing and account management, price negotiating, quality monitoring and liability insurance. It is the information point for (future) parties that certify healthcare service, the logistic process with regards to security and privacy rules and the information process with regards to data storage, continuity and accessibility of information. In this construction, KSYOS is a new business partner for integrated services for health insurers.

Conclusion

With the ageing and more demanding population, healthcare provision is bound to undergo drastic changes. On regional, national and international level, health workers, policy makers and health insurance organisations are addressing issues of how to keep health care accessible for the population in the coming decades despite dramatic changes in demand. Efficiency increase of healthcare delivery and the role of ICT in this process is a recurrent issue in policy documents and grant descriptions. Basic of this efficiency increase is the replacing of the bulk of the work from higher to lower in the health knowledge hierarchy – from medical specialist to general practitioner, from general practitioner to nurse practitioners or from nurse practitioner to the patient – under supervision of the person higher in the hierarchy. Telemedicine is perceived as an excellent tool to achieve this goal, combining innovating techniques, changed working conditions, prevention and education. With the use of telemedicine, conventional general hospitals are able to elaborate on their role as centre of excellence on the top of the knowledge hierarchy in healthcare. On one hand, it enables these hospitals to further focus on highly specialised care, as with the help of telemedicine less routine care will come into their boundaries. On the other hand, telemedicine enables these hospitals to maintain their supervising role in "bulk routine care". In the Dutch setting, KSYOS has taken care of all safety, quality and administrative issues of both general practitioners and has contracted all health insurance organisations for reimbursement. It has therefore enabled hospital to offer this innovative service to their general practitioners and dermatologists without investments, thereby reducing any risk for the hospital.

Apart from the fact that telemedicine in general prepares hospitals for future changes in healthcare delivery, teledermatology has proven to have various immediate positive effects. Teledermatology enables hospitals and dermatologists to influence their waiting lists. This has been mainly due to the positioning of teledermatology in the Netherlands in the growth segment. By doing so, the hospital delivers quicker and better care to general practitioners and patients without cannibalising on their own production. And here is where the second immediate effect has appeared. Teledermatology strengthens the health chain and the contacts between general practitioners and dermatologists. If teledermatology is delivered on a regional basis by a professional institution that stands for safe and user-friendly communication, general practitioners and dermatologists are highly enthusiastic about teledermatology. By offering teledermatology, the hospital firmly strengthens and enlarges its contact area of general practitioners that drain on it. In the Netherlands, teledermatology has proven to be an excellent service tool for hospitals to their regional general practitioners, an issue which has become more and more prominent in the Dutch healthcare system that is planned to be increasingly market driven.

References

1. Central Bureau for Statistics (2010) Centraal Bureau voor de Statistiek. Den Haag/Heerlen: http://www.cbs.nl. Website visited 17 Sep 2010
2. Jaatinen PT, Forsstrom J, Loula P (2002) Teleconsultations: who uses them and how? J Telemed Telecare 8(6):319–324
3. Hailey D, Roine R, Ohinmaa A (2002) Systematic review of evidence for the benefits of telemedicine. J Telemed Telecare 8(Suppl 1):1–30
4. The Dutch Healthcare Authority (2010) Nederlandse Zorg Autoriteit. Utrecht: DBC tarief applicatie http://ctg.bit-ic.nl/Nzatarieven/top.do. Website visited 27 Sep 2010
5. Verheij R, Van Dijk C, Abrahamse H (2010) Landelijk Informatienetwerk Huisartsenzorg. Feiten en cijfers over huisartsenzorg in Nederland. Utrecht/Nijmegen: NIVEL/IQ http://www.linh.nl. Website visited 16 Sep 2010
6. van der Heijden JP, de Keizer NF, Bos JD et al. Teledermatology applied following patient selection by general practitioner in daily practice improves efficiency and quality of care at lower costs. Br.J.Dermatol. 2011

Telederm Australia

4

Jim Muir and Lex Lucas

Core Messages

- A doctor using a teledermatology service needs more skills than one utilising a traditional face-to-face referral.
- Doctors using a telemedicine service face a greater burden of responsibility and an increased workload than with a traditional referral.
- A viable teledermatology service must offer online education alongside its consultation service.
- Telemedicine is an efficient and cost-effective solution to the lack of dermatological services.
- Appropriate remuneration for referring doctors is vital if telemedicine is to become widely adopted.

Introduction

Australia is home to just over 22 million people in a land mass covering an area of slightly under eight million square kilometres [1]. By way of comparison, the United Kingdom has a population almost three times as large in an area of only 244, 820 km^2 [2]. Although predominantly urban, Australia's populace is widely dispersed with many small towns and isolated communities. Delivery of health care to these communities is problematic [3, 4].

In common with the rest of the world, skin disease makes up a significant proportion of the workload of primary care physicians [5–7]. Despite the majority of this being treated without the need for referral to other practitioners, there remains a large unmet demand and need for specialist dermatology services. Unfortunately for reasons of geographic isolation, skilled workforce shortage and costs, many patients have great difficulty accessing such advice.

Most Australian dermatologists are based in the state capitals or large regional centres. Patients in rural and remote areas have to travel vast distances often measured in hundreds rather than tens of kilometres to see a dermatologist. Even then there is often a considerable wait for an appointment. Free access to specialist dermatologists is available through a number of public hospitals but the vast majority of referred patients are seen privately on a fee for service basis. These fees add to the cost burden of travel expenses and lost income for a rural and remote patient seeing an urban dermatologist.

An obvious way to meet the needs of rural patients with skin disease is to have specialist dermatologists perform clinics in regional areas. There are many such services throughout Australia such as the Medical Specialist Outreach Assistance Program (MSOAP) [8]. As with any dermatology service, these suffer from excessive workload. As they supply only an intermittent service, the problem of what

J. Muir (✉)
Dermatology Research Centre, The University of Queensland, School of Medicine, Princess Alexandra Hospital, Woolloongabba, QLD, Australia
e-mail: arnoldmuir@optusnet.com.au

L. Lucas
Australian College of Rural and Remote Medicine, Brisbane, QLD, Australia
e-mail: l.lucas@acrrm.org.au

H.P. Soyer et al. (eds.), *Telemedicine in Dermatology*,
DOI 10.1007/978-3-642-20801-0_4, © Springer-Verlag Berlin Heidelberg 2012

to do with new and review patients needing dermatologist advice between visits remains. The dermatologists providing these services have to absent themselves from their already very busy practices adversely affecting their efficient running. Combined with the need to travel long distances and stay overnight, it can be difficult to gain a long-term service commitment.

Ideally patients in rural and remote Australia and indeed poorly serviced urban regions should be able to access specialist dermatology advice in a timely, efficient and cost-effective manner. The advent of modern telecommunications has meant that telemedicine has become a viable option in health care delivery. Medical advice has long been delivered via the telephone. This purely verbal means of communication suffered from a lack of visual input to aid decision making.

One of the author's first experience of distant diagnosis and management utilising images was in 1992 when he received photographic images and patient history in a letter from a doctor in a hospital over a thousand miles away. The diagnosis of warfarin necrosis was readily made but of course there had been a delay of almost 5 days between its onset and eventual diagnosis due to the time constraints imposed by photographic development and land mail. The advent of digital photography and the Internet has meant that information and images can be delivered over large distances almost instantaneously. This has resulted in telemedicine and teledermatology in particular becoming a viable, effective medical service [9–11].

A teledermatology service has to offer more than just diagnostic and management advice. It needs to educate the medical staff as well. It should provide a resource which can be used when managing patients. The teledermatologist is reliant on the referring medical practitioner to carry out history, examination, photographic documentation, procedures and treatment reliably and competently. To this end educational material needs to be readily available to staff utilising a teledermatology service. This can be delivered along with a consultation service. Each time a doctor refers a patient for a telemedicine consultation, there is a significant educational benefit. This is because the referring doctor is directly involved in all aspects of patient management from diagnosis to follow-up [12].

Tele-Derm National

Tele-Derm National (TN) is a web-based consultational and educational service in clinical dermatology. It is but one resource of a much larger educational platform run by the Australian College of Rural and Remote Medicine (ACRRM) called Rural and Remote Medical Education Online (RRMEO). RRMEO provides online education in multiple medical disciplines including fields as diverse as toxinology and radiology [13].

Established in 2005 TN is an initiative of ACRRM. The site is funded by the Commonwealth Department of Health and Ageing under the Medical Specialist Outreach Assistance Program (MSOAP).

TN provides a free, year-round service to ACRRM members throughout Australia. It was established as a targeted, specific response to the need for rural and remote doctors and their patients to have ready access to specialist dermatology opinion. For many areas the only alternative to a telemedicine service is for the patient to travel often hundreds of kilometres to the nearest large urban centre where Australian dermatologists predominantly base themselves.

The service is designed for and primarily aimed at primary care doctors working in rural and remote Australia. There are 1,226 doctors currently enrolled in the service currently. The majority of these work in either rural Queensland or New South Wales but there are users in all parts of Australia and urban regions [14].

In 2009 the site received over 55,000 hits. In the last three and a half years, 50,000 forum messages have been read across the site. The site is interactive and provides opportunities for practitioners to interact directly and rapidly with the consultant dermatologist and also other users. This is a deliberate policy aimed at reducing professional isolation of isolated and solo practitioners. As medical students are given access to the site, it is hoped that they will incorporate telemedicine into their ongoing clinical and educational lives after they graduate.

The philosophy behind the site is that the vast majority of dermatological problems can be managed in their entirety by non-specialist medical staff provided they have ready access to timely, accurate diagnostic and management advice when needed. To enable and enhance local delivery of dermatology care, the site also provides online education in dermatology and the necessary practical skills such as cryotherapy, cutaneous surgery and use of various specialised dermatological medicaments.

To this end the site offers a variety of features:

Online Consultation

TN provides a 7 day a week consultation service. The turnaround time between submission of a request for advice and reply has been less than 24 h in over 96% of cases. Over 150 cases are submitted per year. Most requests are for help with diagnosis and/or management of inflammatory dermatoses. The store and forward method is used. We receive digital images and an e-mail describing the patient's problem. Initially there was a compulsory proforma detailing the patient's history for the referring doctor to fill in. This was discarded as it was felt to be a disincentive to doctors using the site due to the time involved completing it. We now ask clarifying questions as and when needed.

Uniquely each submitted case can be viewed by all users of the site. This is done to allow cases to have an educational benefit for doctors. To ensure maintenance of patient confidentiality, the site is password protected and no identifying material either written or visual is posted. Patients are informed by the referring doctor of this fact and are free to decline permission for other doctors to view their case.

The site's consultant dermatologist is not provided with any information that can identify the patient. In the majority of cases, the dermatologist is not even aware of the referring doctor's identity.

Many cases are submitted for advice on management rather than help with making a diagnosis. Table 4.1 lists the diagnoses of the last 20 cases submitted for advice.

As can be seen even from this very incomplete list, the conditions submitted cover the entire gamut of dermatology including neoplasia, inflammatory dermatoses, the common and the rare.

Despite attempts we are unable to get comprehensive reliable feedback on patient outcome – a problem common to face-to-face consultation also. In an online survey of users conducted in 2009, 100% of respondents rated their satisfaction as either 'extremely satisfied' or 'satisfied' when commenting on the service they received when submitting cases to TN. In the same survey, 92% of all TN users indicated that TN had 'been of value' to their patients.

Online Education and Resources

Traditionally dermatology has not been given a high priority in undergraduate medical courses in Australia. Informal discussions between the author and medical educators reveal that dermatology is a constantly requested topic at general practice educational meetings. To get the most from a teledermatology consultation, a referring doctor needs some basic dermatological skills. They must be able to submit a consultation of sufficient accuracy and detail for a diagnosis to be made and then have the skills and knowledge to carry out the advice received.

When an Australian doctor refers a patient for a traditional face-to-face consultation with a dermatologist, the management of that patient's skin condition will usually be carried out by the dermatologist. Expanded history, examination of the skin/mucosa/nails/hair, procedures such as skin biopsy, fungal scrapings, cryotherapy, excisions, curettage, explanation and prescription of dermatological treatments will all be performed by the treating dermatologist. This is not the case with teledermatology. If the patient is to be managed in their home community, the referring doctor will have to carry out these tasks and more. Familiarity with digital photography is an essential skill for a doctor referring patients to a teledermatology service.

To enable referring doctors to complete this aspect of a teledermatology consultation, TN has a large and continually expanding educational content. As the

Table 4.1 Recent cases on TN

Twenty recent cases on TN			
Vitiligo	Plant contact dermatitis	Folliculitis	Bier spots
Perioral dermatitis	Delusions of parasitosis	Hidradenitis suppuritiva	Angina bullosa haemorrhagica
Psoriasis	Atopic eczema	Scalp halo naevi	Pyoderma gangrenosum
Dysplastic naevus syndrome	Urticaria	Alopecia areata	Pityriasis rubra pilaris
Adolescent striae	Insect bite reactions	Infective dermatitis	Intertrigo

World Wide Web already contains many readily accessible sites providing didactic, text book style information on dermatology (E medicine, Dermnet NZ, etc.), our approach has been to concentrate on case-based learning. The educational material on the site is designed to enhance the user's ability to perform the tasks which would normally be carried out by the dermatologist when referred a patient for a traditional face-to-face consultation.

To this end we provide the following resources:

- A proforma outlining an ideal dermatological history and examination.
- A guide to the performance of a thorough skin cancer check covering history, examination and pitfalls.
- A guide to digital photography.
- A step-by-step, illustrated guide to punch and shave biopsy, curettage and elliptical excision. These are pitched at the level of a medical student and cover all aspects of these procedures from asepsis to dressings to handling of specimens.
- Techniques such as Marini and pulley sutures, second intention healing, cyst and skin tag removal techniques are also featured.
- A detailed, illustrated guide to cryotherapy is provided. This covers theory and practice including equipment, indications, contraindications, applications and short- and long-term complications. Images show the use of cryotherapy and illustrate the appearance of treatment sites both in the short and long term.
- An illustrated guide to the use of nonsurgical treatments in the management of solar keratosis and skin cancer, i.e. 5% 5 fluorouracil cream, imimiquimod and photodynamic therapy.
- A guide to the use of topical steroids.
- Detailed guides to the diagnosis and management of acne and drug eruptions.
- Streaming video footage covering history taking, skin checks, cryotherapy, eyelid and facial surgery.
- At the time of writing there are 645 case studies.
- A section of the site is devoted to review of interesting articles from the dermatological literature. There are over 70 journal articles reviewed in detail. Articles are selected on the basis of relevance to doctors working in primary care.
- There are discussion forums where site users can discuss matters of concern. All posts are answered by the site's teledermatologist and by any interested user.
- Each week a quiz is sent to all registered users of TN. This is an image accompanied by one or more questions. The answer is posted after a week. During the intervening period users post their answers. If incorrect, clarifying questions are asked or hints given.
- A number of other sites or useful inks (Dermnet NZ, E medicine, Australasian College of Dermatologists, etc.) are listed and can be accessed at a click of a mouse.
- The activity of each user of the site is tracked and recorded. This provides them with a permanent record for the purpose of documenting their continuing professional development requirements.

Case Studies on TN

One of the popular features of TN is ongoing case studies provided by the site consultant dermatologist for users to learn and test their knowledge. Each of the site's case studies is based on a case seen and managed by the site's dermatologist. Each case is presented with illustrative images and a relevant history. This is followed by a series of questions that explore the practical management of that specific case. The initial question is always to describe the clinical features. Further questions explore history, other clinical features, investigations, differential diagnosis, management, prognosis, side effects of treatment and so on. The answers are available at a mouse click. The cases illustrate benign skin lesions, melanoma and nonmelanoma skin cancer including dermoscopy, common and rare inflammatory dermatoses.

Most also have an MCQ at the end. Many have been posted as a result of a direct request from a site user to see a particular condition. New cases are added on a regular basis. There are often multiple examples of a specific condition. Each case is discussed in depth with specific reasons given for the approach to diagnosis and management. Treatment is outlined in detail documenting choice of medication, dosage and duration of use. Where relevant, the management of drug side effects is addressed.

It is hoped that users can adapt the approach taken in the cases to their own patients. Commonly when a telemedicine consultation is received, the inquirer is directed to a posted case study to see how a similar problem was managed. The site avoids text book style, didactic material which is readily available elsewhere in favour of real cases illustrating important clinical principles. These cases can be accessed in a blinded fashion as an exercise in self-assessment. Alternatively they are coded under their diagnoses. This means that if a user wishes to see cases of melanoma, Sweets syndrome, bullous pemphigoid, plant contact dermatitis, drug eruption or sarcoidosis for instance, they have to merely click on that diagnosis and one to often several examples will be available to them. On average, a case study will take 10–20 min to complete.

Many dermatological conditions are readily recognised but management is often not straightforward. As the conditions are coded under diagnosis, these can be used to guide users in managing their own patients without then having to seek advice from the site's dermatologist. To illustrate there are 12 cases of psoriasis, 10 different cases of acne, 7 of tinea incognito, 4 of alopecia areata and 3 of leucocytoclastic vasculitis. The concept is that as these cases are described in detail, doctors can use them as a guide to managing their own patients. A text book for instance may give ten or more options for treating acne. By perusing the cases posted on the site, the enquiring doctor can see how the dermatologist managed them and perhaps apply this specific management or variation thereof to their own patient.

They are also popular as an educational resource when doctors have medical students or trainees in their practice. They are also used by many as a tool for patient education.

As the cases posted on the site are derived from patients seen by the teledermatologist, they reflect the burden of dermatological disease seen in Australia. This means that the majority of conditions are common ones. However, rare conditions such as acrodermatitis enteropathica, mastocytosis, pemphigus foliaceus and many others are available.

Dermoscopy is given special prominence [15–18]. Once again this is explored from a practical basis. Cases are shown with clinical and dermoscopic images as well as relevant history of the lesion and the patient. Dermoscopy is taught in the setting of actual clinical practice and how it impacts on the assessment and management of a specific skin lesion. At the same time, dermoscopic features are illustrated and explained. Each dermoscopy case is explored in detail covering history, clinical and dermoscopic features, management options and how each was finally treated. The reasons why one treatment option was preferred over another are explored. For similar reasons as with inflammatory dermatoses, multiple examples of the various skin lesions are posted. There are over 150 case studies illustrating dermoscopy and subsequent management of skin lesions.

Australia has a very high burden of skin malignancy, and most treatment is carried out by general practitioners [19]. Treatment options are many and the choice of treatment may be determined by multiple independent variables. A superficial basal cell carcinoma on the back of a man in his late eighties will likely be treated completely differently to the same lesion arising on the chest of a woman in her twenties. There are over 80 separate cases of basal cell carcinoma on the site. Each is illustrated in a question and answer format covering everything from diagnosis, dermoscopy to management options to final treatment. There are at least seven available treatment options for BCC (cryotherapy, curettage and cautery, excisional surgery, margin controlled surgery, imiquimod, photodynamic therapy and radiotherapy). Few doctors in rural and remote practice in Australia would have difficulty in diagnosing most basal cell carcinomas. Selection of the best treatment taking into account tumour and patient variables as well as available resources can be difficult. By perusing these posted cases, users expand their knowledge base and at the same time can apply the information gleaned to the specific management of their own patients.

Australia Medical System and Telemedicine

Medicolegal Issues

Before going on line with TN, our two major concerns with the consultational aspect of the service were patient confidentiality and medicolegal issues. Interestingly, no surveyed doctors utilising the service identified medicolegal issues as a concern, and only a few suggested privacy issues were a concern [20, 21].

Doctors are instructed to submit no identifying patient details such as names, addresses or dates of birth. In fact the identity of the doctor submitting the case is restricted to their first name only. The images submitted rarely show identifiable facial features. If this is unavoidable, the doctor submitting the case obtains written consent to use the patient's facial images.

Australia has, at the time of writing, a state-based system of registering doctors. Medical indemnity cover for a consultation only applied to those states within which an individual doctor is registered. Telemedical advice is covered by usual medical indemnity but only when carried out in the state where the doctor is registered. The question arises as to where does a telemedicine consultation take place? Is it in the state where the patient is, where the doctor providing telemedical advice is, in both or neither? With no precedent to go on and no clear ruling available in the relevant legislation, legal advice was sought. The argument was raised that if the patient physically travelled interstate to see the TN dermatologist rather than merely sending their images, the consultation would occur in the dermatologist's home state.

It was felt that a court would likely consider a telemedicine consult based on store-and-forward technology to have occurred in the state where the patient was at the time of the consultation. The practical outcome of this is that any doctor providing an Australia-wide telemedicine service has had to be registered in every state and territory. This means that the dermatologist providing telemedicine advice on TN had to pay eight separate registration fees a year rather than one. Happily national registration is being put in place as of 2010 so this extra cost will no longer be incurred. As there is no technical reason why a teledermatology service could not receive referrals from other countries, the same medicolegal issues would exist in this situation. TN does answer requests for advice from doctors working in foreign lands.

Before submitting a case the referring doctor has to agree to an acknowledgement and disclaimer*. This form confirms that:

- The doctor is currently registered and insured for practice in Australia.
- That TN is designed to assist the doctor in diagnosis and management of their patient's condition. The referring doctor remains responsible for making the diagnosis and managing the patient.
- The referring doctor recognises that a face-to-face consultation may carry less risk of diagnostic error than telemedicine.
- That their insurer will cover them when seeking telemedicine advice.
- That they have obtained written, informed consent from their patient to use TN to help manage their case.
- The patient understands that the referring doctor is responsible for their management.
- The patient is given the option of referral for a face-to-face consultation.
- The patient agrees to their deidentified information and images being viewed by other doctors using the site for educational purposes. This is not a condition of using the service.
- The patient has signed the TN patient consent form*.
- That the doctor will not submit any material that could identify the patient.
- Lastly that the organisations and individuals responsible for providing TN are not liable for the information or guidance provided by TN and that although every effort is made the site cannot be guaranteed to be secure.

As in the rest of the world the fallout from medical negligence cases that involve a teledermatology consultation is unknown. The main reason for this is that so far and fortunately there have been no cases of medical negligence brought before an Australian court involving teledermatology that we know of. There is a great deal of evidence supporting the use of telemedicine in the management of dermatological disease [22–27]. Without telemedicine many patients in rural and remote Australia can only access specialist advice by travelling to urban areas which greatly increases the burden on these patients in terms of expense and time. In some rural areas, there is a visiting dermatology service but this can still mean long delays.

We hope that our consent, acknowledgement and disclaimer forms allow doctors and patients to be able to make informed decisions on whether or not they choose to use our service. Naturally we strive to give the best advice possible with the information we receive. It is quite common that we need to request additional images and history to ensure optimal results.

Reimbursement

Australia has a government-run universal health insurance program, 'Medicare'. Doctors receive remuneration from this for medical services rendered. Thus, when a doctor sees a patient for a consultation or performs a

*Copies of these forms are in Appendices 4.1 and 4.2.

surgical procedure, Medicare will reimburse a set amount of money for the service delivered. At the moment teledermatology does not attract a Medicare reimbursement for either the doctors utilising, or those providing, a teledermatology service. This is despite the fact that utilising a telemedicine service places a considerable burden of time and effort on the referring practitioner especially when compared to referral for a traditional face-to-face consultation. By using a telemedicine service to assist in managing their patients, the referring doctor is also undertaking far greater responsibility for the patient's management then with a traditional referral.

A recent survey of doctors using TN found that submitting a case for consultation took between 20 and 30 min of their time. Combining this with the considerable savings to the individual patient and indeed society in terms of not needing to take time off work, no need to travel, lack of delay in receiving a specialist opinion and earlier intervention, it would seem obvious that the use of teledermatology should attract reimbursement for the referring practitioner in the same way as any other medical service.

Conclusion

'Tele-Derm National' is one part of a larger online education and consultation service directed at the needs of practitioners and their patients in rural and remote Australia. It is also used by urban doctors, doctors in training and medical students. Its aim is to provide practical and readily accessible education in dermatology as well as a rapid turnaround consultation service. We feel that one cannot exist without the other.

Appendix 4.1. Submit a Case to Tele-Derm

Acknowledgement and Disclaimer

Before using the TELE-DERM service you must agree to the following terms:

1. I am a doctor registered to practice in Australia and hold current medical indemnity insurance.
2. I acknowledge that the TELE - DERM service is intended to assist me in diagnosing and managing my patient's condition. A consultation with a TELE - DERM dermatologist *is not a substitute for my clinical judgement. I continue to be responsible at all times for the diagnosis and management of my patient's* condition.
3. I acknowledge that there is less margin for error in a face to face consultation compared with an internet consultation such as the TELE - DERM service.
4. I have written confirmation from my medical indemnity insurer that the existing policy of medical indemnity insurance issued to me covers my use of the TELE - DERM service.
5. I have obtained my patient's informed consent to using the TELE - DERM service. In doing so, I explained to my patient that I would be using the internet to consult a TELE - DERM dermatologist on the patient's condition but that all decisions regarding diagnosis and management would be made by me. I also explained to my patient that the consultation would necessitate e-mailing information and images relating to my patient's condition and that there could be an increased potential for unauthorised disclosure or error in diagnosis or management arising from use of an internet service as compared to a face to face consultation. As an alternative, I offered my patient referral to a dermatologist.
6. Unless specifically indicated by me, my patient has also given informed consent to his or her case being posted on the TELE - DERM website for educational purposes. My patient was made aware that this is not a condition to my using the TELE - DERM service.
7. My patient has signed the TELE - DERM consent form. I have included this in my patient record.
8. *I will not include in any material submitted to a TELE - DERM dermatologist any information from which my patient could be identified. In particular no names, addresses or dates of birth will be included. The images of the condition submitted are such that the patient cannot be identified by his or her physical features.*
9. I acknowledge that the TELE-DERM service is hosted by the Australian College of Rural and Remote Medicine ("ACRRMquot") and funded by the Commonwealth Government as represented by its Department of Health and Ageing, with the fundholder being Queensland Divisions of General Practice. The Department and ACRRM, and their respective directors and other officers and employees, partners, agents and sub-contractors make

no representations or warranties and do not accept any liability from any person for the information or guidance (or the use of such information or guidance) which is provided on the TELE-DERM web site or as part of the TELE-DERM service.

10. Although every effort is made by ACRRM and its contractors to ensure the integrity of TELE-DERM web site, ACRRM cannot guarantee the safety of computer systems of site users. ACRRM does not accept liability for any damage to any computer system which has been connected to the TELE - DERM web site. Users enter the web site at their own risk.

Appendix 4.2. Patient Consent Form for Use of TELE-DERM Service

I ...., acknowledge that my doctor is seeking information and guidance on the diagnosis and management of my condition from a qualified dermatologist at TELE–DERM. This involves transmission of details of my case, including images over the internet. I have checked with my doctor that no details or images sent can reveal my identity. I acknowledge that the internet is not a totally secure medium and third parties may be able to gain unauthorized access to my TELE-DERM consultation. I realize that a face to face consultation with a dermatologist is less likely to result in an error of diagnosis or management.

I understand that I can instead be referred to a dermatologist for a face to face consultation if I wish.

I understand that dermatologists at TELE–DERM are merely giving my doctor information and guidance. They will not be responsible for the diagnosis and management of my condition.

I understand that all decisions on the diagnosis and management of my condition will be made by my doctor, [insert referring doctor's name].

I understand that I may still need to see a dermatologist face to face if my condition cannot be managed by my doctor after consultation with a TELE–DERM dermatologist.

I consent to my case being posted on the TELE – DERM web site for educational purposes. [Delete if consent not given].

I acknowledge that the TELE-DERM service is hosted by the Australian College of Rural and Remote Medicine ("ACRRM") and funded by the Commonwealth Government as represented by its Department of Health and Ageing. The Department and ACRRM, and their respective directors and other officers and employees, partners, agents and sub-contractors make no representations or warranties and do not accept any liability from any person for the information or guidance (or the use of such information or guidance) which is provided on the TELE-DERM web site or as part of the TELE-DERM service

This Consent may be relied upon by the Doctor, Queensland Division of General Practice, the TELE – DERM dermatologists, the Commonwealth Government and ACRRM (including their directors and other persons mentioned above).

Signed..............Date ....

Witness..................... [referring doctor]

References

1. Australian Bureau of Statistics, Australian Demographic Statistics, Sep 2009 (2010) http://www.abs.gov.au/Ausstats/abs@.nsf/mf/3101.0. Last updated 30 Mar 2010; Accessed June 2010
2. Encyclopedia of the Nations (2010) http://www.nationsencyclopedia.com/Europe/United-Kingdom.html. Accessed June 2010
3. Lim AC, See AC, Shumack SP (2001) Progress in Australian teledermatology. J Telemed Telecare 7(Suppl 2):55–59
4. Smith AC, Gray LC (2009) Telemedicine across the ages. Med J Aust 190:15–19
5. Kerr OA, Tidman MJ, Walker JJ, Aldridge RD, Benton EC (2010) The profile of dermatological problems in primary care. Clin Exp Dermatol 35(4):380–383
6. Davila M, Christenson LJ, Sontheimer RD (2010) Epidemiology and outcomes of dermatology in-patient consultations in a Midwestern U.S. University hospital. Dermatol Online J 16(2):12
7. Ludwick DA, Lortie C, Doucette J, Rao J, Samoil-Schelstraete C (2010) Evaluation of a telehealth clinic as a means to facilitate dermatologic consultation: pilot project to assess the efficiency and experience of teledermatology used in a primary care network. J Cutan Med Surg 14(1): 7–12
8. Australia Government Department of Health and Ageing (2010) http://www.health.gov.au/internet/main/publishing.nsf/Content/ruralhealth-services-msoap. Page last modified: 03 Dec 2009; Accessed June 2010
9. Wootton R, Oakley A (eds) (2002) Teledermatology. The Royal Society of Medicine Press, London
10. Wurm EM, Hofmann-Wellenhof R, Wurm R, Soyer HP (2008) Telemedicine and teledermatology: past, present and future. J Dtsch Dermatol Ges 6(2):106–112
11. Whited JD (2010) Economic analysis of telemedicine and the teledermatology paradigm. Telemed J E-Health 16(2): 223–228

12. van der Heijden JP, Spuls PI, Voorbraak FP, de Keizer NF, Witkamp L, Bos JD (2010) Tertiary teledermatology: a systematic review. Telemed J E-Health 16:1–7
13. Australian College of Rural and Remote Medicine (2010) http://www.acrrm.org.au/rrmeo. Assessed June 2010
14. Muir J, Lucas L (2008) Tele-dermatology in Australia. In: Latifi R (ed) Current principles and practice of telemedicine and e-health. Rifat Latifi Publisher, Amsterdam; Washington, DC, pp 243–253
15. Katz BJ, Oliviero M, Rabinovitz H (2010) Dermoscopy and its impact on skin cancer diagnostics. J Drugs Dermatol 9(2):129–130
16. van der Rhee JI, Bergman W, Kukutsch NA (2010) The impact of dermoscopy on the management of pigmented lesions in everyday clinical practice of general dermatologists: a prospective study. Br J Dermatol 162(3):563–567
17. Massone C, Brunasso AM, Hofmann-Wellenhof R, Gulia A, Soyer HP (2010) Teledermoscopy: education, discussion forums, teleconsulting and mobile teledermoscopy. G Ital Dermatol Venereol 145(1):127–132
18. Johr R, Soyer HP, Argenziano G, Hofman-Wellenhof RMD, Scalvenzi M (2004) Dermoscopy: the essentials. Mosby, Edinburgh
19. Dixon A, Rosengren H, Connelly T, Dixon J (2009) Education in skin cancer management – assessing knowledge and safety. Aust Fam Physician 38(7):557–560
20. Leung ST, Kaplan KJ (2009) Medicolegal aspects of telepathology. Hum Pathol 40(8):1137–1142
21. Stanberry B (2006) Legal and ethical aspects of telemedicine. J Telemed Telecare 12(4):166–175
22. Lim AC, Egerton IB, See A, Shumack SP (2001) Accuracy and reliability of store-and-forward teledermatology: preliminary results from the St George Teledermatology Project. Australas J Dermatol 42:247–251
23. Levin YS, Warshaw EM (2009) Teledermatology: a review of reliability and accuracy of diagnosis and management. Dermatol Clin 27(2):163–176
24. Whited JD, Hall RP, Simel DL, Foy ME, Stechuchak KM, Drugge RJ (1999) Reliability and accuracy of dermatologists' and clinic-based and digital image consultations. J Am Acad Dermatol 41(5, pt 1):693–702
25. Burdick AE (2007) Teledermatology: extending specialty care beyond borders. Arch Dermatol 143(12):1581–1582
26. See A, Lim AC, Le K, See JA, Shumack SP (2005) Operational teledermatology in Broken Hill, rural Australia. Australas J Dermatol 46:144–149
27. Tait CP, Clay CD (1999) Pilot study of store and forward teledermatology services in Perth, Western Australia. Australas J Dermatol 40:190–193

Teledermatology in Pakistan

5

Shahbaz A. Janjua, Ijaz Hussain, Arfan Bari,
Sadia Ammad, and Rahila Naz

Core Messages

- Pakistan like other developing countries is facing problems in addressing the issues of availability of health care services to its growing population, which is concentrated in the villages and remote areas. On the contrary, telecommunication connectivity all over the country improved remarkably in the last decade. In this scenario, telemedicine can be utilized to provide health care to the remote and underserved areas. Telemedicine has also played a major role in bridging the gap between primary and tertiary health care facilities during disaster relief operations. Dermatology is undoubtedly the most suitable specialty for telemedicine. Therefore, teledermatology has been an integral part of various telemedicine projects and networks in Pakistan. However, to meet the challenge of integrating teledermatology into the current health care system of the country, major issues need to be addressed.

A Preview of Existing Health Care Services

Pakistan is a densely populated country of Southeast Asia. More than 75% of its population lives in villages and small towns. There is a major rural-urban disparity in the delivery of health care services because most of the well equipped hospitals and clinics are located in big cities where most of the physicians prefer to reside and practice. The current health care infrastructure supervised by the ministry of health, consists of basic health units, rural health centers, tehsil headquarter (THQ) hospitals, district headquarter (DHQ) hospitals, and teaching medical institutions. A large number of private clinics and hospitals established in the urban areas also contribute to the delivery of health care services to the urban population. On the contrary, health care services in the rural areas remain far from sufficient. The people living in the rural and remote areas often have to travel long distances to get medical treatment in big cities. This incurs both expenditure and inconvenience of transporting sick patients, which is further complicated by the deficient road network and the low per capita income of an average Pakistani.

S.A. Janjua (✉) • R. Naz
Teledermatology Unit, Ayza Skin & Research Center, Lalamusa, Pakistan
e-mail: shahbaz.janjua@telederm.org; rahilanaz01@gmail.com

I. Hussain
Department of Dermatology, Sheikh Zayed Medical College, Rahimyar Khan, Pakistan
e-mail: drijazhussain@gmail.com

A. Bari
Department of Dermatology, Combined Military Hospital, Peshawar, Pakistan
e-mail: albariul@gmail.com

S. Ammad
Aesthetic dermatology division, DermaCosmo Care, Lahore, Pakistan
e-mail: sadia0027@gmail.com

H.P. Soyer et al. (eds.), *Telemedicine in Dermatology*,
DOI 10.1007/978-3-642-20801-0_5, © Springer-Verlag Berlin Heidelberg 2012

The situation is even worse for the remote Northern areas of Pakistan where difficult mountainous terrain hampers mobility and access to modern health care services. A high morbidity rate is a direct consequence of this situation [1].

To summarize, Pakistan like other developing countries is facing problems in addressing the issues of availability of health care services to its growing population, which is concentrated in the villages and remote areas. Moreover, junior doctors serving in these areas feel isolated as they are unable to consult senior or specialist doctors in case of any difficulty regarding diagnosis or treatment of complicated cases.

Telecommunication Infrastructure

The telecommunication industry in Pakistan underwent a rapid development in the last decade, as a result of which the communication connectivity all over the country improved remarkably. The number of fixed telephone lines in the country is now well over four million, and the Internet is increasingly becoming a popular medium with about 170,000 broadband subscribers and 3.7 million dial-up users [2]. In this scenario, telemedicine holds great promise as an alternative means of health care delivery to the underserved rural and remote areas [3]. The concept of moving information instead of people has been the basis of all telemedicine efforts in developing countries like Pakistan.

Existing Telemedicine/Teledermatology Scenario

In a country like Pakistan with poorly developed basic health infrastructure and major rural-urban disparity regarding provision of health care services, the need and importance of telemedicine cannot be denied [4]. Various private and governmental organizations have pioneered implementation of telemedicine in Pakistan, and a number of telemedicine projects have recently been launched. These projects offer a great opportunity for the people living in underserved rural areas to have access to improved healthcare services. Telemedicine is now being utilized in a growing number of medical specialties including dermatology, oncology, radiology, surgery, cardiology, psychiatry, and gynecology [5]. Dermatology, because of its inherent visual nature, has been considered the most suitable specialty for telemedicine by various telemedicine networks and projects presently working in Pakistan [6]. In addition to providing specialist dermatologic care to the underserved areas of the country, teledermatology has the potential to lessen the feeling of isolation experienced by the doctors serving in rural and remote areas. In the sections to follow, we will discuss the present status and future prospects of various telemedicine projects in Pakistan with special emphasis on teledermatology. It would be important to note here that the teledermatology services have been launched in Pakistan either as part of various telemedicine projects or as separate and independent teledermatology projects. Preliminary results of these projects have shown a number of potential benefits not only to the patients and the doctors but also to the health care system of the country (Fig. 5.1).

Telemedicine Networks Involving Teledermatology

TelemedPak

Elixir Technologies, a software development company based in the US, introduced the concept of telemedicine for the first time in Pakistan in 1998 as a philanthropic project, TelemedPak [7]. The website of TelemedPak (http://www.telmedpak.com) serves as the largest Pakistan-based medical web interface which provides public information concerning all types of health problems.

TelMedPak worked in collaboration with major universities in Pakistan including Rawalpindi Medical College, Agha Khan University, and the National University of Science & Technology, offering various training programs in telemedicine for the medical students.

In addition to the training programs, TelemedPak successfully completed two telemedicine pilot projects – the Taxila and Gilgit projects to assess the applicability of telemedicine in Pakistan. The hospitals were equipped with computers, Internet access, and scanners, and were required to email case reports of difficult cases for expert medical opinion to the specialist doctors at the Holy Family Hospital, Rawalpindi, which served as the hub of all telemedicine activities for these projects.

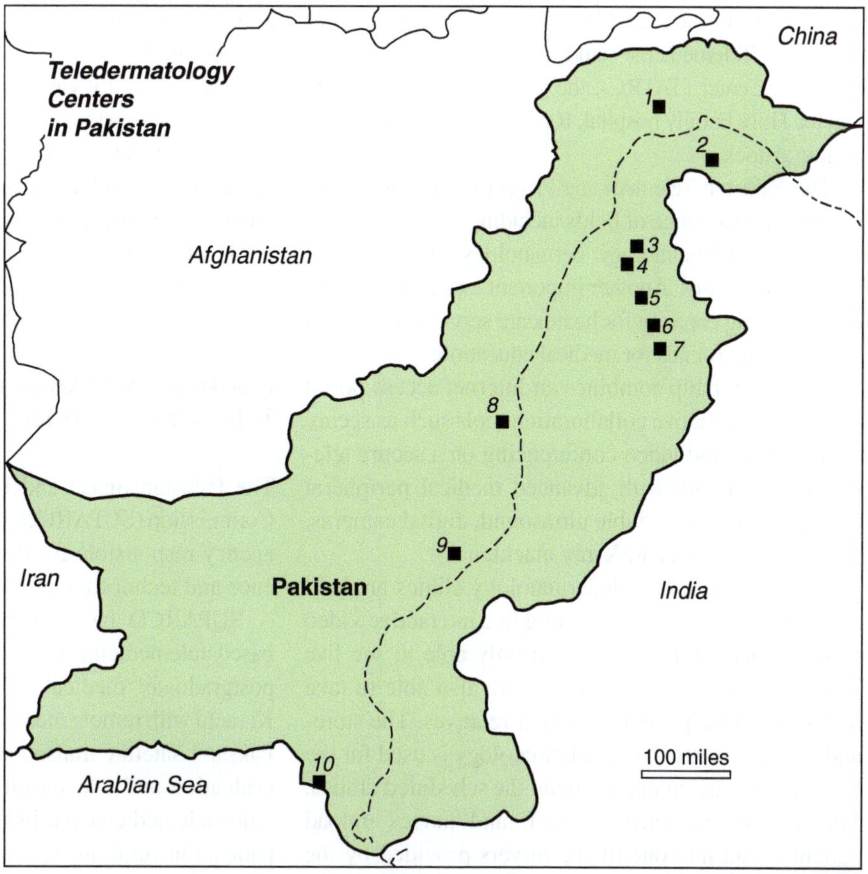

Fig. 5.1 Teledermatology centers in Pakistan; Gilgit *1*, Sakardu *2*, Islamabad *3*, Rawalpindi *4*, Gujar Khan *5*, Lalamusa *6*, Lahore *7*, Dera Ghazi Khan *8*, Shikarpur *9*, Karachi *10*

The success of these projects proved that telemedicine was not only possible in Pakistan but it could also potentially uplift the health status of the remote areas by provision of the specialist care in areas where conventional face-to-face consultation with the specialists may not be possible.

Teledermatology has been the integral part of these projects providing teleconsultation, tele-assistance, and distance learning to the junior doctors working in remote areas of Gilgit and Taxila. Telemedicine centers established in THQ hospitals of Gujar Khan, Pind Dadan Khan, Pindi Ghaib, Fateh Jang, and Jhand were linked with the main co-ordinating centers in Holy Family and DHQ hospitals in Rawalpindi.

A study to compare the store-and-forward method of teledermatology with the conventional face-to-face consultation was conducted with technical support of TelemedPak [8]. Patients were selected from the dermatology department of Pakistan Institute of Medical Sciences (PIMS), Islamabad. Images along with a short history and clinical findings were stored in a computer and sent via email to the department of dermatology of King Edward Medical College, Lahore, for teleconsultation. Diagnoses made by face-to-face consultations at PIMS were then compared with the diagnoses made after teleconsultation. The study showed that diagnoses made through teleconsultations were similar to the diagnoses reached after conventional face-to-face consultation.

The Pakistan Telemedicine Project

The U.S. Department of State and IBM are leading a partnership bringing telemedicine to northern areas of Pakistan [9]. The partnership has helped to improve technology at a central coordinating hospital, the Holy Family Hospital, Rawalpindi, with more limited resources at a "spoke" hospital in District Attock [10, 11]. Other members of the partnership include Wateen Telecom, Motorola

Inc., Medweb Inc., USAID, the U.S. Department of Defense, Telemedicine and Advanced Technology Research Center (TATRC), the government of Pakistan, and the Holy Family hospital, Rawalpindi, and DHQ hospital in Attock.

The Pakistan Telemedicine Project offers teleconsultation in a wide range of fields including general surgery, cardiology, ophthalmology, dermatology, radiology, and infectious diseases. Another important aspect of the project is building capacity for healthcare services via virtual clinical grand rounds for medical education.

The partnership combines an Internet access portal providing interactive collaboration tools such as secure email, voice, and video conferencing on a secure telemedicine network with advanced medical peripheral devices including portable ultrasound, digital cameras, EKG, stethoscope, and X-ray machine.

Weekly scheduled teledermatology clinics are held at the Holy Family hospital using live interactive video method. Dermatologists are not only able to see live images of the skin disorders but are also able to take history from the patients and their relatives. The store-and-forward method of teledermatology is used for the patients who are unable to attend the scheduled clinics. The doctors, paramedical staff, and nurses upload patient's data into one of the servers provided by the Medweb. The consultants can view the cases and respond by logging into the server at leisure.

Telemedicine/e-Health Training Center

The telemedicine/e-health training center is a joint Pak-US collaboration [12]. This center consists of a teaching laboratory in the surgical Unit II of the Holy Family Hospital, Rawalpindi, and a remote consulting unit at THQ hospital in Pindi Gheb. This center has high bandwidth telecommunication link with collaborating institutions in the US, Virginia Commonwealth University (VCU), Richmond, and Telemedicine & Advanced Technology Research center (TATRC), Fort Detrick.

The telemedicine/e-health course is designed to train doctors and nurses from both tertiary care hospitals and primary care centers in telemedicine. The main objective is to train primary referring doctors and nurses as well as doctors and nurses responding to the referrals at the tertiary care hospital. In the initial phase, 45 doctors and nurses from Rawalpindi region were trained.

Teledermatology remains a widely used application and focus of various telemedicine projects of the center. Twice weekly teledermatology clinics are held at the center providing teleconsultations to the patients attending teledermatology clinics in remote DHQ hospitals of Gujrat, Attock, Pindi Gheb, and Khushab using live interactive video method.

Pakistan Space Organization (SUPARCO) Telemedicine Project

The Pakistan Space and Upper Atmosphere Research Commission (SUPARCO) is the country's national space agency responsible for the execution of the space science and technology programs in the country.

SUPARCO has launched Pakistan's first satellite-based telemedicine network. It has connected Jinnah postgraduate medical college hospital (JPMC) in Karachi with remote medical center at Shikarpur through Paksat-1 satellite transponder for the purpose of patient evaluation and teleconsultations [13]. Live interactive video telemedicine has linked specialists in JPMC to the patients in rural areas, thus providing specialist health care services to the rural areas. The next step is the development of satellite-based telemedicine centers at Holy Family hospital, Rawalpindi, in Punjab province and primary care centers in Muzaffarabad keeping in view the geographical isolation of northern areas.

Role of Telemedicine in Natural Disaster Management

Earthquake 2005

Telemedicine/e-health training center played a remarkable role in providing telemedicine service to the disaster-stricken northern areas of Pakistan during the earthquake of October 2005. This was a high magnitude earthquake which left at least 86,000 people dead, 69,000 people injured, and 4 million people homeless. This also heavily damaged the physical infrastructure of the area that included all major hospitals in the government and private sector (Fig. 5.2). Soon after the earthquake, outbreaks of infectious, parasitic, viral, and fungal skin

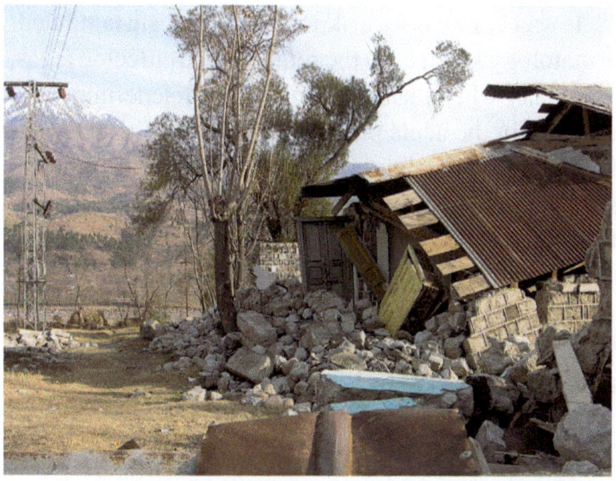

Fig. 5.2 A hospital completely demolished by the October 2005 earthquake in Muzaffarabad

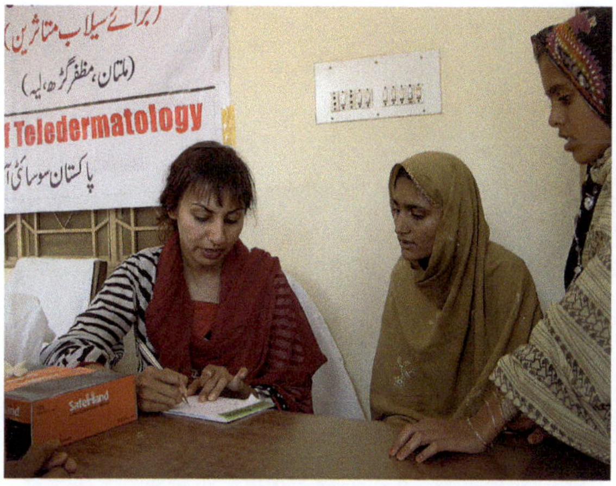

Fig. 5.3 Dr. Aisha Sethi recording a patient's history for teleconsultation at an outreach skin clinic in a remote flood-affected village

diseases occurred due to unhygienic living conditions in overcrowded camps. Telemedicine/e-health training center promptly responded to the disaster providing telemedicine services with the help of the ministry of information technology, International Telecommunications Union, Pakistan Software Board, and INTEL [14]. A telemedicine center was established at the Holy Family Hospital in Rawalpindi which customized telemedicine software for disaster relief, to train volunteers, to respond to teleconsultations from relief camps at disaster site, to coordinate relief activities with Prime Minister Relief Cell in Islamabad, and to address daily needs of the earthquake victims. Mobile telemedicine centers were established in the most heavily affected areas including Muzaffarabad, Hattian Bala, Shoal Najaf, and Balakot. "Telemedicine for disaster relief" also worked in collaboration with the foreign missions, NGOs, and government relief missions. Most of the teleconsultations were provided in dermatology, orthopedics, pediatrics, and gynecology utilizing both real-time and store-and-forward modalities. The patient's data including history, examination, and images of the patients was collected and stored in the main server by the trained doctors and health workers in the affected areas. This was later sent to the consultant dermatologists via Internet or satellite. The consultants promptly responded to these requests with diagnosis and treatment plans. In the live video interactive teleconsultations, the consultants were able to communicate directly with the patients and their treating physicians [15]. These teleconsultations resulted in speedy treatment and minimized hospital stay of the patients.

Floods 2010

Pakistan faced the worst flooding of its recorded history in July 2010. The flooding continued for 2 months devastating a large part of the country and displacing millions of people. The extent of damage to the already compromised and poor physical infrastructure was huge. The roaring flood waters washed away almost everything including houses, livelihoods, schools, hospitals, roads, and the bridges. At one point about one-fifth of the country was under water. People in the affected areas were isolated and stranded with no access to shelter, clean drinking water, food, and medicines (Fig. 5.3).

Medical implications of the floods were also immense. In addition to the physical and psychological trauma caused by heavy large-scale flooding, the incidence of food- and water-borne diseases, malaria, and skin diseases increased due to damage to the drainage systems and contamination of water supplies. Hundreds of medical camps were established in various parts of the country by the NGOs and the government-supervised health sector to meet the medical needs of the people displaced by the floods. According to one survey every third patient reporting to these medical camps had a skin problem. Although the commonly reported skin diseases were scabies and

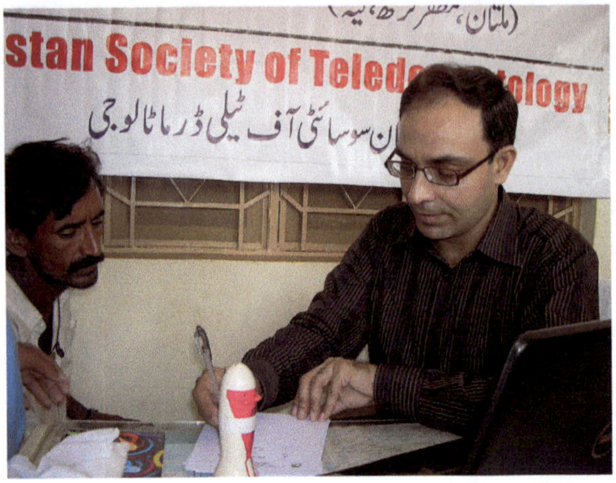

Fig. 5.4 Dr. Janjua providing teledermatology services in a remote flood-affected area during an outreach skin clinic organized by the Pakistan Society of Teledermatology

bacterial and fungal skin infections, complicated skin disorders were also reported. Unfortunately, most of the doctors and health workers serving in the medical camps had little or no training to deal even with common skin diseases. In this difficult time, the Pakistan Society of Teledermatology arranged outreach mobile skin clinics in various remote flood-stricken areas of the country to meet the dermatologic needs of the affected communities. Expert dermatologists from Pakistan and the United States volunteered to work in the outreach mobile skin clinics providing dermatologic care to the affected people [16]. Thousands of patients presenting to the outreach mobile skin clinics were treated and provided medicines free of cost (Fig. 5.4). The society also collaborated with the already established medical camps and offered to provide necessary basic training to the doctors and health workers in general dermatology. To continue the delivery of expert dermatologic care, teledermatology was introduced to the doctors and the health workers in base medical camps. Initially, five such medical camps established in remote flood-hit areas were selected, and connected to the dermatology departments of teaching institutions and privately working dermatology centers to provide expert dermatologic care through store-and-forward method of teledermatology. Over 800 teleconsultations were made during 2 months (Fig. 5.3).

The e-Health Association of Pakistan, Swinfen charitable trust, and iCons in Medicine also played significant role in providing teledermatology/telemedicine services to the flood-affected areas.

It was not an easy task to initiate and sustain teledermatology services to the remote flood-affected areas, especially when there was no planned teledermatology network in the acute phase [15]. Other limiting factors included low voltages, frequent power shutdown, shortages of the necessary equipment, inadequate funding, and large number of patients.

Independent Teledermatology Networks and Projects

Teledermatology Units in Teaching Institutions

The ministry of science and technology realizing the potential of telemedicine in Pakistan established "National Telemedicine Task Force" in September 2001. The following were the main objectives of the task force [17]:

- To identify telemedicine pilot projects of national interest including telemedicine education of doctors, tele-psychiatry, and teledermatology
- To create awareness about telemedicine in the country by arranging seminars and conferences at the national level

National Telemedicine Conference 2002 was organized by the forum on June 22, 2002. Live telemedicine sessions were demonstrated during the conference showing teleconsultations between the doctors and the specialists and also between the patients and the specialists.

Teledermatology had always been the main focus of national telemedicine task force. Teledermatology units were therefore established all over the country in the dermatology departments of almost every teaching institution. These institutions have been connected with the district headquarter (DHQ) hospitals employing both store-and-forward and real-time modalities. The DHQ hospitals have been provided with high-resolution digital cameras, computers, and a high-speed Internet connection. The medical staff including doctors, nurses, and paramedical staff at the point of care is trained how to use the equipment. Teleconsultation and tele-assistance regarding diagnosis and treatment of various dermatologic disorders is provided to the doctors and paramedical staff in the DHQ hospitals. These teledermatology projects also involved some degree of tele-education providing continuing medical education for the doctors who submitted their cases. Although there have not yet been any large studies focusing on the clinical outcomes of teledermatology in Pakistan, the preliminary results of a few small-scale studies comparing the conventional face-to-face consultations with teledermatology consultations have shown several benefits of teledermatology including easy extension of dermatologic services to remote areas with few or no dermatologists at all [18].

Teledermatology Project of Ayza Skin & Research Center

This project was initiated in the private sector by the Ayza Skin & Research Center (AS & RC) in a small town of central Punjab in 2004 [19]. The scope of the project was to connect general practitioners working in small towns and villages with the specialist dermatologists in teaching institutions and dermatology centers in big cities. The project utilized email-based store-and-forward teledermatology. Difficult and challenging cases presenting at the center or sent by the general practitioners and dermatologists from other parts of the country are reviewed, processed, and then sent to a pool of expert dermatologists from Pakistan, Austria, Australia, India, and the United States using the store-and-forward modality.

The project also uses telederm.org (http://www.telederm.org) web application which is world's largest online discussion forum [20]. Cases are submitted to a pool of selected international experts for discussion. A prompt specialist opinion is therefore obtained, leading to more accurate diagnosis and treatment outcomes. Through this initiative, scientific cooperation has been established with a large number of expert dermatologists from renowned institutions worldwide.

Teledermatology Project of COMSATS, Islamabad

COMSATS Institute of information technology, Islamabad, launched a telemedicine pilot project in 2006 with the aim of providing teleconsultation to the patients in Sakurdu, a remote town in the Himalayan mountainous region of Pakistan [21]. The project was initiated with the collaboration of COMSATS, Association of Physicians of Pakistani Descent of North America (APPNA), and Digital Vision program of Stanford University in Boston. Initially a telemedicine project soon turned into a teledermatology project because 77% of the teleconsultations were for various dermatologic disorders. Store-and-forward method was preferred over live video sessions mainly because of time difference between the remote facility and the US. A simple format was selected to collect medical records. Images of the skin problems along with short history and clinical findings were sent to Stanford University in Boston, US, where specialist dermatologists responded to the queries. The following tasks were accomplished by the project team during the project which lasted from April 2006 to October 2006:

- Local medical health professionals at the point of care were assisted to gather proper medical records for dermatology cases.
- The doctors were educated to better understand dermatologic disorders.
- They were assisted in providing better diagnosis for treatment in the rural community.
- The quality of care provided to the rural community was improved.
- The software interface was improved and its features were tested.
- The system was devised to facilitate store-and-forward method of teledermatology.

Pakistan Society of Teledermatology

The Pakistan Society of Teledermatology was founded in 2004 in Lahore by a few devoted dermatologists from renowned teaching institutions and dermatology centers with the prime objective of creating awareness among dermatologists, family practitioners, and general public regarding the need and importance of providing specialist dermatology services through telecommunication to the remote and rural areas of Pakistan [22]. Other aims and objectives of the society include:

- To review existing teledermatology networks and projects in the country
- To assess current status of telecommunication and to identify technology that best meets the demands
- To assess the ability of existing teledermatology networks and projects to meet the needs and willingness of the general practitioners and dermatologists
- To optimize teledermatology services in the country
- To plan and distribute basic information regarding practice of teledermatology to all health professionals involved in various teledermatology projects
- To provide an online discussion forum to discuss difficult and challenging cases submitted by family practitioners and dermatologists from various parts of the country

- To provide online educational resource of dermatology curriculum, and access to online dermatology atlases for the continuing medical education of residents, dermatologists, and medical students
- To arrange seminars and workshops for the education and training of dermatologists, family physicians, medical students, and paramedical health workers regarding the use of teledermatology system
- To provide a center for coordination among various teledermatology projects
- To collaborate with various international teledermatology projects

The society is presently working in collaboration with the International Society of Teledermatology based in Austria, and Dr. Ian McColl's web-based educational program for medical students, family physicians, and dermatologists [23].

Limitations and Cultural Issues

Despite general consensus supporting the increased diagnostic accuracy, reliability, and effectiveness of teledermatology, unfortunately, the technique has not yet become the integral part of the existing health care system of Pakistan. Since available resources are mostly allocated to the prevention and treatment of serious medical conditions rather than to nonlethal skin disorders, dermatology therefore is not the main focus of health policies of the country [4].

Generally, the following problems are being faced by the health care professionals involved in various teledermatology projects in the country explaining the limited use of teledermatology.

- Poor quality or low-resolution images
- Insufficient clinical information
- Lack of proper training of the doctors and paramedical staff
- Patient loss to follow-up
- Inadequate medical record system
- Technological problems from failure of computer hardware, software, telecommunications, and peripheral equipment
- Inadequate privacy and confidentiality of identifiable health information
- Medical liability issues
- Cultural barriers
- Political barriers
- Language barriers
- Distrust in the safety and privacy of the technique
- Economic issues

Suggestions and Future Prospects

To meet the challenge of integrating teledermatology into the current health care system of the country, the authors recommend addressing the major issues already discussed in the previous section [24].

We suggest that health professionals involved in various teledermatology projects be adequately trained to take good quality, high-resolution images and taught how to properly send their cases for teleconsultation using the store-and-forward method.

It is also advisable to follow certain rules and regulations to maintain privacy and confidentiality of all identifiable health information of the patients.

Internet services need to be widely and readily accessible in the rural and remote areas.

It has been observed that people who are educated and well acquainted with the computers and Internet are usually open to the use of teledermatology. Therefore, to overcome cultural and language barriers, the literacy level of the people needs to be raised by establishing educational institutions in remote and rural areas.

It is also crucial to engage the dermatology departments of the hospitals and medical centers in the process of introducing teledermatology as soon as possible. Comprehensive training programs and seminars need to be arranged emphasizing the potential advantages of teledermatology.

The health policy makers should weigh the economic value of various teledermatology projects against potential benefits of extending specialist dermatology services to remote underserved areas through telecommunication.

Both implementation and sustainability costs need to be considered before planning new teledermatology centers. The services can be cost effective with subsidized funding from the provincial and federal health sector.

With further development of telecommunication infrastructure in near future, Internet services will soon be within the reach of rural and remote northern areas of Pakistan resulting in improvement of the teledermatology services to these areas [5].

It is hoped that teledermatology will ultimately become an increasingly mainstream activity for all the telemedicine projects discussed above, but it would not be possible without the whole-hearted involvement of physicians and dermatologists of the country in various national and international teledermatology initiatives.

References

1. World Health Organization/Pakistan/Country health profile. Available at: http://www.who.int/countries/pak/en/ (January, 22, 2010)
2. Pakistan telecommunication authority/achievements 06–07. Available at: http://www.pta.org.pk (July 20, 2010)
3. Ahmad S, Gilani S, Malik AZ (2006) Telemedicine software for a developing country. In: Proceedings 4th APT telemedicine workshop, Rawalpindi, 2006, p 189
4. Country Telemedicine Report of Pakistan. (2005) Published in proceedings of APT workshop in Malaysia, 2005. http://www.pta.gov.pk (Feb 2005)
5. Murad F (2003) Telemedicine in Pakistan: current status and potential. In: 8th annual international meeting and exposition of American telemedicine Association, Florida, 2003
6. Lipozencić J, Pastar Z, Janjua SA (2007) Teledermatology. Acta Dermatovenerol Croat 15(3):199–201
7. TelemedPak. Available at: http://www.telmedpak.com (March 12, 2010)
8. Rashid E, Ishtiaq O, Gilani S, Zafar A (2003) Comparison of store and forward method of teledermatology with face-to-face consultation. J Ayub Med Coll Abbottabad 15(2): 34–36
9. U.S. Department of State Taps IBM to Extend Telemedicine's Reach to Remote Regions of Pakistan. Available at: http://www-03.ibm.com/press/us/en/pressrelease/25355.wss (March 4, 2010)
10. The Pakistan telemedicine project. Available at: http://technhealth.blogspot.com/2008/10/pakistan-telemedicine-project.html (May 6, 2010)
11. U.S. bringing telemedicine to northern Pakistan. Available at: http://www.ibm.com/news/us/en/2008/10/09/n119153n03440s73.html (March 4, 2010)
12. Telemedicine and eHealth training center. Available at: http://www.telemedicine.pk/index.html (January 18, 2010)
13. SUPARCO Tele-medicine Pilot Project. Available at: http://www.suparco.gov.pk/pages/tele-medicine.asp?telelinksid=1 (February 18, 2010)
14. Malik AZ (2007) Role of satellite communications in telemedicine during earthquake in Pakistan. In: 12th annual international meeting and exposition of American Telemedicine Association, Nashville, 2007
15. Merrell RC, Cone SW, Rafiq A (2008) Telemedicine in extreme conditions: disasters, war, remote sites. Stud Health Technol Inform 131:99–116
16. Mobile Skin Clinic in Muzaffar Garh. Available at: http://paktelederm.blogspot.com/2010/10/mobile-skin-clinic-in-muzaffar-garh.html (October 14, 2010)
17. Khoja S, Scott R, Gilani S (2008) E-health readiness assessment: promoting "hope" in the health-care institutions of Pakistan. World Hosp Health Serv 44(1):36–38
18. Shoaib SF, Mirza S, Murad F, Malik AZ (2009) Current status of e-health awareness among healthcare professionals in teaching hospitals of Rawalpindi: a survey. Telemed J E Health 15(4):347–352
19. Ayza Skin & Research Center. Available at: http://www.asrc.blogspot.com (August 3, 2010)
20. Soyer HP, Hofmann-Wellenhof R, Massone C, Gabler G, Dong H, Ozdemeir F, Argenziano G (2005) Telederm.org: freely available online consultations in dermatology. PLoS Med 2(4):e87, Epub 2005 Apr 26
21. Jaroka Telehealth Care: pilot project. Available at: http://www.tele-healthcare.org/projects/pilot-project.html (July 24, 2010)
22. Pakisan Society of Teledermatology. Available at: http://www.paktelederm.blogspot.com (February 5, 2010)
23. McColl I (2003) Dermatology education on the Web. J Telemed Telecare 9(Suppl 2):S33–S35
24. Siddiqui U, Salman S, Gilani N, Murad F, Malik AZ (2006) Standards and best practices for implementing telemedicine networks in Pakistan. In: Proceedings 4th Apt telemedicine workshop, Rawalpindi, 2006, p 196

Teledermatology in Developing Countries

6

Jennifer Weinberg, Steven Kaddu, and Carrie Kovarik

Core Messages

- Teledermatology can facilitate access to high-quality, cost-effective health care in developing countries, as well as play an essential role in clinician education, foster distribution of educational materials, and promote independence in clinical practice as well as improving patient care.
- Store-and-forward technology is the most commonly utilized method in developing countries, given the availability of the Internet, general ease of use, level of familiarity for clinicians, and affordability; however, mobile teledermatology may be another feasible option with the rapid scale up of sophisticated cellular networks around the world.
- Certain challenges exist with the use of teledermatology in developing countries, including technical and systems problems, as well as economic, legal, and cultural limitations.
- There are many examples of systems that are in place and available for use, including the Swinfen Charitable Trust (http://www.swinfencharitabletrust.org/), the African Teledermatology Project (africa.telederm.org), Proyecto Latinoamericano de Teledermatología (latinoamerica.telederm.org), the Community for Teledermatology (www.telederm.org), and the Telepathology network of the University of Basel (http://telemed.ipath.ch/ipath/).
- Teledermatology programs hold the potential for extending much-needed health care services to remote and resource-poor areas in developing countries, and an important feature of these programs must be that they are sustainable and can positively contribute to the community over an extended period of time.

J. Weinberg
Department of Dermatology, Perelman School of Medicine at the University of Pennsylvania,
Philadelphia, PA, USA
e-mail: jenniferlweinberg@alumni.upenn.edu

S. Kaddu
Department of Dermatology, Medical University of Graz, Graz, Austria
e-mail: steven.kaddu@medunigraz.at

C. Kovarik (✉)
Departments of Dermatology, Dermatopathology, and Infectious Diseases, Perelman School of Medicine at the University of Pennsylvania, Philadelphia, PA, USA
e-mail: carrie.kovarik@uphs.upenn.edu

Rationale for Use of Teledermatology in Developing Countries

Many nations in the developing world have a dire shortage of doctors, especially specialists, such as dermatologists. Disparities in access to all facets of health care exist, especially in rural areas, with several factors contributing to the disproportionate impact of disease in these resource poor settings: poverty, disease stigma, cultural and social barriers to testing and treatment, insufficient health care infrastructure to support the large patient pool, lack of health literacy, limited provider

H.P. Soyer et al. (eds.), *Telemedicine in Dermatology*,
DOI 10.1007/978-3-642-20801-0_6, © Springer-Verlag Berlin Heidelberg 2012

training, inadequate medical equipment, scarce manpower to distribute health care throughout the region, and few qualified laboratory facilities exist amongst many complex factors [1]. Therefore, affordable, easy-to-use technologies like teledermatology are imperative for facilitating specialty patient care and providing much needed health care worker educational opportunities.

One significant resource-limitation in the provision of dermatologic care is a dearth of trained providers in many developing countries. In 2004, 7.7 million physicians were practicing worldwide, distributed such that half of these physicians were practicing in areas with less than one-fifth of the world's population [2]. Furthermore, an estimated 3.4 billion people in over 300 developing countries are living in regions with little to no access to basic dermatological care [3, 4]. For example, it has been reported that Sub-Saharan Africa has as few as 10 doctors per 100,000 inhabitants, with many areas having no dermatologists at all [5]. Even in countries which have a supply of dermatologists, there is frequently a rural-urban distributional imbalance of such providers. For example, the majority of the nearly 6,000 dermatologists in the Indian Association of Dermatologists, Venerologists and Leprologists practice in large cities, while 72% of the 1.2 billion people live in rural villages, creating a scarcity of skin care for many throughout the country [6].

Due to this shortage of physicians, especially specialists, poor infrastructure, and lack of resources, rural health care workers who serve the majority of the population in many developing nations are isolated from specialist support and current information. Around 90% of cutaneous conditions in tropical developing countries are diagnosed and managed by care providers who have no formal dermatologic training [4]. A shortage of elementary skills in the management of skin diseases is a further confounding problem, with several studies assessing success in the management of skin diseases in primary care settings in the developing world reporting that treatment failure rates of over 80% are common [7]. In developing countries where skin diseases are highly prevalent but misdiagnosis and treatment failure rates for such diseases remain significant, there is terrific potential for increasing local health care workers' knowledge and skills in treating skin disease through the use of teledermatology while also improving patients' access to quality skin care. Local workers can learn through participation in a teleconsultation service, garnering information about diagnosing and managing skin disease through submission of consultations and expert feedback. It has been established that providing feedback to remote health providers regarding the patients they are caring for is an effective educational method through which these providers may significantly increase their competency in dermatological diagnosis, management, knowledge and differential diagnosis [8, 9]. Additionally, electronic learning resources can be incorporated into teledermatology programs and targeted to commonly seen dermatological conditions, circumventing the limitations of time and distance often encountered by health workers in developing countries when attending courses, conferences, or training programs in person. Online databases facilitate continued acquisition and revision of knowledge with these educational opportunities contributing to an increased understanding and independence in clinical practice and improved clinical care.

A means for an accessible, cost-effective and accurate diagnosis and treatment of skin conditions in developing countries should be met for a number of important reasons. Skin diseases are very common, with patients presenting in large numbers in primary care settings, such that ignoring patients with skin disease is not a viable option. Up to 80% of the population living in developing countries suffers from cutaneous disease, with over 30% of the health issues dealt with in rural health clinics of developing countries involving cutaneous diseases [7, 4]. Children and the immunocompromised, in particular, tend to be affected, adding to the burden of disease amongst already vulnerable groups. Some estimates suggest that 75% of children in developing countries have skin diseases, with most lacking access to dermatologic care [4]. Significantly, morbidity and mortality due to skin diseases are substantial, with skin diseases ranking amongst the five most frequent causes among rural populations for loss of working capacity and/or death [4]. Furthermore, morbidity from cutaneous disease is significant through disfigurement, disability, and symptoms such as intractable itch, contributing to a reduction in quality of life. Also significant is the relative economic cost to families of even trivial skin complaints, which limits patients' ability to access many therapies and leads to a potential reduction of income due to an inability to work secondary to cutaneous disease. Very importantly, the need for effective recognition and management of mucocutaneous conditions cannot be ignored given that many systemic diseases, such as HIV/AIDS and leprosy, have presenting skin manifestations, yet a basic knowledge of the simple features of diseases whose presenting signs occur in the skin is often lacking at the primary care level [10].

Teledermatology can facilitate access to high-quality, cost-effective health care and play an essential role in clinician education, fostering distribution of educational materials to the local workers in an effort to promote increased understanding and independence in clinical practice as well as improving patient care. Benefits to patients are many, including a reduction of waiting and travel time for appointments with skin specialists, expanded and more rapid access to screening for skin diseases and more accurate and efficient diagnosis and management of cutaneous diseases [11]. Similarly, teledermatology technology can be seen as a practical and effective manner to distribute information to local health care workers with the hope of significantly improving their ability to recognize, diagnose and treat cutaneous conditions while decreasing health inequalities in resource-limited settings. Local providers in developing countries can benefit from the use of teledermatology via improved and efficient access to specialized dermatology consultation, increased opportunities for continued medical education, enhanced professional collaboration, greater research exposure and collaboration, more efficient screening of patients with skin conditions and better follow-up of such patients [11]. Additionally, local health systems in developing nations can benefit from the use of teledermatology due to a reduction in health care costs, fewer hospital admissions and shorter hospital stays, increased efficiency of human and other resources, a compilation of online databases and increased and effective support for local health care professionals [11]. Therefore, teledermatology is an ideal technology for increasing and improving care for skin disease in developing countries.

Methods of Use (Live Interactive Versus Store and Forward – Internet Based System, Email Based System, Mobile Phone Based)

Fortunately, dermatologic disease can frequently be recognized visually, making teledermatology a feasible method to employ in the care of skin disease. Teledermatology merges medical expertise and communication technology to allow for patient examination, monitoring and management by a dermatologic expert in a distant location, facilitating provision of clinical support services to remote, isolated and rural regions which lack access to higher level medical expertise. It involves the electronic transfer of information which may be done in several ways. One form of telemedicine technology is video teleconferencing, during which patients, specialists and, sometimes the referring clinician, interact via a real-time video link with dynamic visual images [12]. Currently, the most common type of teledermatology is store-and-forward or asynchronous teledermatology, which involves the transfer of digital images across locations, allowing consultation to occur at a later time when the situation does not necessitate immediate feedback [12]. Store-and-forward technology involves transfer of patient history, clinical examination findings, and digital images via email or on a web-based interface to a consulting dermatologist who later evaluates the information and returns his impressions and recommendations [13]. This method is more commonly utilized due to its lesser technological requirements and affordability [11]. Internet-based store-and-forward teledermatology is commonly utilized as it allows for worldwide reach, constant availability, general ease of use and a level of familiarity for clinicians and the public [14]. As technology expands, mobile telephones are being employed for the transfer of teledermatology data. Mobile teledermatology may be useful when neither a specialist nor equipment for Internet-based store-and-forward telemedicine consultations is available, such as in emergency situations, in remote or under-served locations, or while traveling [15]. These various formats of teledermatology programs commonly involve providing assistance with diagnosis and management via teleconsultation services as well as discussion forums and educational databases.

Evidence of Efficacy of Teledermatology in Developing Countries

Teledermatology systems must be efficient, reliable, and easy to use. While there have been several studies investigating teledermatology outcomes, they have mainly focused on projects in industrialized countries. The accuracy of teledermatology is reflected by the degree of concordance between teledermatology and face-to-face diagnoses. Several studies show that store-and-forward teledermatology consultations produce similar clinical outcomes when compared with conventional clinic-based consultations. For example, Lim et al. [16] found a concordance of 88% for primary diagnosis and 96% for differential diagnoses between store-and-forward versus face-to-face dermatologic consultations in Australia. Several other studies have confirmed the accuracy of teledermatology in industrialized nations with diagnostic agreement between face-to-face dermatologists and teledermatologists ranging from 81% to 89% and agreement on management decisions ranging from 90% to 96% [17, 18].

Only a few studies have looked at the use of teledermatology in developing countries. For example, Rashid et al. [19] showed that 81% ($p<0.05$) of store-and-forward teledermatology consultation cases resulted in the same diagnosis as face-to-face diagnosis of patients with skin conditions in Islamabad, Pakistan. Similarly, Lepe et al. [20] report a high concordance of diagnoses obtained via face-to-face versus filmed evaluation of skin lesions in Mexican patients. Trindade et al. [21] examined the use of an Internet-based store-and-forward teledermatology service in the diagnosis of patients with suspected leprosy at public health clinics in outlying areas of Sao Paulo, Brazil. They found an overall agreement in the diagnosis of cutaneous leprosy in 74% of the 106 cases [21]. Caumes et al. [22] investigated the use of store-and-forward teledermatology to diagnose skin disease in patients in Burkina Faso (both travelers and Burkinabese nationals) and to enhance local general practitioners knowledge of skin disease. They found a 49% diagnostic agreement (64 of 130; 95% CI 41–58) between the local general practitioner and the remote consulting dermatologists based in France, with the percentage agreement between the local health worker and the consulting dermatologists improving significantly over time ($p<0.05$) [22]. Therefore, research suggests that when health care providers are trained to take appropriate photographs of the skin and provide relevant clinical information, the teledermatology encounter produces similar diagnoses as a live patient encounter and can also serve as an effective means of education for enhancing local health care workers knowledge of mucocutaneous disease. Furthermore, a study investigating the use of teledermatology in India found that teleconsultation was the first contact for the patient with a dermatologist in over 90% of the cases, suggesting that teledermatology is a means to increase access to specialty skin care in areas with a shortage of dermatologists [23]. The dearth of studies looking at the use of teledermatology in developing countries may be due to problems in obtaining funding or in assessing clinical outcomes due to a loss of patient follow-up and inadequate medical record systems in resource-limited settings. Large studies investigating the economic value, clinical benefit and sustainability of teledermatology in developing countries remain to be conducted.

Challenges with Using Teledermatology in Developing Countries

Certain challenges exist with the use of teledermatology in developing countries. These include technical and system problems along with cultural and economic limitations. For example, several factors may lower diagnostic accuracy in teledermatology consultations including poor image quality, insufficient clinical data supplied, difficulty in appreciating the three-dimensional quality of skin lesions and the loss of information gained by hands-on patient examination. While some of these factors (i.e. inability to physically examine the patient) are inherent to the nature of telemedicine technology, others (i.e. poor image quality) have the potential to be ameliorated through the provision of up-graded equipment and/or increased training of personnel in taking and submitting appropriate photographs and clinical information. To help address this aspect, materials detailing the proper technique for taking clinical photographs and successfully submitting consultations should be provided to participating clinicians (for example, see the Africa Teledermatology project website) [24].

Economic, legal, cultural and technical limitations may also arise when establishing teledermatology programs in developing countries. Although skin diseases have been shown to occur with substantial frequency and inflict significant morbidity, dermatological health care is often overlooked in the allocation of medical resources. This is especially true in resource-limited settings already significantly impoverished by epidemic levels of deadly diseases such as HIV/AIDS, which are often considered to be more pressing. This lack of recognition has resulted in limited financial, technological and manpower resources at many health centers providing dermatological care. Even when external funding is available to establish teledermatology programs, implementation and ongoing utilization of these programs can be challenging, as the services place an increased burden on already scarce financial and human resources. Sustainability of such programs is limited by political, economic, technical and cultural barriers. For example, modern communication systems including Internet services in hospitals and remote health clinics must be maintained by governments of developing nations to ensure the sustainability of telemedicine programs [11].

Additionally, social structures and cultural beliefs often limit the implementation of teledermatology services, with some patients, providers and local institutions expressing unease with the technology secondary to a lack of trust in security or privacy concerns. Others may feel that the technology will not improve their health care experience or outcomes. Similarly, local health care workers may also adopt negative attitudes toward the use of teledermatology services due to a variety of concerns. They may not feel comfortable submitting consultations in English, believe that teledermatology will not improve the care of their patients, distrust the safety and privacy of the technology, prefer to refer patients to face-to-face consultations, or feel that teledermatology is time-consuming and generates extra work [11]. These attitudes may result from inadequate information due to political and economic differences, cultural viewpoints, language barriers and varied perceptions of health and wellness. These beliefs can potentially be addressed via increased education about the technology and its potential benefits, with the provision of translation services to allow consultations to be submitted in the providers' native language and assurance of adequate privacy and security. Further, listening to the communities' concerns and involving them in the incorporation of this technology in local health care may help increase the acceptability of the services.

Another issue which may arise with the use of teledermatology technology in developing countries is the presence of new and challenging legal problems. These issues generally relate to problems concerning the privacy and security of identifiable health information, the reliability and quality of health data and medical liability issues arising in distance consultation. Consulting experts are commonly located in remote locations, necessitating that they investigate the potential risks concerning medical liability in the respective countries where the patients are located. The medicolegal position of remote expert dermatologists is similar to that when telephone, fax, letter or email is used for consultation; therefore normal standards of care and skill should apply [11]. Submitting health care providers have an obligation to provide accurate clinical information, submit quality, appropriate images and administer recommended treatments with the patient's permission. Additionally, developing countries must adopt rules and regulations to address legal aspects of teledermatology technology including safeguards regarding data forwarding, data security, confidentiality and the responsibilities of the involved providers, in order to protect patients' rights [11].

While most teledermatology projects in developing countries receive subsidized funding from external governments, NGOs or foreign universities and hospitals, financial constraints can contribute to the challenge of providing care via teledermatology programs and sustaining these programs over time. While some have demonstrated financial advantages of teledermatology versus face-to-face consultations in terms of advantages for patients including reduced time missed from work, decreased loss of income and diminished time and expense for traveling, there is a lack of information about the cost-effectiveness and sustainability of such services. This may result in part from the fact that economic analysis of teledermatology services is complicated due to the presence of a number of hidden costs and benefits which are difficult to quantify, including the cost of patients' time and the intangible benefit of earlier correct diagnoses [11]. Implementation costs for the establishment of teledermatology programs mainly consist of the costs for equipment, such as digital cameras and accessories, computers, image editing software, back-up systems and printers; equipment maintenance; telecommunication services; and staff time and training [11]. On the other side of these programs, expert consultant dermatologists are not generally reimbursed for their time and efforts.

Another obstacle to the implementation of teledermatology programs relates to infrastructure and resource limitations. Power supplies in many areas of developing countries are frequently unreliable and telephone and/or Internet networks may also be inconsistent or lack widespread data coverage. In many areas of the developing world, workers experience difficulty uploading images onto a computer network, which is necessary for use of store-and-forward teledermatology using digital cameras and a computer with Internet connection. Many remote medical workers do not have access to traditional Internet, using a computer connection, however, they may have access to cellular phone data connections, making mobile teledermatology a potential solution. Mobile teledermatology also has an economic advantage over traditional store-and-forward teledermatology using digital cameras and Internet-connected computers [25].

Examples of Systems in Place Available for Use

The Swinfen Charitable Trust

Lord and Laby Swinfen established the Swinfen Charitable Trust (http://www.swinfencharitabletrust.org/) in 1998 in order to "assist poor, sick and disabled people in the developing world" through consultation services allowing for the provision of access to expert medical advice from consultants around the world [11, 26]. Clinicians in developing nations are able to submit cases to specialists worldwide via an email telemedicine system which employs an automatic email messaging service, developed by the Centre for Online Health at the University of Queensland, Brisbane, Australia, that directs email messages about each case to all involved parties. The Swinfen Charitable Trust has 163 hospital links with 448 consultants in 59 countries in the developing world and in disaster and post conflict situations, including Afghanistan, Cambodia, East Timor, Iraq, Nepal, Papua New Guinea and Sri Lanka. Services are provided in many specialty areas including dermatology, dentistry, pediatrics, obstetrics and gynecology, oncology, orthopedics, ophthalmology, neurology, plastic surgery and trauma. This service provides users with high-resolution digital cameras and tripods and trains the local medical staff in the proper use of the equipment, allowing remote hospitals in developing countries to receive assistance free of charge [11].

African Teledermatology Project (africa.telederm.org)

The African Teledermatology Project (http://africa.telederm.org/) is an effort to utilize store-and-forward teledermatology technology to connect various medical institutions in Sub-Saharan Africa to more specialized dermatology units in the USA, Europe and Australia [24]. It was initially conceived as the *Uganda Tele-Dermatology-and E-Learning-Project* in February 2007 under the sponsorship of the Kommission für Entwicklungsfragen (KEF) der Österreichischen Akademie der Wissenschaften [11]. The scope of the project was expanded with the collaboration between the Departments of Dermatology at the University of Pennsylvania, USA and the Medical University of Graz, Austria with the eventual additional inclusion of a number of other medical centers in eastern, central and southern Africa, leading to the formation of the Africa Teledermatology Project. The goal of the project is to create a network for dermatologic teleconsultation and e-learning, providing medical support to local physicians, dermatologists, and health care workers in hospitals and clinics throughout Africa. Utilizing the telederm.org application, the consultation services allow for individual discussions pertaining to diagnosis and management of patients with skin diseases, links to educational resources, and access to a dermatologic curriculum. This curriculum has been created specifically for African sites in an effort to foster increased understanding and independence in clinical care and increase access to information and care in resource-limited areas [11, 27].

The network allows users to register as clients or experts. Clients can submit cases via the Internet to experts who review cases, write comments, suggest diagnoses, make management recommendations and/or discuss cases with other experts within the system. The web-based application allows store-and-forward medical cases to be uploaded with digital photographs and transferred via a password protected Internet connection to an expert teledermatologist for feedback and suggestions. Clients may choose to send a request for consultation to a selected expert or for discussion in an open forum. Automatic email notifications are sent to selected experts when a case is submitted for their review. Notifications are also sent via email to clients when a comment is posted to one of their cases. Expert answers and interactions remain in a private field for viewing only by the submitting client unless the case has been submitted for an open "discussion view." In the first year of the program, 160 teledermatology-supported patient cases have been processed via the project, with 35% of these cases involving children and 25% of these cases relating to HIV-associated skin conditions [11]. The project website also includes a curriculum with educational materials. These include a "discussion forum" for interesting or complex cases, exemplary cases with comprehensive discussions, a list of dermatology literature resources and a dermatology curriculum tailored to the most common conditions seen at participating sites. Additionally, detailed instructions are provided as to how to join the project as a consultant or submitting site.

Proyecto Latinoamericano de Teledermatología (latinoamerica.telederm.org)

The Proyecto Latinoamericano de Teledermatología (http://latinoamerica.telederm.org/) utilizes a Spanish version similar to the africa.telederm.org system in order to provide remote dermatology consultation services and facilitate the exchange of information between health care providers in various parts of Latin America and dermatology experts. The program was created through a collaboration between the Department of Dermatology at the University of Pennsylvania, Philadelphia, USA; the Servei de Dermatologia Hospital Clinic in Barcelona, Spain; the Department of Dermatology at the Medical University of Graz, Austria; and the Dermatology Research Centre, University of Queensland, Brisbane, Australia. The project incorporates a store-and-forward teledermatology platform, discussion forums, and Internet based educational resources. The website is currently being used to increase access to specialty dermatology consultations by linking local dermatologists to clinicians in rural Mexico; however, any Spanish-speaking health care workers in Latin America may submit cases to be answered by expert dermatologists that are registered on the site [28].

Amazonas – Brazil Teledermatology and Teledermatopathology Project (piel.telederm.org)

Amazonas-Brazil teledermatology and teledermatopathology project (http://piel.telederm.org/) is a web application utilizing the telederm.org system which was created through a collaboration between the Department of Dermatology at the Medical University of Graz, Austria; the Unit of Social Dermatology at the National Reference Center for Hansen's Disease (NRCHD), San Martino University Hospital, University of Genoa, Italy; the Dermatology Group of the University of Queensland School of Medicine, Brisbane, Australia; and the Foundation of Tropical Medicine of Amazonas (FMTAM) in Manaus, Amzaonas-Brazil. It allows dermatologists, dermatopathologists, pathologists, infectious disease specialists and other health care workers to discuss interesting cases in clinical dermatology of tropical diseases, with a special emphasis on leprosy, at no cost. Registered users can submit case information and digital images to a moderated forum for discussion with other users, and the site has been created to function in English, Spanish, or Portuguese [29].

The Community for Teledermatology (www.telederm.org)

The Community for Teledermatology was established in 2002 by the Department of Dermatology of the Medical University of Graz, Austria with the goal of developing a software application to facilitate worldwide exchange of expertise and knowledge in dermatology and dermatopathology [11]. The program allows for the transmission of store-and-forward medical cases with attached clinical images via several teledermatology networks, some of which are active in developing countries. These include the telederm.org project and the Africa Teledermatology Project [11].

The telederm.org project was initiated in April 2002 as a non-profit venture under the auspices of the International Society of Teledermatology in partnership with the Department of Dermatology, Medical University of Graz, Graz (Austria) and the Dermatology Group, School of Medicine, University of Queensland, Brisbane (Australia) [11]. The telederm.org project teledermatology network currently has over 1,300 participating physicians from over 90 countries worldwide who participate in a teleconsultation service to seek dermatology diagnostic and treatment advice as well as in an online discussion forum for the examination of challenging cases [11]. Clinicians from different medical specialities and regions of the world are matched with dermatologists with a range of experience and expertise. Approximately 30–40 new users join this network each month and around 20–30 new cases are submitted via the project each month [11].

India's Telemedicine Initiative of the Indian Space Research Organization (ISRO)

The Indian Space Research Organization (ISRO) has created a telemedicine initiative linking super-specialty hospitals with rural and remote hospitals across the county via its geo-stationary satellites and through mobile telemedicine units. The ISRO's telemedicine pilot program began in 2001 and has currently expanded to connect over 330 hospitals, 280 remote/rural district health centers and hospitals with at least 50 super specialty hospitals in major Indian cities, including 13 mobile telemedicine units. These mobile telemedicine units consist of medical equipment, telemedicine hardware and software and a connection to the satellite communication system mounted in a van, allowing for the establishment of a mobile telemedicine center at any location which can be used for teledermatology, tele-ophthalmology, diabetic screening, mammography, childcare and community health [30]. Over 300,000 patients have been served with teleconsultation and management through the ISRO telemedicine network. Additionally, the ISRO's telemedicine program provides a means for continuing medical education and training of health care providers as well as regular monitoring of emergency and intensive care and disaster management support [31, 32, 33].

Institute of Tropical Medicine, in Antwerp, Belgium Telemedicine for HIV Care (http://telemedicine.itg.be)

In 2003 the Department of Clinical Sciences at the Institute of Tropical Medicine in Antwerp Belgium initiated this project to facilitate the introduction of antiretroviral therapy and guide AIDS care delivery in resource-limited settings. This site provides training, distance support, case discussions, and education for health care providers working in these areas [11, 34]. Users from many countries are able to register, log on, and submit questions and patient consultations by uploading a clinical scenario, which may include information on the history, physical examination, laboratory findings, and/or clinical images. The users receive advice via email messages from a server list and through a discussion forum on this telemedicine website (http://telemedicine.itg.be/) [11, 34].

University of Washington/University of Cape Town Initiative in South Africa

The Teledermatology Network for Underserved Areas of South Africa is a collaborative project between the University of Washington, USA and the University of Cape Town, South Africa. The program connects rural primary-care clinics via a teledermatology network to specialists and clinicians at the University of Cape Town and the University of Washington in order to provide dermatology consultation and educational services. Consultations are sent via a secure email system for review to a distant dermatologist [35].

Operation Village Health at Harvard

Operation Village Health began in 2001 as a means to allow Harvard-affiliated physicians in the Partners HealthCare system (now the Center for Connected Health) to support Cambodian health care workers. Local providers are able to send point-of-care clinical data including digital images via email to volunteer physicians in Boston, USA and Phnom Penh, Cambodia for consultation and recommendations. The program also provides resources on the ground such as basic point-of-care laboratory supplies and relevant clinical guidelines to supplement the telemedicine support [36].

Telepathology Network of the University of Basel (iPath)

The Department of Pathology of the University Hospital Basel developed the iPath software as an open source framework for building web- and email-based tele-medicine applications (http://telemed.ipath.ch/ipath/) [37, 38, 11]. This system is currently in use on all continents, including in many developing countries, as a means to store medical cases with attached images and other supporting documents in closed user groups in which users can review cases, suggest diagnoses and submit feedback and comments [38, 11]. Membership is open to anyone, and users are organized into one or more discussion group with moderators who can assign group members and edit erroneous data.

Several telemedicine networks serving developing countries, including some which involve teledermatology, are currently hosted by iPath. These include the Solomon

Islands National Telemedicine Network, a partnership between the National Referral Hospital in Honiara, South Pacific Medical Projects and the University of Basel which strives to improve health care delivery in provincial hospitals in the Solomon Islands with a focus on dermatology, radiology, orthopedics and pediatrics [39]. Another telemedicine network which utilizes iPath is the LT Telepatologija network of pathologists and other medical specialists in the Baltics which serves to support clinicopathological case discussions, consultations and education [40]. RAFT-Forum, a telemedicine platform of the Réseau de Téle-enseignement et de Télémédicine Francophone, utilizes the iPath host to provide a forum for webcasting of interactive courses for health care workers in French-speaking regions of Africa to encourage knowledge sharing amongst participating institutions [41]. iPath also hosts the Telemedicine Sur platform for medical discussions, education and consultations for health care practitioners in Latin America involving mainly dermatology, pathology, pediatrics and venerology [42]. The West Africa Doctors and Healthcare Professionals Network is also based on the iPath software and aims to enhance communication capabilities of physicians for continuing medical education, information access and diagnosis and management support in various specialties [43]. In Nepal, the iPath platform is used to provide low-cost email, Internet access and a range of medical and public health resources via the HealthNet Nepal program which enables health care providers through Nepal to communicate and exchange knowledge [44]. Another telemedicine program which utilizes iPath is the Teledermatology project in Port St Johns, South Africa. This project strives to improve access to dermatological care for patients while also increasing practitioner's skills and knowledge [45].

ClickDiagnostics – Mobile Phone Based

ClickDiagnostics, Inc. is a global tele-health company headquartered in Cambridge, Massachusetts, USA. The ClickDiagnostics mobile telemedicine service has been developed with resources from the MIT Media Lab, MIT Sloan School of Management, Harvard Kennedy School of Government, Harvard Medical School, University of Pennsylvania Department of Dermatology, and africa.telederm.org. It provides a mobile technology-based infrastructure to connect community-based health-workers to remote medical specialists. Remote health care workers are able to gather information and digital images with a mobile camera phone and upload this information to a central server via mobile phone software whenever connectivity is available. Successful programs for dermatology and oral medicine have been initiated in Botswana, and a teledermatology pilot has been completed in Ghana. Additionally, educational resources can be provided via a mobile-phone interface [46].

What Is Needed to Get Started for a Store and Forward Versus a Live Interactive (Real-Time) Program

Participants in teledermatology programs require some basic equipment. For participation in store-and-forward teledermatology projects, a computer with necessary software, a digital camera of adequate resolution, an uninterruptible power supply and access to the telephone and or Internet network are needed [14]. Digital clinical and/or pathological images can be provided via a digital camera, video camera, and/or a flatbed or slide scanner [14]. Mobile teledermatology based on the store and forward method involves the use of mobile devices such as mobile camera phones or personal digital assistants which are equipped with digital cameras with sufficient resolution to capture good quality digital images and transmit them via a wireless network directly to remote experts' cellular telephones or computers. Mobile phones which incorporate digital cameras are currently available around the world at an affordable price and allow for data and image capture, transfer and storage, with high mobility and portability [47].

Live interactive, or real-time, teledermatology consultation utilizes a video-conferencing monitor to allow a distant dermatologist to visualize and directly interact with the patient in a manner similar to a traditional clinic-based encounter. This platform requires more expense and sophisticated video-conferencing technology as well as wide bandwidth communication lines for an adequate quality of streaming video [48].

Conclusion

The use of teledermatology is increasing in developing countries and shows promise for enhancing provider educational opportunities, increasing access to specialized dermatology care and improving patient care. With these various benefits and the growing number of programs targeted at developing nations, teledermatology may soon become an integral part of the health care system in some countries. With the incorporation of such technology into the health care systems, health policy makers and health care workers in developing countries must consider standards and regulations relating to the use of telemedicine [21]. Additional attention must be focused on the ethical, legal, economic and technical issues arising with the use of teledermatology to ensure acceptance, security, economic viability and efficacy of such programs thus leading to sustainability. Research efforts to expand the understanding of teledermatology programs in developing countries is also needed to confirm the clinical benefits and cost-effectiveness of such technology in this setting [21]. The growing use of mobile-phone based teledermatology may help overcome some of the technical and economic challenges of store-and-forward or live video teledermatology platforms and potentially allow for such services in more remote areas. Additionally, teledermatopathology programs could refine teledermatology services by assisting with confirmation of diagnoses and contributing to training and collaborative research [21].

Teledermatology programs hold the potential for extending much-needed health care services to remote and resource-poor areas in developing countries. An important feature of these programs must be that they are sustainable and can positively contribute to the community over an extended period of time. For teledermatology to become integrated into health care in developing countries, all participants must be satisfied and comfortable with the technology.

References

1. Charles M, Boyle B (2002) Excess and access: the continuing controversy regarding HIV and health care in Africa. AIDS Read 12:288–292
2. Worldmapper. Physicians working. Map No. 219. Available at: accessed on Oct 4, 2009 http://www.worldmapper.org/display.php?selected=219
3. International Foundation for Dermatology (IFD) About IFD: Who needs our help? Available at: accessed on Oct 4, 2009 http://www.ifd.org/about2.html
4. Morrone A (2007) Poverty, health and development in dermatology. Int J Dermatol 46(Suppl 2):1–9
5. Schmid-Grendelmeir P, Doe P, Pakenham-Walsh N (2003) Teledermatology in sub-Saharan Africa. Curr Probl Dermatol 32:233–246
6. Indian Association of Dermatologists, Venerologists and Leprologists (IADVL) Welcome to IADVL. accessed on Oct 4, 2009 http://www.iadvl.org/site/?q=node/14
7. Figueroa JI, Fuller LC, Abraha A et al (1996) The prevalence of skin disease among schoolchildren in rural Ethiopia: a preliminary assessment of dermatologic needs. Pediatr Dermatol 13:378–381
8. Aas IH (2002) Learning in organizations working with telemedicine. J Telemed Telecare 8(2):107–111
9. Shaikh N, Lehmann C, Kaleida P et al (2008) Efficacy and feasibility of teledermatology for paediatric medical education. J Telemed Telecare 14:204–207
10. World Bank (2006) Disease control priorities project: skin diseases. The World Bank Web Site: http://www.dcp2.orq/pubs/DCP/37/FuliText. Updated 2006. Accessed 20 Sept 2008
11. Kaddu S, Kovarik C, Gabler G et al (2009) Teledermatology in developing countries. In: Wootton R, Patel N, Scott R, Ho K (eds) Telehealth in the developing world. Royal Society of Medicine Press/IDRC, London, pp 112–124
12. Myers MR (2003) Telemedicine: an emerging health care technology. Health Care Manag 22:219–223
13. Dill S, Digiovanna J (2003) Changing paradigms in dermatology: information technology. Clin Dermatol 21:375–382
14. Wootton R, Oakley AM (2002) Teledermatology. Royal Society of Medicine Press Ltd, London
15. Ebner C, Wurm EM, Binder B et al (2008) Mobile teledermatology: a feasibility study of 58 subjects using mobile phones. J Telemed Telecare 14:2–7
16. Lim AC, Egerton IB, See A et al (2001) Accuracy and reliability of store-and-forward teledermatology: preliminary results from the St George Teledermatology Project. Australas J Dermatol 42(4):247–251
17. Eedy DJ, Wootton R (2001) Teledermatology: a review. Br J Dermatol 144:696–707
18. High WA, Houston MS, Calobrisi SD et al (2000) Assessment of the accuracy of low-cost store-and-forward teledermatology consultation. J Am Acad Dermatol 42:776–783
19. Rashid E, Ishtiaq O, Gilani S et al (2003) Comparison of store and forward method of teledermatology with face-to-face consultation. J Ayub Med Coll Abbottabad 15(2): 34–36
20. Lepe V, Moncada B, Castanedo-Cázares JP et al (2004) First study of teledermatology in Mexico: a new public health tool. Gac Med Mex 140(1):23–26
21. Trindade MA, Wen CL, Neto CF et al (2008) Accuracy of store-and-forward diagnosis in leprosy. J Telemed Telecare 14(4):208–210
22. Caumes E, Le Bris V, Couzigou C et al (2004) Dermatoses associated with travel to Burkina Faso and diagnosed by means of teledermatology. Br J Dermatol 150:312–316
23. Kaliyadan F, Venkitakrishnan S (2009) Teledermatology: clinical case profiles and practical issues. Indian J Dermatol Venerol Leprol 75(1):32–35
24. African Teledermatology Project: accessed on Oct 4, 2009 http://africa.telederm.org/
25. Chung P, Yu T, Scheinfeld N (2007) Using cellphones for teledermatology, a preliminary study. Dermatol Online J 13(3):2
26. Swinfen Charitable Trust Website: accessed on Oct 4, 2009 www.swinfencharitabletrust.org
27. Kaddu S, Soyer P, Gabler G et al (2009) The Africa Teledermatology Project: preliminary experience with a sub-Saharan teledermatology and e-learning program. J Am Acad Dermatol 61(1):155–157

28. Proyecto Latinoamericano de Teledermatología: accessed on Oct 4, 2009 http://latinoamerica.telederm.org/default.htm
29. Amazonas-Brazil teledermatology and teledermatopathology project: accessed on Oct 4, 2009 http://piel.telederm.org.
30. Kanthraj GR, Srinivas CR (2007) Store and forward teledermatology. Indian J Dermatol Venereol Leprol 73(1):5–12
31. Bagchi S (2006) Telemedicine in rural India. PLoS Med 3(3):e82
32. Bhaskaranarayana A, Satyamurthy LS, Remilla M (2009) Indian Space Research Organization and telemedicine in India. Telemed J E Health 15(6):586–591
33. Indian Space Research Organization (ISRO) Telemedicine: accessed on Oct 4, 2009 http://www.isro.org/scripts/telemedicine.aspx
34. Telemedicine: Online support for HIV/AIDS care: accessed on Oct 4, 2009 telemedicine.itg.be/telemedicine/site/Default.asp
35. Teledermatology South Africa: accessed on Oct 4, 2009 http://faculty.washington.edu/rcolven/teledermatology.shtml
36. Operation Village Health: accessed on Oct 4, 2009 http://www.connected-health.org/programs/remote-consultations/center-for-connected-health-models-of-care/operation-village-health.aspx
37. Brauchli K, O'Mahony D, Banach L et al (2005) iPath – a telemedicine platform to support health providers in low resource settings. Stud Health Technol Inform 114:11–17
38. ipath Association Home page. Available at: accessed on Oct 4, 2009 http://ipath.ch/site/en/verein
39. Solomon Islands Telemedicine Network: accessed on Oct 4, 2009 telemed.ipath.ch/solomons
40. LT Telepatologija – Lithuania: accessed on Oct 4, 2009 ipath.ch/site/node/441. Also, in Lithuanian, at: telemed.ipath.ch/lithuania
41. RAFT: accessed on Oct 4, 2009 raft.hcuge.ch
42. Telemedicina Sur: accessed on Oct 4, 2009 telemed.ipath.ch/tmsur
43. West Africa Doctors and Healthcare Professionals Network: accessed on Oct 4, 2009 www.wadn.org
44. HealthNet Nepal: accessed on Oct 4, 2009 www.healthnet.org.np
45. Teledermatology in Port St Johns, South Africa: accessed on Oct 4, 2009 ipath.ch/site/node/22
46. Click Diagnostics: accessed on Oct 4, 2009 http://www.clickdiagnostics.com/index.html
47. Tsai HH, Pong YP, Liang CC et al (2004) Teleconsultation by using the mobile camera phone for remote management of the extremity wound: a pilot study. Ann Plast Surg 53:584–587
48. Whited J (2006) Teledermatology research review. Int J Dermatol 45:220–229

Part II

Clinical Practice

Teledermatopathology

7

Cesare Massone, Alexandra Maria Giovanna Brunasso,
Terri M. Biscak, and H. Peter Soyer

Core Messages

- Teledermatopathology can be performed with three options: (a) the static store-and-forward (SAF) option involves the single file transmission of subjectively preselected and captured areas of microscopic images by a referring physician, (b) the real-time transmission of images from distant locations to consulting pathologists by the remote manipulation of a robotic microscope, (c) the hybrid virtual slide systems (VSS) that involves the digitization of whole slides at high resolution thus enabling the user to view any part of the specimen at any magnification.
- VSS overcomes those major limitations concerning SAF teledermatopathology (i.e. "field selection error," image quality).
- VSS has various applications: telediagnosis in daily routine work, second opinion consultation, quality assurance service, teleteaching, tele-education and Virtual Slide Congresses.
- Already several specific web sites are present in Internet.
- Despite SAF teledermatopathology being the most frequently used and less expensive approach to teledermatopathology, VSS represents the future in this discipline.
- Anyhow, expertise of the teleconsultants and a sophisticated clinico-pathologic correlation remains of upmost importance to finalize a correct diagnosis with teledermatopathology.

Introduction

Teledermatopathology is the application of modern advances in communication to dermatopathology for the distant diagnosis of skin specimens. This diagnostic approach involved in the beginning two major systems: the dynamic real-time transmission of images from distant locations to consulting pathologists via

C. Massone (✉)
Division of General Dermatology, Department of Dermatology, Medical University of Graz
Graz, Austria
e-mail: cesare.massone@klinikum-graz.at

A.M.G. Brunasso
Division of Environmental Dermatology and Venereology, Department of Dermatology, Medical University of Graz, Graz, Austria
e-mail: alexandra.brunasso-vernetti@medunigraz.at

T.M. Biscak
Dermatology Research Centre, The University of Queensland, School of Medicine, Princess Alexandra Hospital, Brisbane, QLD, Australia
e-mail: t.biscak@uq.edu.au

H.P. Soyer
Dermatology Research Centre, The University of Queensland, School of Medicine, Princess Alexandra Hospital, Brisbane, QLD, Australia
e-mail: p.soyer@uq.edu.au

H.P. Soyer et al. (eds.), *Telemedicine in Dermatology*,
DOI 10.1007/978-3-642-20801-0_7,

the remote manipulation of a robotic microscope or alternatively, a static store-and-forward (SAF) option in which each image is captured and transmitted as a single file [1–3].

Analyzing the number of publications in telermatopathology and in telepathology in Pub Med, it is a matter of fact that after the initial enthusiasm that followed the general development of telemedicine in general and specifically of teledermatology more than 15 years ago, interest of dermatopathologists for teledermatopathology decreased during the last years. On the contrary, research and innovation in telepathology increased and nowadays telepathology is a florid reality. This makes that new systems are firstly tested and implemented for telepathology and afterwards translated to teledermatopathology, as happened for the recently developed Virtual Slide Systems (VSS) and the Virtual Microscope (VM) [4, 5].

The Technological Equipment

Even if the technological bases of teledermatopathology are a suited microscope, a digital camera, a computer and an Internet connection, each of the three systems requires completely different hardware and software from low cost systems to high expensive ones. Moreover, a more than basic IT knowledge is required for optimal results. Last, but not least, independently from the system applied, the final result depends directly to the quality of the original HE slide.

SAF Teledermatopathology

The SAF-system is currently the most common application used in teledermatopathology. Recently, DeAgustín et al. reviewed hardware and software currently available for SAF systems [6]. Each image is captured by a conventional camera/video camera adapted on a normal microscope. Images are saved on a smart card and then downloaded on a personal computer where editing can be done using image specific software (i.e. Photoshop, Adobe Systems GmbH, Saggart, Republic of Ireland). These are then transmitted as a single file by e-mail or File Transfer Protocol (FTP) to one or more teleconsultants individually for evaluation. Compression of the files using the current standard compression format called Joint Photographic Experts Group (JPEG) can solve transmission problems due to large image size. Upon arrival, the images are saved on the teleconsultant's personal computer but would need to be sent along to other teleconsultants in order to seek further opinions [1, 7, 8].

SAF teledermatology presents both advantages and disadvantages. The application is relatively easy and fast to use, requiring only basic informatics knowledge. In fact, most modern microscopes today are already equipped with a photographic camera adaptor, reducing any additional costs. A photographic digital camera and a personal computer with Internet connection that can be associated to specific image software are the minimum equipment requirements.

An important issue of SAF teledermatopathology is that of image quality and selection. The former is dependent upon two basic points: image acquisition and photo-editing. The currently available digital photo-cameras can acquire high-resolution images and produce excellent images even at high magnifications. At low magnification (scanning, ×2), however, the image quality is not satisfactory and does not compare to conventional microscopy. Interestingly enough, none of the previously mentioned studies attributed their errors to image quality [1, 7–15]. The process of photo-edition using specific image software can enhance the image quality, but requires special skills and experience in order to obtain quality results.

Secondly, image selection is critical in achieving correct histopathologic diagnosis, even for expert observers. A referring pathologist who correctly establishes a reliable differential diagnosis will be able to identify which morphologic elements require expert interpretation. On the other hand, one who does not formulate a plausible differential diagnosis will most likely hinder the correct expert assessment. Indeed, the selection issue becomes crucial when particular subtle features are clues for diagnoses. Incorrect diagnoses due to the lack of relevant image capture are termed "field selection error." This type of error was reported in three of the above-mentioned studies and is an important issue not only in skin pathology but also in many others organ systems [1, 8].

Even highly experienced dermatopathologists encounter serious difficulties in performing diagnoses in difficult cases; this premise can also be applied for SAF teledermatopathology. It is therefore important that expert teleconsultants be mindful of the individual limitations regarding particular cases. In some cases the result will simply refute or confirm the baseline proposal. If a diagnosis is done by exclusion of other diseases, SAF teledermatopathology will require more images, a detailed clinical background and an accurate follow-up of the patient in order to achieve a conclusive diagnosis.

Real-Time (Dynamic) Teledermatopathology

This approach attempts to reproduce a dynamic screening via live, full-motion, remotely controlled video microscopy. Real-time teledermatopathology is more appealing to most pathologists because it closely resembles the established technique of traditional pathologic examination. However, it requires a high quality and flexibility of communication in order to transmit video images and carries economical limitations associated with software and hardware applications, in addition to availability of high fidelity telecommunication [1, 8]. A further limitation of this option is the requirement of synchronicity between the consultant and the referring physician. It can prove difficult to coordinate each person's availability and indeed time-zonal differences create a further challenge.

Virtual Microscope Teledermatopathology

In the last several years hybrid systems that combine limited robotic capabilities with high resolution images have been introduced in telepathology and are known as Virtual Slide Systems (VSS) (i.e. see also www.aperio.com). These new VSS are large, single file, digital facsimiles of the visual content of glass microscope slides acquired at high magnification using a ×20 or ×40 objective lens [2, 16]. This file can then be viewed on any computer at any location with a virtual microscope interface where a user can alter the magnification during virtual assessment [2, 16]. VSS image quality is influenced by the quality of the H&E slide, presence on the H&E slide of the whole section and the positioning of the image, where an orthogonal disposition of the tissue in the slide border becomes mandatory in order to ensure correct image orientation [17]. VSS overcomes those major limitations concerning SAF teledermatopathology and combines the advantages with those of the real-time method. This technique has enormous potential with the introduction of an automatic slide feeder that allows the user to produce slides in digital format that can be used in daily routine diagnostic work (Fig. 7.1).

The initial concerns of VSS regarding the time needed to scan the slides have been overcome by the development of ultrarapid virtual slide processor (DMetrix) [5]. The application of this technique however, is hindered by economical concerns (cost of equipment) and by slow transmitting connections related to the present scarcity of broadband lines [1, 16, 18]. Some web-based versions of a virtual microscope have been developed in an effort to reduce transmission problems by only transmitting those fields which are immediately required by the viewer (see next section) [15, 18, 19]. Images stored on a VS server are accessible to multiple users simultaneously, and are of diagnostic quality that could be used for many purposes from routine work to education for medical students or self assessment courses [3, 4].

The Literature Background in Teledermatopathology

A number of studies have investigated the feasibility of *SAF teledermatopathology* application predominantly on nonmelanoma skin cancers or melanocytic lesions and all have indicated a significant level of diagnostic agreement [9–13]. A diagnostic concordance of 100% was achieved in studies by Weinstein et al. and Dawson et al. who evaluated margin assessment in frozen sections of nonmelanoma skin cancer and cutaneous Basal cell and Squamous cell carcinomas respectively [9, 10]. Okada et al. achieved this same value through comparison of pathologic and dermatopathologic techniques for investigations of melanocytic lesions while Ferrara et al. found a diagnostic accuracy of 100% for the combined dermoscopic-pathological approach towards these lesions [11, 12]. Della Mea et al. observed a *K* statistic of 0.79 between two pathologists also examining melanocytic lesions [13]. Piccolo et al. demonstrated an improvement of telepathologic concordance when combined with conventional microscopy, an outcome also seen by Berman et al. who additionally found improvements with the provision of clinical history [14, 15]. These studies also revealed that diagnostic efficacy and accuracy in teledermatopathology may be particularly weak when examining entities that require the identification of subtle architectural arrangements

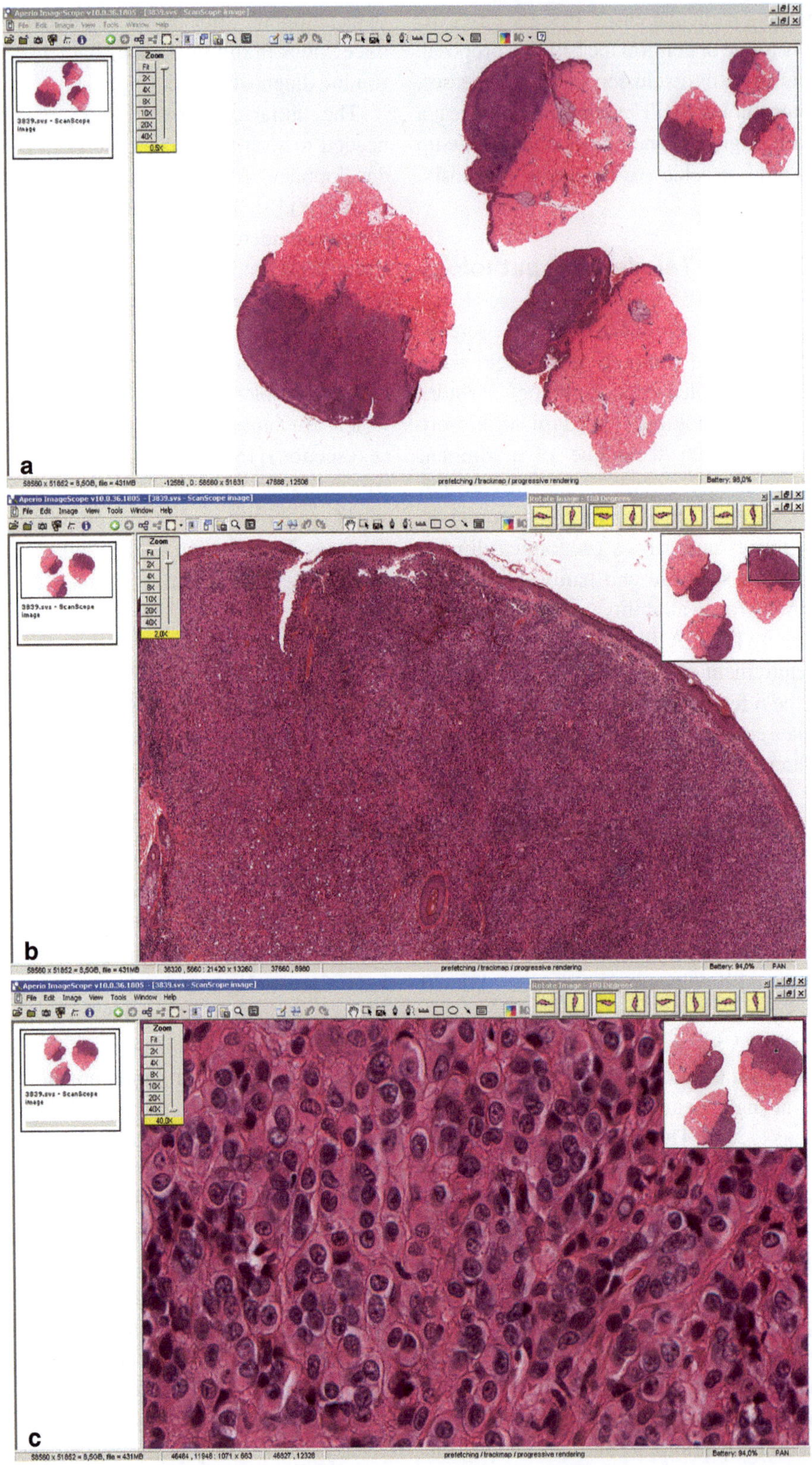

Fig. 7.1 (**a–c**) Images from a virtual microscope image (Aperio, Aperio Technologies, Inc., Vista, CA, USA). Starting from the single image file (which is a svs file 431 MB in size) a user can change the magnification from an overall low-power (**a**), to medium-power (**b**), till to the maximal resolution at which the specimen was scanned (×40) (**c**). The image resolution does not decrease when the magnification increases. The "rotate tool" allows to turn the image as desired. The "hand tool" allows to move and to look the digital image exactly as a normal glass slide

as in inflammatory skin diseases or delicate cytologic features as in dysplastic nevi [1, 7–15].

Morgan et al. studied the efficiency and reproducibility of *dynamic teledermatopathology* through comparison of diagnoses on 100 specimens (25 melanocytic lesions, 50 non-melanoma skin cancers, 25 inflammatory dermatoses) rendered by two independent, board certified dermatopathologists using a double-headed microscope and teledermatopathology from two remote sites (approximately 64 km apart) [1]. The image was sent through T1 line and was received through a reciprocal personal computer running the identical V-TEC code and software. It was then processed and sent at a resolution of 640×480 active lines. A separate voice-transmittal speakerphone line was present at each facility and in this setting the pathologists were able to generate remote telediagnoses in less than 1 min per slide for random, unselected cases. The agreement for teledermatopathology (κ=0.76) was good, but still below that of the conventional two-headed microscopy (κ=0.93) and the video assessed diagnosis took longer. It was concluded however, that dynamic teledermatopathology does not appear to present a serious time limitation in clinical practice given the proper equipment and expertise of the operators [1].

Concerning *VSS*, a high level of diagnostic concordance between microscope diagnosis and remote telediagnosis of gastrointestinal specimens based on VSS was achieved by Molnar et al. and China Li et al. demonstrated feasibility in surgical pathology [20, 21]. In addition to showing that VSS are a realistic alternative to conventional pathology, Costello et al. developed an online pathology software tool (ReplaySuite) based on a VSS that presents archived virtual slide examinations to pathologists in an accessible video-like format [22, 23]. Studies by Gilbertson et al. established that the VS images are sufficient for pathologists to make reliable diagnostic decisions and compose diagnostic reports [24]. Furness et al. found that the only significant difference between diagnoses proffered on the basis of VSS and conventional slides, was that using VSS took pathologists considerably longer [25].

Few experiences have been reported concerning the use of VSS specifically in teledermatopathology. Leinweber et al. focused on the technical requirements for achievement of a correct diagnosis on digital histopathologic images [26]. A collection of 560 melanocytic lesions was selected from the files of the Department of Dermatology, Medical University of Graz, Austria. From each lesion one entire histologic slide was digitally scanned with a robotic microscope, a second generation virtual slide processor of "Class 4A" (according to the classification of Weinstein et al. on telepathology systems) [3, 27]. Apart from scanning, focusing, recording and storing, the software also allowed a reproduction of images in different magnifications. Digital pictures were reviewed by four dermatopathologists using a presentation program, which recorded the number of image calls, applied magnifications, overall time needed and amount of transmitted bits during the digital sign-out. One month later, the four microscopists had to review the corresponding slides and render a direct diagnosis on each case. Telepathologic diagnoses corresponded with the original diagnoses in a range from 90.4% to 96.4% of cases (K = 0.80–0.93). The transmission time correlated to about 1 min and the median time needed for achievement of a diagnosis was 22 s (being significantly higher for melanomas compared with nevi). The authors concluded that minimal time exposure is needed for correct reporting on digital histopathologic images and that ISDN lines are sufficient for adequately fast transmission following JPEG compression [26].

Massone et al. performed the first specific study in teledermatopathology using VSS focusing only on inflammatory skin diseases [28]. Twelve teleconsultants from six different countries were asked to report on 46 cases recruited from the routine collection of the Research Unit for Dermatopathology, Medical University of Graz, Austria. Digitalized images of each slide were obtained by scanning at ×20 optical magnification with a second generation virtual slide processor of "Class 4A" that allows performing a high-resolution automatic acquisition of tissue sections [2, 3]. The image software integrated and created digital high-resolution images of the whole skin specimen in JPEG format with a compression ratio of 80%. The digital images in original format were uploaded to a server of a specific web application suited for telepathology (http://telederm.org/research/dermatopath/default.asp) which was login and password protected and only available to the participants of this study [29, 30]. This web application integrates an image viewer software (WebScope©) and works in a manner that closely resembles a light microscope. Sample images of this study are available on the Internet at http://telederm.org/research/dermatopath/. For each case histopathologic images and limited clinical data were available directly on the web application.

Even taking into consideration the differences between this study and those among the literature it is obvious that the result of 73% correct telediagnosis is significant low [1, 7–15]. As the teleconsultants in the studies were highly experienced, it is believed that intrinsic diagnostic difficulties associated with cutaneous inflammatory pathology as well as the availability of complete clinical data influenced this loss of diagnostic accuracy. Other plausible explanations include the unfamiliarity of the consultants to the device where the slide analysis setting is very different to that which they are accustomed. Rather than viewing slides through a circular plane via the microscope eyepiece, the consultants are now seeing the image on a rectangular plane presented via the computer screen which will no doubt require a period of adjustment. Another limitation of VSS is the failure to identify microorganisms in the virtual images despite their documented histologic presence (personal experience). Cerroni et al. confirmed that both clinical picture and data can improve the diagnosis of telepathologists of 16.6% [31].

Nielsen et al. recently tested VSS feasibility for skin tumors, proving an accuracy of 89.2% for VSS and 92.7% for conventional microscopy. All κ coefficients expressed very good intra- and interobserver agreement among the four telepathologists [32].

VSS in Telepathology

VSS has various applications and apart from telediagnosis in daily routine work and second opinion consultation, teleteaching and tele-education represent two major alternatives with high potentiality. In a telepathology education setting, Lundin et al. developed a digital atlas of breast histopathology based on a web based virtual microscope application (http://www.webmicroscope.net/breastatlas) [33] while Helin et al. applied VSS in teaching and standardizing Gleason grading in prostate carcinoma [18]. Schrader et al. developed a unique software capable of combining the histological virtual slide and the text information of the dictation process: this "diagnostic path" can be used for image retrieval, quality assurance or for educational purposes [34]. Boutonnat et al. received positive feedback from students of two French medical schools that were taught histopathology using VSS, where overall student interaction also improved [35]. Analogous good results in the educational setting were obtained by Kumar et al. [36]. Fujita et al. developed a VSS to create and viewing clinico-pathologic cases [37]. Della Mea et al. developed an open source software system for whole slide imaging (eSlide suite) [38]. Web conferencing systems using Skype and MSN have been tested by Klock and Gomes [39]. An innovative telemedicine-enabled rapid breast care service that bundles telemammography, telepathology, and teleoncology services into a single day process has been implemented by Lopez et al. [40] Successful experiences in Virtual Congresses of Pathology and Virtual Slide Congresses have been reported [41].

Teledermatopathology on the Web

Different web applications shares dermatopathology images with free access for educational purposes.

- Dermpedia: http://www.dermpedia.org/
- Diagnostic Image Forum: http://www.uninet.edu/copat/dermopat.html
- Derm-Path India: http://www.histopathology-india.net/dermpath.htm
- Atlas of dermatopathology: http://atlases.muni.cz/atlases/kuze/atl_en/sect_main.html
- Dermatopathonline.com: http://www.dermatopathonline.com/
- Pathowiki: http://www.pathowiki.org/pathowiki/index.php/Kategorie:Haut

Other websites where cases are presented for second opinion consultations have a limited access to registered users only.

- The Community for Teledermatology: www.telederm.org
- piel.telederm.org: http://piel.telederm.org/default.asp

The advantage of these SAF application is that images are available to a number of teleconsultants simultaneously. The security and privacy of the web application is guaranteed by a personal login and password used by each teleconsultants to access to patients data [29, 30].

SAF web applications specifically have been also used for specific teledermatopathology studies (i.e. http://telederm.org/research/dermatopath/default.asp)[28].

Some web-based versions of a virtual microscope have been developed in an effort to reduce transmission problems by only transmitting those fields which are immediately required by the viewer (i.e. http://www.webmicroscope.net/, http://telederm.org/research/dermatopath/default.asp, http://alf3.urz.unibas.ch/vmic/list.cfm, http://interpath1.uio.no/telemedisin/WebInterPath/interpathindex.htm).

Limitations of Teledermatopathology

In dermatopathology the detailed knowledge of skin pathology and semiotics should always be integrated with the clinical background in order to arrive at a correct diagnosis. Two examples of dermatopathologic entities that might be particularly problematic in routine dermatopathology are inflammatory dermatoses, characterized by subtle pattern-arrangements of inflammatory cells and dysplastic nevi revealing subtle changes in architectural and cytologic appearance that lead easily astray to a more malignant behavior. These lesions are also of major concern for achieving correct diagnoses in teledermatopathology [28, 31]. Earlier studies focusing on nonmelanoma skin cancers or melanocytic lesions have successfully demonstrated the feasibility of both real time and SAF teledermatopathology [1, 12–15]. However, it was already observed that examination of lesions requiring identification of subtle architectural arrangements or delicate cytologic features as in examples just described, may significantly weaken the diagnostic efficacy and accuracy in teledermatopathology [1, 12–15, 28]. Also the recent applications of VSS in teledermatopathology both on melanocytic lesions and inflammatory skin diseases have confirmed the intrinsic difficulty of dermatopathology and teledermatopathology [26, 28, 31]. Further development of the VSS, new studies using the new virtual slide processor and training with the virtual microscope might improve the diagnostic performance of teleconsultants. Suffice to say that expertise of the teleconsultants and a sophisticated clinico-pathologic correlation remains of upmost importance [32, 42–45].

Prospects for the Future

The virtual microscopy is widely accepted in pathology for educational purposes and teleconsultation [46, 47]. The recent pilot studies suggest that the use of remote expert consultants in diagnostic pathology can be integrated into the daily routine [5, 16, 45–50]. A recent study investigated a randomized comparison of virtual microscopy and traditional glass microscopy and showed that residents in dermatology and pathology performed similarly in diagnosing dermatopathology disorders using virtual slides or glass slides [51]. VSS telepathology definitively offers the possibility to break the limitations of conventional static telepathology. The complete histological slide may be investigated instead of sets of images of lesions sampled by the presenting pathologist. The benefit is demonstrated by the high diagnostic security of 95% accordance between first and second diagnosis [46]. Open issues still remain medicolegal and reimbursement that will have to be clarified and specified [48], but definitively VSS possesses high potentiality not only in teleconsultation and tele-education, but also in quality assurance service and remote routine diagnosis [50].

Also in teledermatopathology, VSS technology would enable rapid and reproducible diagnoses, even though problems exist in the intrinsic difficulty of interpreting dermatopathology of inflammatory and neoplastic skin diseases particularly in the context of lack of complete clinical data. In fact, Massone et al. concluded that despite its usability, the performance in teledermatopathology seemed to have also been influenced by the availability of complete clinical data [28]. As stated above, clinico-pathologic correlation will be the gold standard also for teledermatopathology [28, 31].

Despite SAF teledermatopathology being the most frequently used and less expensive approach to teledermatopathology, VSS represents the future in this discipline. As technology continues to be refined, the problems reported in previous literature will be overcome. While presently the economical investment for VSS or real time teledermatopathology equipment may be beyond the reach of most dermatopathology practices, high resolution devices will become accessible for most of us in the not too distant future [42–45].

Conclusions

The clinical reading environment for the twenty-first century pathologist looks very different than it did even a few short years ago. Glass slides are quickly being replaced by digital "virtual slides," and the traditional light microscope is being replaced by the computer display [45, 49]. Improvements in the diagnostic facility will no doubt follow on from further development of the VSS, the slide processor and of course training in the use virtual microscope. Undoubtedly as technology becomes even more sophisticated, in the future VSS will overcome the present drawbacks and find its place specifically in the field of teledermatopathology.

References

1. Morgan MB, Tannenbaum M, Smoller BR (2003) Telepathology in the diagnosis of routine dermatopathologic entities. Arch Dermatol 139:637–640
2. Cross SS, Dennis T, Start RD (2002) Telepathology: current status and future prospects in diagnostic histopathology. Histopathology 41:91–109
3. Weinstein RS, Descour MR, Liang C et al (2001) Telepathology overview: from concept to implementation. Hum Pathol 32:1283–1299
4. Glatz-Krieger K, Glatz D, Mihatsch MJ (2003) Virtual slides: high-quality demand, physical limitations, and affordability. Hum Pathol 34:968–974
5. Weinstein RS, Descour MR, Liang C et al (2004) An array microscope for ultrarapid virtual slide processing and telepathology. Design, fabrication, and validation study. Hum Pathol 35:1303–1314
6. DeAgustín D, Sanmartín J, Varela-Centelles P et al (2008) Technological bases for teledermatopathology: state of the art. Semin Cutan Med Surg 27:25–31
7. Pak HS (2002) Teledermatology and teledermatopathology. Semin Cutan Med Surg 21:179–189
8. Black-Schaffer S, Flotte TJ (2001) Teledermatopathology. Adv Dermatol 17:325–338
9. Weinstein LJ, Epstein JI, Edlow D et al (1997) Static image analysis of skin specimens: the application of telepathology to frozen section evaluation. Hum Pathol 28:30–35
10. Dawson PJ, Johnson JG, Edgemon LJ et al (2000) Outpatient frozen sections by telepathology in a Veterans Administration medical center. Hum Pathol 31:786–788
11. Okada DH, Binder SW, Felten CL et al (1999) "Virtual microscopy" and the internet as telepathology consultation tools: diagnostic accuracy in evaluating melanocytic skin lesions. Am J Dermatopathol 21:525–531
12. Ferrara G, Argenziano G, Cerroni L et al (2004) A pilot study of a combined dermoscopic-pathological approach to the telediagnosis of melanocytic skin neoplasms. J Telemed Telecare 10:34–38
13. Della Mea V, Puglisi F, Forti S et al (1997) Expert pathology consultation through the Internet: melanoma versus benign melanocytic tumours. J Telemed Telecare 3(suppl 1):17–19
14. Piccolo D, Soyer HP, Burgdorf W et al (2002) Concordance between telepathologic diagnosis and conventional histopathologic diagnosis: a multiobserver store-and-forward study on 20 skin specimens. Arch Dermatol 138:53–58
15. Berman B, Elgart GW, Burdick AE (1997) Dermatopathology via a still-image telemedicine system: diagnostic concordance with direct microscopy. Telemed J 3:27–32
16. Weinstein RS (2005) Innovations in medical imaging and virtual microscopy. Hum Pathol 36:317–319
17. Glatz-Krieger K, Glatz D, Mihatsch MJ (2006) Virtual microscopy: first applications. Pathologe 27:469–476
18. Helin H, Lundin M, Lundin J et al (2005) Web-based virtual microscopy in teaching and standardizing Gleason grading. Hum Pathol 36:381–386
19. Dee FR, Lehman JM, Consoer D et al (2003) Implementation of virtual microscope slides in the annual pathobiology of cancer workshop laboratory. Hum Pathol 34:430–436
20. Molnar B, Berczi L, Diczhazy C et al (2003) Digital slide and virtual microscopy based routine and telepathology evaluation of routine gastrointestinal biopsy specimens. J Clin Pathol 56:433–438
21. Li X, Liu J, Xu H et al (2007) A feasibility study of virtual slides in surgical pathology in China. Hum Pathol 38: 1842–1848
22. Costello SS, Johnston DJ, Dervan PA, O'Shea DG (2003) Development and evaluation of the virtual pathology slide: a new tool in telepathology. J Med Internet Res 5:e11
23. Johnston DJ, Costello SP, Dervan PA, O'Shea DG (2005) Development and preliminary evaluation of the VPS ReplaySuite: a virtual double-headed microscope for pathology. BMC Med Inform Decis Mak 5:10
24. Gilbertson JR, Ho J, Anthony L et al (2006) Primary histologic diagnosis using automated whole slide imaging: a validation study. BMC Clin Pathol 6:4
25. Furness P (2007) A randomized controlled trial of the diagnostic accuracy of internet-based telepathology compared with conventional microscopy. Histopathology 50: 266–273
26. Leinweber B, Massone C, Kodama K et al (2006) Teledermatopathology: a controlled study about diagnostic validity and technical requirements for digital transmission. Am J Dermatopathol 28:413–416
27. KS400 Imaging System Release 3.0. CarlZeissVision, Munich; 1997
28. Massone C, Soyer HP, Lozzi GP et al (2007) Feasibility and diagnostic agreement in teledermatopathology using a virtual slide system. Hum Pathol 38:546–554
29. Massone C, Soyer HP, Hofmann-Wellenhof R et al (2006) Two years' experience with Web-based teleconsulting in dermatology. J Telemed Telecare 12:83–87
30. Soyer HP, Hofmann-Wellenhof R, Massone C et al (2005) Telederm.org: freely available online consultations in dermatology. PLoS Med 2:e87
31. Cerroni L, Argenyi Z, Cerio R et al (2010) Influence of evaluation of clinical pictures on the histopathologic diagnosis of inflammatory skin disorders. J Am Acad Dermatol 63: 647–652
32. Nielsen PS, Lindebjerg J, Rasmussen J et al (2010) Virtual microscopy: an evaluation of its validity and diagnostic performance in routine histologic diagnosis of skin tumors. Hum Pathol 41:1770–1776
33. Lundin M, Lundin J, Helin H, Isola J (2004) A digital atlas of breast histopathology: an application of web based virtual microscopy. J Clin Pathol 57:1288–1291
34. Schrader T, Niepage S, Leuthold T et al (2006) The diagnostic path, a useful visualisation tool in virtual microscopy. Diagn Pathol 1:40
35. Boutonnat J, Paulin C, Faure C et al (2006) A pilot study in two French medical schools for teaching histology using virtual microscopy. Morphologie 90:21–25
36. Kumar RK, Velan GM, Korell SO et al (2004) Virtual microscopy for learning and assessment in pathology. J Pathol 204:613–618
37. Fujita K, Crowley RS (2003) The virtual slide set – a curriculum development system for digital microscopy. AMIA Annu Symp Proc: 846
38. Mea VD, Bortolotti N, Beltrami CA (2009) eSlide suite: an open source software system for whole slide imaging. J Clin Pathol 62:749–751

39. Klock C, Gomes Rde P (2008) Web conferencing systems: Skype and MSN in telepathology. Diagn Pathol 15(3 suppl 1):S13
40. López AM, Graham AR, Barker GP et al (2009) Virtual slide telepathology enables an innovative telehealth rapid breast care clinic. Hum Pathol 40:1082–1091
41. Góngora Jará H, Barcelo HA (2008) Telepathology and continuous education: important tools for pathologists of developing countries. Diagn Pathol 15(3 suppl 1):S24
42. Massone C, Brunasso AM, Campbell TM, Soyer HP (2008) State of the art of teledermatopathology. Am J Dermatopathol 30:446–450
43. Massone C, Wurm EM, Soyer HP (2008) Teledermatology. G Ital Dermatol Venereol 143:213–218
44. Massone C, Wurm EM, Hofmann-Wellenhof R, Soyer HP (2008) Teledermatology: an update. Semin Cutan Med Surg 27:101–105
45. Weinstein RS, Graham AR, Richter LC et al (2009) Overview of telepathology, virtual microscopy, and whole slide imaging: prospects for the future. Hum Pathol 40:1057–1069
46. Wienert S, Beil M, Saeger K et al (2009) Integration and acceleration of virtual microscopy as the key to successful implementation into the routine diagnostic process. Diagn Pathol 9(4):3
47. Dee FR (2009) Virtual microscopy in pathology education. Hum Pathol 40:1112–1121
48. Leung ST, Kaplan KJ (2009) Medicolegal aspects of telepathology. Hum Pathol 40:1137–1142
49. Krupinski EA (2009) Virtual slide telepathology workstation of the future: lessons learned from teleradiology. Hum Pathol 40:1100–1111
50. Graham AR, Bhattacharyya AK, Scott KM et al (2009) Virtual slide telepathology for an academic teaching hospital surgical pathology quality assurance program. Hum Pathol 40:1129–1136
51. Koch LH, Lampros JN, Delong LK et al (2009) Randomized comparison of virtual microscopy and traditional microscopy in diagnostic accuracy among dermatology and pathology residents. Hum Pathol 40:662–667

Teledermoscopy

8

Dougal F. Coates and Jonathan Bowling

Core Messages

- Dermoscopy images are easy to capture and transmit.
- A teledermoscopy service implemented in the correct clinical setting has the potential to save health systems considerable money.
- Teledermoscopy needs to be used as an adjunct to a thorough history and full examination rather than to view single lesions in isolation.
- Legal waters are nebulous and without precendent.
- Mobile phones and portable USB microscopes are interesting future developments in image acquisition and relay.
- Rigorous evaluation is still required before widespread implementation of teledermoscopy.

Telemedicine and Teledermatology

The twenty-first century has ushered in an ever expanding network of medical communication modalities. Subsequently Telemedicine, a now well established component of modern medicine, is used internationally, with the goal of optimizing diagnosis, treatment, and teaching. Dermatology, perhaps the most visual of medical specialities, is uniquely positioned to take advantage of this field of medicine.

Despite the relative age of telemedicine and the potential for dermatology to take advantage of this medical modality, quite surprisingly teledermatology as a subdivision has only recently evolved. Dermatologists in the USA were the first to begin exploring the area. In response to Dermatological isolation, Perednia and Brown [1] first utilized teledermatology in rural Oregon in 1995. Two years later in Minneapolis, Zelickson and Homan [2] found a diagnostic concordance of 88% between face-to-face diagnosis and teledermatology on nursing home patients, albeit on a mere 29 subjects. Teledermatology has become far more widespread subsequent to this early experience, particularly in restricted areas with a paucity of dermatologists, where it provides an invaluable resource for a wide range of doctors and their patients.

Teledermoscopy

Dermoscopy (dermatoscopy) is a non-invasive, in-vivo technique which allows the clinician to examine cutaneous micro-features not visible under macroscopic examination. It is proven to be a more accurate tool in the diagnosis of melanoma than naked-eye examination [3]. Considerable time passed between the initial descriptions of dermoscopy as a valuable technique to diagnose skin tumors and its incorporation into everyday practice – some believed it was difficult to learn and not worth their while as established clinicians, whilst others questioned its accuracy and clinical utility. Only relatively recently has it become incorporated into the mainstream practice of

D.F. Coates (✉) • J. Bowling
Department of Dermatology,
Churchill Hospital, Oxford Radcliffe Health,
Oxford, UK
e-mail: dougalfc@yahoo.com; jonathan.bowling@orh.nhs.uk

H.P. Soyer et al. (eds.), *Telemedicine in Dermatology*,
DOI 10.1007/978-3-642-20801-0_8, © Springer-Verlag Berlin Heidelberg 2012

dermatologists, particularly in the USA. Once considered an area of high specialization, dermoscopy is now the fasted growing method used to image skin and an integral part of the initial consult for many patients.

Teledermoscopy represents a rapidly evolving field of teledermatology. Through 'store and forward systems' or less commonly 'real-time systems' a remote teleconsultant can give an opinion on the diagnosis and management of images. Dermoscopic images are obtained digitally through the use of a consumer camera with a special lens or adaptor. These images are then easily sent, typically via secure email, to experts in a remote location. Resultantly, most practitioners with access to a matched dermoscope/digital camera and internet access have the facility to participate in teledermoscopy.

Within 24 h of receiving images, the teleconsultant will typically send a reply email offering their provisional diagnosis, any differential diagnoses, and a preferred course of action. The referral system is therefore extremely convenient, as the interaction is not hampered by different time zones or the time restraints of a busy practice.

Teledermoscopy Versus Teledermatology

Teledermatology has already gained widespread acceptance; It is however easy to envisage a time when teledermoscopy becomes far more popular amongst GPs, dermatologists inexperienced in dermoscopy, and patients alike. Clearly the major pressure driving telemedicine and teledermatology is the lack of regional dermatologists to cover a huge burden of disease in remote locations. This rural patient:doctor ratio is ever-expanding, and in concert with the high proportion of pigmented skin lesions amongst consultations, makes teledermoscopy an attractive concept in this medical context. Patients can be reassured that an expert will be examining their lesion within 24 h, as opposed to travelling huge distances after waiting several months for an appointment.

Additionally, teledermoscopy is not burdened by limitations which make accurate diagnoses difficult in many medical teledermatology consultations, such as a preference for 3D images. Dermoscopic images can be sent with color and image calibration, and in the majority of cases the image, which is projected on a large computer screen, is equivalent to that which the clinician would see in person.

Provost and colleagues compressed digital dermoscopic images and transmitted them over telephone lines in 1998, finding that an accurate diagnosis could be made using this modality [4]. Comparing teleconsultation with face-to-face diagnosis of pigmented skin lesions, Piccolo et al. [5] later found a diagnostic concordance of 91%. In another study of 43 pigmented skin lesions by Piccolo [6], the diagnostic accuracy was related to the experience of the teleconsultant and the intrinsic level of diagnostic difficulty of the lesion, with a concordance of between 77% and 95% (mean 85%) compared to face-to-face diagnosis. Interestingly, image quality did not seem to affect accuracy in these studies.

Expert dermoscopists do however excel in making accurate diagnoses by recognizing subtle morphological features not otherwise appreciated by those less experienced in the technique. Subsequently, it seems logical that providing the teledermoscopist with consistent images that are calibrated to standardize color/brightness etc and transmitted effectively would be a crucial component of correctly diagnosing lesions. The ultimate goal therefore is standardization of image documentation and transmission.

It seems intuitive that a crucial component of any successful doctor-patient relationship is the connection made during face-to-face consultation. Despite this, in a nurse-led study on teledermatology by Williams et al. [7], 93% of surveyed patients were happy with the teleconsultation, and 86% found it more convenient than attending an out-patient clinic. Studies are yet to be published to date that assess the patient acceptance of teledermoscopy.

In a medical age dominated by bottom lines and financial viability, few studies have analyzed the public health ramifications and potential cost reduction in utilizing a teledermatology service. A recent publication by Moreno-Ramirez and colleagues [8] addressed this issue, and found a €49.59 per patient saving in favor of teledermatology over conventional care (GP referral to dermatologist). 2009 patients presenting to GPs with suspicious skin growths had digital photos sent via an intranet service to dermatologists, and those diagnosed with benign appearing lesions were managed in primary care without the need for in-person dermatology assessment.

It is tempting to extrapolate from this data that teledermoscopy would be an even more financially advantageous tool for the health system, given teledermoscopic analysis of skin tumors is potentially more accurate than macro-image teledermatology [9, 10], meaning fewer suggested referrals by teleconsultants, who are more certain of the benign nature of lesions.

Image Capture and Relay

More recently, teledermoscopy by personal digital assistants (PDAs) and mobile phones has been proposed as a potential candidate for triaging pigmented skin lesions [11]. Wireless communication via Global Positioning Radio System (GPRS) or a Universal Mobile Telecommunications System (UMTS) enables an image to be transmitted where internet connection is not available, allowing the previously undiagnosed lesions of patients with poor access to services an opportunity to have their concerns addressed.

Inherent in mobile telemedicine and mobile teledermoscopy is the advantage of all doctors having access and being familiar with mobile phones. Such devices are not a burden to carry and are easy to use, meaning if the quality was to reach parity with digital cameras, as a technology it has the potential to be more warmly received. A study looking into the potential for using 2-megapixel phone cameras to diagnose melanomas found that, with the images being captured by directly applying a cellular phone on a pocket dermoscope, only 2/18 had suboptimal image quality with the potential to influence telediagnosis [12]. Regardless of these statistics, when dealing with melanoma and triaging patients with potentially fatal skin tumors, one cannot be overly conservative, and therefore although this technology holds promise, until images are of higher quality its use is likely to be reserved for areas without dermoscopically trained doctors and internet access.

Digital portable/USB microscopes, as used in the printing industry, may also serve to bridge the technological gap. If these devices were constructed with inbuilt software, images could be easily captured and exported directly for e-mail. This may simplify the process of image acquisition and export.

Teledermoscopy Forums

The more recent widespread use of dermoscopy as a diagnostic tool amongst dermatologists and GPs alike, in addition to the quality of captured images, ease of transmitting teledermoscopic photos, and ever expanding research in the field has seen the birth of a number of active discussion forums in which enquiring doctors and interested experts come together to discuss diagnoses and dermoscopic concepts. Examples of more active forums include

- http://www.dermoscopy-ids.org/discussion
- http://www.dermoscopyatlas.blogspot.com
- http://dermoscopic.blogspot.com

Pitfalls

With pigmented lesions forming the backbone of teledermoscopy consults, the overwhelming concern in the field lies in the misdiagnosis and subsequent mismanagement of malignant melanoma.

Despite the findings of early studies [7, 8], a recent paper by Warshaw et al. [9] conducted in a war veteran's hospital in Minneapolis was not as reassuring. Aggregated diagnostic rates for teledermoscopy were found to be inferior compared to clinic dermatology. Of particular concern, 7 of 36 index melanomas would have been mismanaged by teledermoscopy as opposed to one in the clinic. Three teledermoscopists were enrolled, each a recognized expert dermoscopist with more than five years experience. Most of the mismanaged melanomas were rated with moderate confidence and moderate photograph quality by the teledermoscopists. Although the study population was almost entirely elderly Caucasian males (96%), it could be argued this is the population with the greatest incidence and mortality secondary to melanoma, and even perhaps the demographic most likely to be isolated in a regional area and utilizing an available teledermoscopy service. One must keep in mind however, that teledermoscopy was compared against trained clinic dermatologists and not general practioners, and therefore these findings have less relevance in the setting of limited access health care.

The same group also analyzed the accuracy of teledermoscopy in the diagnosis and management of nonpigmented neoplasms. 728 patients were studied, and although in-patient clinic dermatology was statistically more accurate than teledermoscopy overall, the aggregated diagnostic accuracy rates (percent correct matches of any of chosen diagnoses with histopathology) for malignant lesions were equivalent. Management plan appropriateness was also equivalent for most groups, with the exception of benign lesions viewed by the teleconsultant without the aid of dermoscopy (macro only), where clinic dermatology was superior to teledermatology.

Another significant pitfall in teledermoscopy is in regards to the problematic pink/hypomelanotic lesions, where correlation with the fundamental principles of medicine are essential, including

1. A thorough tumor history, with emphasis on the patient's previous sun exposure, history of tumors, and family history of skin disease.
2. Clinical examination of all melanocytic lesions and consideration of associated skin type.
3. Dermoscopy as the final clinical adjunct to a comprehensive history and clinical examination.

These hypomelanotic or amelanotic lesions are very challenging to diagnose by the clinic dermatologist, and they therefore represent a high-risk group in the teledermoscopy consult.

Legal Hurdles

Another concern for teledermoscopists, especially those working internationally, regards the legislature surrounding teledermoscopy, which is nebulous at best and without precedent. Teledermoscopists rarely hold professional licensure outside their country of residence, and the potential to be charged in a legal case abroad without insurance exists, particularly given the potential consequences of misdiagnosing malignant melanoma.

Additionally, at this point in time teledermoscopists are relying on their medical indemnity cover as a dermatologist to cover any malpractice suits filed against them in teledermoscopy, but it is not yet established whether legal cover as a dermatologist extends to include this form of work.

Intrinsic to the medical legislature of any country is an attempt to protect its citizens from unknown, underqualified, or incompetent doctors. All of these legal questions therefore assume that international doctors would even be officially endorsed by foreign Governments to receive and correspond to teledermoscopic images. Teledermoscopy has, until now, almost entirely been the domain of internationally recognized experts. Resultantly, the well-established precedent in medicine and dermatology, whereby world experts give opinions requested from oversees consultants on challenging cases has largely been the validation for its legality and use. With the aforementioned increased use of dermoscopy throughout dermatology, married to an increased acceptance of telemedicine, this paradigm is likely to shift significantly, bringing these previously under-recognized legal problems to the fore. Lastly, the nature of teledermoscopy means that all images and correspondence are stored, meaning these legal issues are particularly relevant and easily tracked, and the transmission of these images over the internet means that encryption protocols and protection of private patient information are crucial issues which are still yet to be fully resolved.

Financial Considerations

To date, most teledermoscopy projects have been pilot studies or between friends, and accordingly lacked financial reimbursement. As teledermoscopy grows and emerges out of this realm, these financial issues in addition to problems with referral pathways cloud its progression.

Increasingly, High Street clinics are developing teledermoscopy services as financial ventures. Teledermoscopic images are taken by underqualified staff that often lack the training to take a valid history or identify appropriate lesions to capture. Current lack of evidence to support this practice and reports of misdiagnosis are of particular concern. If teledermoscopy is used for commercial gain rather than as an adjunct to medical care, a potential for real patient harms exists, and further evaluation of this business model is needed.

As a concept, teledermoscopy works well where geography dictates the patient has poor access to a local dermatologist who is trained in dermoscopy. Continuing to pursue such a consult when a competent and appropriately timely local service exists carries the very real potential for disrupting established referral pathways and fragmenting professional relationships. Furthermore, notwithstanding the accuracy of teledermoscopy relative to face-to-face consultation, a thorough history and full examination by a trained dermatologist still represents the gold-standard of patient care. A teleconsultant can gather little information about patient concerns and conceptions, and has no facility to probe patient answers or explore further pockets in the history. Moreover, they are provided with a only one or a selection of lesions as opposed to having the opportunity to examine the entire patient, and are denied the opportunity to examine lymph node basins and palpate internal organs etc.

Of particular concern is reassuring a patient based on a small number of lesions selected by an untrained eye, when a malignant lesion may lie elsewhere unnoticed.

Future Challenges and Direction

Telemedicine has become increasingly accepted as a part of modern medicine as technology is integrated into the everyday lives of society. "Computerization" of interpersonal relationships is a billion-dollar industry not restricted to medicine but rather inherent in twenty-first century society. Although societal and generational chasms exist within this cultural re-orientation, its ongoing development and acceptance paves the way for the smoother transition of all forms of telemedicine, including teledermoscopy.

Despite this, the "mechanization" that it represents is likely to remain a concern for a subset of the population, particularly the elderly who may not be as "tech savy" or trusting of an unknown doctor in a displaced location. Counterbalancing this concern, especially in remote areas, is the convenience of a rapid service, a lower cost of consultation, and in the case of teledermoscopy, potentially equivalent diagnostic capabilities.

Dermoscopy is an accurate and effective clinical tool because the experienced user can correlate subtle morphological changes with corresponding histological changes, and in doing so make an accurate diagnosis. Expert dermoscopists are particularly skilled in making this connection. In addition, the accuracy of histological diagnoses of pigmented skin lesions has been shown to be enhanced when the clinician indicates a specific area of concern [12]. An exciting prospect therefore exists whereby a clinician could send a specimen for histological examination, accompanied by a teledermoscopic image and a comment indicating a particular focus of concern. A pathologist could then compile a report with dermoscopic-histologic correlates, including the original image of the suspicious lesion attached, and in doing so improve the understanding of dermoscopy amongst pathologists, and the dermoscopy–pathology relationship amongst dermatologists.

A common stumbling block in the everyday application of teledermoscopy is the bulkiness and cumbersome nature of dermoscopes and camera attachments. Digital portable/USB microscopes offer the potential of a single, easy device for acquiring images, and with direct JPEG uploading and easy forwarding via e-mail, are a practical solution to image capturing and forwarding. This technology however still requires evaluation before consideration can be given to implementation.

Conclusion

Teledermoscopy holds the promise of delivering convenient, cost-effective, and competent care to remote areas not easily accessed by expert dermoscopists. Given these attractive features it is likely to be well accepted by patients. Furthermore, an ever expanding and accepting technological society dictates that capturing and transmitting dermoscopic images becomes increasingly simple, and combined with the rising medico-legal stakes involved with managing pigmented skin lesions makes GPs increasingly likely to utilize such a service.

Before widespread implementation however, it is important to ensure its use is appropriate, and in particular not in preference to face-to-face consultations with local, trained dermatologists. Even without discounting the importance of the doctor-patient relationship, evidence exists which questions the accuracy of teledermoscopy in diagnosing and managing malignant melanoma. Moreover, in an increasingly litigious society there exist numerous legal concerns which are a distance from being resolved. Ongoing, rigorous evaluation is therefore still required before we can be sure of the role teledermoscopy will play for the next generation of doctors and their patients alike.

References

1. Perednia DA, Brown NA (1995) Teledermatology: one application of telemedicine. Bull Med Libr Assoc 83:42–47
2. Zelicksin BD, Homan L (1997) Teledermatology in the nursing home. Arch Dermatol 133:171–174
3. Vestergaard ME, Macaskill P, Holt PE, Menzies SW (2008) Dermoscopy compared with naked eye examination for the diagnosis of primary melanoma: a meta-analysis of studies performed in a clinical setting. Br J Dermatol 159:669–676
4. Provost N, Kopf AW, Rabinovitz HS et al (1998) Comparison of conventional photographs and telephonically transmitted

compressed digitised images of melanomas and dysplastic naevi. Dermatology 196:299–304
5. Piccolo D, Smolle J, Wolf IH et al (1999) Face-to-face diagnosis vs telediagnosis of pigmented skin tumours: a teledermoscopic study. Arch Dermatol 135:1467–1471
6. Piccolo D, Smolle J, Argenziano G et al (2000) Teledermoscopy – results of a multicentre study on 43 pigmented skin lesions. J Telemed Telecare 6:132–137
7. Williams T, May C, Kelly S et al (2001) Patient satisfaction with store-and-forward technology. J Telemed Telecare 7:45–46
8. Moreno-Ramirez D, Ferrandiz L, Camacho F et al (2009) Economic evaluation of a store-and -forward teledermatology system for skin cancer patients. J Telemed Telecare 15:40–45
9. Warshaw E, Lederle F, Nelson D et al (2009) Accuracy of teledermatology for pigmented neoplasms. J Am Acad Dermatol 61(5):753–765
10. Warshaw E, Lederle F, Nelson D et al (2009) Accuracy of teledermatology for nonpigmented neoplasms. J Am Acad Dermatol 60:579–588
11. Massone C, Brunasso A, Soyer HP et al (2009) Mobile teledermoscopy – melanoma diagnosis by one click? Semin Cutan Med Surg 28(3):203–205
12. Soyer HP, Kenet RO, Wolf IH et al (2000) Clinicopathological correlation of pigmented skin lesions using dermoscopy. Eur J Dermatol 10:22–28

Tele-Reflectance Confocal Microscopy

9

Caterina Longo, Paul Hemmer, and Giovanni Pellacani

Core Messages

- Reflectance confocal microscopy (RCM) is a revolutionary diagnostic tool that enables rapid non-invasive imaging of skin tissue at nearly histologic resolution without biopsy.
- In the field of dermato-oncology, RCM has been successfully applied on melanoma and non-melanoma skin cancers for diagnostic purposes, even in equivocal dermoscopic lesions where subtle cyto-architectural atypia is present.
- RCM provides the clinicians with a combination of clinical, dermoscopic and in vivo pathologic information that greatly increase the diagnostic confidence.
- RCM application in clinical centers dealing with challenging skin cancers, could be of great value for both clinicians and patients. However, the need of intense confocal training and expertise could represent an impediment for its successful application.
- Tele-RCM has been created to solve the issue of personnel training (e-learning) and also to offer a tele-consult among scientific community while improving diagnostic knowledge.

C. Longo (✉)
Department of Dermatology,
Arcispedale Santa Maria Nuova, Reggio Emilia, Italy
e-mail: longo.caterina@gmail.com

P. Hemmer
Software Engineering, Lucid. Inc, Rochester, NY, USA
e-mail: phemmer@lucid-tech.com

G. Pellacani
Department of Dermatology and Venereology,
University of Modena and Reggio Emilia, Modena, Italy
e-mail: giovanni.pellacani@unimore.it

Introduction

First described by Marvin Minsky in 1957 [1], reflectance confocal microscopy (RCM) has been applied in clinical settings only in the past decade. RCM is an emerging noninvasive diagnostic tool that rapidly provides in vivo tissue images at nearly cellular histological resolution [2, 3]. Because of its great capability to explore tissue with high resolution, RCM has found its application in many different skin entities and clinicians pioneered using RCM to characterize cellular and architectural morphology of inflammatory and other skin diseases [4]. Later on, diagnostic algorithms and features specific for melanoma (MM) were defined as well as the characterization of non-melanoma skin cancers. Here, we aimed to describe current applications of RCM and future directions regarding the potential application of RCM for tele-consultation and e-learning.

Instruments

In reflectance confocal microscopy, a low power laser beam illuminates a point inside the object. RCM works by detecting single back-scattered photons from the

H.P. Soyer et al. (eds.), *Telemedicine in Dermatology*,
DOI 10.1007/978-3-642-20801-0_9, © Springer-Verlag Berlin Heidelberg 2012

illuminated in-focus section. A pinhole-sized filter rejects the light reflected from out-of-focus portions of the object. The name "confocal" derives from the fact that the point source of light, the illuminated spot in the sample, and the pinhole aperture lie in optically conjugate "focal" planes. With the laser beam (wavelength of 830 nm) a scan on the horizontal plane is performed, producing two-dimensional pictures representing parallel sections of the skin. Contrast is provided by differences in refraction indices of organelles, melanin, melanosomes and other microstructures that are bright, contrasting with the dark background. Commercial instruments (Vivascope 1500®, Lucid Inc, Henrietta, NY) produce black and white images with a lateral resolution of 0.5–1.0 μm and an optical sectioning thickness of 1.0–5.0 μm, reaching a depth of 200–300 μm in healthy skin, corresponding to the papillary dermis.

Image Acquisition

A metal ring is placed onto the skin by a double-side adhesive window, with a drop of water or oil as contact medium between the skin and the plastic window. A dermoscopic image is acquired by means of a handheld dermoscope. The camera provides a 24-bit, full–color, 1,000 by 1,000 pixel image of the site within a 10 × 10 mm field of view. After dermoscopic image acquisition, the ring is filled with gel and the probe is placed onto it. A sequence of montage images ("block" images, 500 × 500 μm) can be automatically acquired on the examined lesion area at the selected depth level resulting in a mosaic of single high resolution images covering an area up to 8 × 8 mm ("cube"). Moreover, an automated stepper permits the acquisition of subsequent confocal sections, beginning at the stratum corneum and ending inside the papillary dermis, with a step interval of minimum 2 μm ("stack"). Live audio-video interlave (AVI) files can be recorded at the DEJ or superficial dermis to evaluate vessel morphology.

RCM Applications in Dermato-Oncology

RCM permits exploration of skin tissue, enabling the global evaluation of the architecture and cytological details of a given lesion. Therefore, RCM is as an effective method for the early diagnosis of diseases such as melanoma and non-melanoma skin cancer, enabling diagnosis, margin assessment (even in amelanotic tumors [5]), and detection of residual disease after topical/surgical therapies [6]. Currently, the main applications of RCM are diagnosis of melanocytic lesions, basal cell carcinoma (BCC), squamous cell carcinoma (SCC) and actinic keratosis (AK). Typical findings of BCCs in RCM include elongated nuclei of tumor cells oriented along the same axis ("polarization"), presence of well-circumscribed trabeculae/cordlike structures or round to oval islands or nodules surrounded by dark nonrefractile cleftlike dark spaces, scattered bright oval, plump to stellate-shaped structures with indistinct borders, corresponding to melanophages, admixed with or between tumor cords and islands in the papillary dermis, bright dendrites or dendritic cells and presence of tortuous vessels. The assessment of specific confocal features of BCC is useful not only for difficult-to diagnose cases, but also to monitor the efficacy of topical treatments [7] or to help clinicians in surgical margin detection [8]. Even thought limited laser depth penetration hinders the exploration of hyperkeratotic lesions, RCM findings for SCC have been recently described [9]. Analyzing 38 cases including SCCs and AK, the presence of atypical honeycombed or disarranged pattern, round cells at spinous-granular layer and round blood vessels in the superficial dermis, emerged as key features for SCC diagnosis.

Undoubtedly, RCM plays a major role in melanoma diagnosis and many efforts have been directed to clearly define specific confocal criteria and their value in real clinical setting [10]. Moreover, RCM has been applied to evaluate specific cyto-architectural aspects of melanocytic lesions that correlate well with dermoscopic features and conventional histological findings [11].

Melanomas are characterized by architecture disarray (so called "non edged papillae") [12] and irregular nested proliferations forming "sparse" nests and sheet-like structures [13] whereas benign nevi show an edged papillary contour and "dense" nests. Cytologically, large bright cells with hyporeflective prominent nuclei, scattered through epidermal layers, are commonly found in MMs, often presenting an extensive distribution on the lesion [14]. Although pagetoid cells can be present also in benign nevi and Spitz nevi, in these lesions, they tend to have a focal distribution and a mild cellular atypia [15]. However, confocal diagnosis of in situ MMs or very thin malignancies can be very challenging especially when facing with atypical nevi presenting architecture disarray and cytologically atypical cells [15]. The presence of atypical melanocytes and nests surrounding adnexal openings, sheets of mainly dendritic melanocytes, cord-like rete ridges at the DEJ and an infiltration of adnexal structures by atypical melanocytes are considered to be striking confocal features of facial lentigo maligna [16], and these features seems efficient in differentiating lentigo maligna from benign freckles of the face.

Advantages/Promises of RCM Application

The advantage of RCM application in a clinical setting lies in a great diagnostic accuracy that help clinicians in decision making for dermoscopically atypical lesions. On the basis of confocal features that distinguish MM from nevi, clinical studies have analyzed the potential of RCM in diagnosis of melanocytic lesions [15]. Moreover, the role of RCM as a second-level examination of difficult to diagnose lesions has been elucidated [17]. In fact, in a blind setting, diagnostic accuracy for MM was far superior for RCM than for dermoscopy, particularly for the greater specificity of the former [17].

The great advantage of RCM lies in the possibility to combine clinical-dermoscopic data with confocal aspects that enable the clinicians to rapidly explore in vivo pathologic details while considering the patient-related information. This is the same diagnostic path applied by a trained dermo-pathologist in front of a specimen under conventional light microscope, but it happens in real time and at patient's bedside. Additionally, RCM imaging doesn't modify the architecture of the tissue, avoiding the artifacts that occur during sample handling for routine H&E staining. Moreover, the possibility to horizontally scan the lesion (*en face*) gives us the opportunity to extensively explore a large tissue area while marking the foci of concern to direct pathological sectioning. It is particularly useful in case of facial lentigo maligna that may display skip areas, where RCM can be applied for biopsy site selection.

Although RCM is a powerful and versatile tool in the hands of clinicians, it has a limited depth penetration that hinders the exploration of hyperkeratotic or mostly dermal lesions. In addition to technical impediments, the RCM application in a diagnostic center requires a specific confocal training and expertise. To overcome the issue of personnel training, tele-RCM may represent a suitable and low cost tool that can offer the advantage of specific training and "at distance" consult.

E-Learning and Tele-Consult

RCM represents a revolutionary technique in the field of dermato-oncology that requires a specific expertise in evaluation of lesions for the presence of confocal criteria and diagnosis assessment. The possibility to use a web platform for teaching purposes has been recently explored. In 2007, a dedicated web-platform (www.skinconfocalmicroscopy.org) was developed for training purposes and with the aim to test the reproducibility of RCM descriptors and parameters by means of inter- and intra-observer agreement [18]. Trained observers were asked to evaluate high resolution single images (500 × 500 μm) for the presence of specific RCM criteria. Interestingly, a good reproducibility resulted for most of the evaluated parameters, in particular for the ones previously proposed within diagnostic algorithms [15].

The growing interest in confocal microscopy application, resulted in the need to have a free on-line tutorial for new users. For this reason, the web-site and the images employed in the aforementioned study of reproducibility were made available as an open source for users interested in testing their capability in recognizing confocal features. Later, a new interactive web-platform has been developed and it is operative after subscription (www.skinconfocalmicroscopy.net). The e-learning platform comprises a "tutorial" and a "training" section. The tutorial section describes the major confocal aspects in different layers, and aspects of architecture and aggregates by use of example images together with definitions of the parameters and diagnostic examples. The training session is constituted by series of cases to be explored and evaluated for pattern identification and diagnostic challenge. At least one dermoscopic image of the case, along with two complete "mosaics" of the lesion (superficial layer, DEJ level and, in some cases, a third level corresponding to the superficial dermis), and not only high resolution single images, were provided to the users in order to mimic what happens during a real-life examination at the patient's bedside. To overcome the slow uploading of large size images, a dedicated software was implemented enabling the rapid navigation and zooming within the mosaic image. Essential clinical data are also included with description of clinical appearance of the lesion. This training section provides a set of cases testing the users diagnostic ability, is intended to transfer the know-how of expert centers to distant users aiming to learn the method. In fact, the user is asked to fill in specific forms with his/her diagnostic suspect and the identified RCM features. Separate lists of features for epidermal and junctional-dermal layers are displayed below the corresponding mosaics. The user is first required to submit the evaluation of each case, after which he/she is able to visualize the correct diagnosis and to compare his/her evaluation with that proposed by an expert in a real-time feedback. This real-time feedback is designed to assist the participants in learning the criteria for RCM diagnosis and to improve the confidence in the decision making process. A recent study, which included six residents as users, has demonstrated the efficacy of e-learning web platform in MM diagnosis assessment for people not previously skilled in the use of confocal microscopy (*data not published*). Moreover, it was possible to evaluate the "e-learning curve" that resulted in an improvement of diagnostic accuracy and confidence over the first 50 cases analyzed.

VivaNet®

Issues concerning image storage, retrieval and privacy of information should be taken in consideration when applying tele-RCM. In fact, it is imperative as well that the quality or content of the acquired images is not altered or irreversibly compressed in any way. Equally important is the protection of patient privacy. In view of these needs, a new net system, called VivaNet®, has been developed. It is a DICOM and HIPPA compliant server for the storage, retrieval, and transfer of medical images that does not digitize, print, display, process, or irreversibly compress the medical images. From a high-level perspective, VivaNet® is little more than a group of high performance computers, all speaking the same language and securely connected to each other over a Virtual Private Network (VPN) in a manner that protects data, prevents intrusion and ensures consistency in presentation while allowing for the seamless sharing of information between medical professionals using the system. By linking VivaNet® computers to each other over a secure, private and high speed connection, VivaNet® users are able to share and evaluate these large image sets quickly and effortlessly. Like a tree, VivaNet® has a root server which is responsible for permanently and securely archiving medical records. The branches and leaves of the tree represent the connections to imaging and reading workstations. As is often the case, a primary care physician may have colleagues he or she is accustomed to working with for the examination of excised tissue samples. VivaNet® will allow for these collaborations to continue and flourish while opening up a world of additional resources for second opinions and consent based information sharing to the benefit of all those involved. In some cases, VivaNet® imaging workstations may be directly connected to the expert who will be performing the evaluation. In other cases where a direct connection between the primary care physician and confocal expert is not possible due to any number of geographic, political or economic limitations, the remote VivaNet® workstations can still communicate with each other by way of the root VivaNet® server. Up to day the Vivanet® implementation is going on, being in an experimental phase in Europe and US in order to test its applicability and efficiency.

Conclusions

The use of an e-learning platform may be very useful to provide continuing medical education and also to exchange difficult cases among scientist community while improving diagnostic knowledge.

Tele-reflectance confocal microscopy is thought with the aim of linking a broad range of medical private and public institutions involved in skin cancer diagnosis to more specialized dermatology units owing a specific expertise in confocal use. In this setting, tele-reflectance confocal microscopy can offer prompt expert diagnosis that is helpful in improving management of many skin cancers resulting in an increase of diagnostic confidence.

References

1. Minsky M (1957) Microscopy apparatus. US Patent 3013467
2. Rajadhyaksha M, Grossman M, Esterowitz D et al (1995) In vivo confocal scanning laser microscopy of human skin: melanin provides strong contrast. J Invest Dermatol 104:946–952
3. Rajadhyaksha M, Gonzalez S, Zavislan JM et al (1999) In vivo confocal scanning laser microscopy of human skin II: advances in instrumentation and comparison with histology. J Invest Dermatol 113:293–303
4. Gonzalez S, Sackstein R, Anderson RR et al (2001) Real-time evidence of in vivo leukocyte trafficking in human skin by reflectance confocal microscopy. J Invest Dermatol 117:384–386

5. Braga JC, Scope A, Klaz I et al (2009) The significance of reflectance confocal microscopy in the assessment of solitary pink skin lesions. J Am Acad Dermatol 61:230–241
6. Richtig E, Ahlgrimm-Siess V, Koller S et al (2010) Follow-up of actinic keratoses after shave biopsy by in-vivo reflectance confocal microscopy – a pilot study. J Eur Acad Dermatol Venereol 24(3):293–298
7. Torres A, Niemeyer A, Berkes B et al (2004) 5% imiquimod cream and reflectance-mode confocal microscopy as adjunct modalities to Mohs micrographic surgery for treatment of basal cell carcinoma. Dermatol Surg 30:1462–1469
8. Goldgeier M, Fox CA, Zavislan JM et al (2003) Noninvasive imaging, treatment, and microscopic confirmation of clearance of basal cell carcinoma. Dermatol Surg 29:205–210
9. Rishpon A, Kim N, Scope A et al (2009) Reflectance confocal microscopy criteria for squamous cell carcinomas and actinic keratoses. Arch Dermatol 145:766–772
10. Pellacani G, Cesinaro AM, Seidenari S (2005) Reflectance-mode confocal microscopy of pigmented skin lesions – improvement in melanoma diagnostic specificity. J Am Acad Dermatol 53:979–985
11. Guitera P, Li LX, Crotty K et al (2008) Melanoma histological Breslow thickness predicted by 75-MHz ultrasonography. Br J Dermatol 159:364–369
12. Pellacani G, Cesinaro AM, Longo C et al (2005) Microscopic in vivo description of cellular architecture of dermoscopic pigment network in nevi and melanomas. Arch Dermatol 141:147–154
13. Pellacani G, Cesinaro AM, Seidenari S (2005) In vivo assessment of melanocytic nests in nevi and melanomas by reflectance confocal microscopy. Mod Pathol 18:469–474
14. Pellacani G, Cesinaro AM, Seidenari S (2005) Reflectance-mode confocal microscopy for the in vivo characterization of pagetoid melanocytosis in melanomas and nevi. J Invest Dermatol 125:532–537
15. Pellacani G, Guitera P, Longo C et al (2007) The impact of in vivo reflectance confocal microscopy for the diagnostic accuracy of melanoma and equivocal melanocytic lesions. J Invest Dermatol 127:2759–2765
16. Ahlgrimm-Siess V, Massone C, Scope A et al (2009) Reflectance confocal microscopy of facial lentigo maligna and lentigo maligna melanoma: a preliminary study. Br J Dermatol 161(6):1307–1316
17. Guitera P, Pellacani G, Longo C et al (2009) In vivo reflectance confocal microscopy enhances secondary evaluation of melanocytic lesions. J Invest Dermatol 129(1):131–138
18. Pellacani G, Vinceti M, Bassoli S et al (2009) Reflectance confocal microscopy features of melanocytic lesions: an internet-based study of the reproducibility of terminology. Arch Dermatol 145(10):1137–1143

Mobile Teledermatology

10

Elisabeth M.T. Wurm and H. Peter Soyer

Core Messages

- Mobile telemedicine refers to telemedicine applications that do not depend on stationary equipment.
- Small portable devices such as mobile phones/smart phones and PDAs or portable PCs are showing potential for telemedicine applications.
- Mobile phone ownership and subscriptions are increasing exponentially world-wide, including underserved areas and developing countries.
- Practical applications of mobile telemedicine include emergency services, triage, routine screening and telehomecare services.
- Other mobile teledermatology services comprise prevention and follow up via text messaging and mobile phone application software for patients and physicians.

Introduction

The term mobile telemedicine is nowadays widely used and encompasses a wide range of telemedicine applications. As telemedicine is also frequently called eHealth, some authors prefer to use the term mHealth [1] (mobile Health). For the purposes of this chapter, the term mobile telemedicine is used to describe telemedicine applications that do not use stationary equipment, but enable exchange of medical information over a distance without location-dependence of the participants. For this, small portable devices such as mobile phones, PDAs or portable PCs that are connected wirelessly to telecommunication services are used. Of note, this concept of mobile telemedicine differs mobile telemedicine as a distinct entity from 'traditional' telemedicine, although they often overlap in reality. An increasing percentage of telemedicine work is becoming mobile based – i.e. it relies on portable devices to collect patient data using wireless methods of communication.

Mobile telemedicine enables health care of patients on travels or in disaster stricken areas as well as monitoring of patients at home, work, school and during transport. Mobile technologies can be used widespread in numerous medical specialities from telecardiology to teleneurology, for example. It enables emergency patient data to be sent during ambulance transport ahead to the hospital. Mobile devices are applied to monitor vital parameters such as pulse and blood pressure, breathing patterns, of electrocardiograms (ECGs) and electroencephalograms (EEGs). In the hospital, mobile videoconferencing systems that are brought to the patient's bedside can be applied to make a telemedical ward round [2].

These mobile applications seem to have great benefit for the management of patients in a non-hospital environment. This particularly applies to the management of patients with chronic disease who require long-term care and often find it difficult to travel to and

E.M.T. Wurm (✉) • H.P. Soyer
Dermatology Research Centre, The University of Queensland, School of Medicine, Princess Alexandra Hospital, Brisbane, QLD, Australia
e-mail: e.wurm@uq.edu.au, lissy.wurm@gmail.com; p.soyer@uq.edu.au

H.P. Soyer et al. (eds.), *Telemedicine in Dermatology*,
DOI 10.1007/978-3-642-20801-0_10,

from their health service provider. Furthermore, follow up and drug prescriptions could be enabled conveniently at home by dedicated application software for mobile phones to assist people with disease self-management. Especially telephone messages and text messaging technologies have been recently adopted for disease prevention and management [3]. Potential applications of short messaging (SMS) and multimedia messaging (MMS) services comprise use as a home monitoring and surveillance tool, that offers a two way communication [4] (Table 10.1).

Mobile teledermatology refers to the use of mobile telemedicine in dermatology. In mobile teledermatology, primarily mobile devices such as mobile phones and PDAs with built-in cameras are used to transmit images of skin lesions with accompanying patient data. There are more applications in mobile teledermatology using asynchronous (store-and-forward) methods, although mobile real-time video and audio transmission are also enabled.

Mobile end devices that are very appealing for the usability in teledermatology are small portable devices such as mobile phones comprising so-called smart phones and PDAs as well as portable PCs with wireless Internet connection with built-in cameras. Due to constant technological improvement there is a vast variety and constant change in commercially available devices.

Table 10.1 Applications of mobile telemedicine expand the services offered by the conventional health care system. Overlap between the given categories often occurs

Purpose	Example
Administrative/alerting	Appointment reminder Automatic notification of diagnosis Regain prescription
Health status improvement/ disease prevention	Smoking cessation reminder Sunscreen use reminder
Screening	Application for mole triage on mobile phone
Emergency services	Emergency data sent to hospital from ambulance
Access to medical information for patients	Advise to prevent sexual transmitted diseases
Mobile diagnosis and management	Store-and-forward and real-time mobile teledermatology
Clinical improvement/ follow up	Homecare of chronic diseases (psoriasis, leg ulcers)
Communication between professionals	Teledermatology consultation on a ward round
Continuous education for health care professionals	Drug databases Diagnostic algorithms

Mobile phones with text messaging service are ubiquitous in the hands of millions of people and easy to apply for most people as they are already part of their daily lives. A personal digital assistant (PDA) is a small, lightweight portable device that shares the features of a computer, such as basic word processing, databases, web browsing and transmission of email [5]. Newer models offer audio capabilities for mobile telephony thus overlapping with the features of 'smart' phones. The not well defined term "smart phone" refers to a mobile phone with computing capabilities [5]. Smart phones and PDAs allow for installation of customized software – or Apps [1] (short form of Application software), i.e. specialized software programs with various features, comprising medical databases for example.

Each device has advantages and disadvantages regarding user-friendliness, equipment for digital imaging, screen size or memory, and cost to name a few. Screen size and display features and integrated digital cameras are especially important for applicability in teledermatology.

It is not only the end devices but also the transmission technologies that undergo a continuous change [6]. Wide-range telephony technologies comprise satellite connections and the mobile telephone network. Satellite connections where the end device connects to an orbiting satellite can provide mobile telephony in areas where terrestrial telecommunication networks are rare to nonexistent. Geostationary satellites enable almost worldwide Internet access, including ships and moving land vehicles. WLAN (Wireless local area network) allows mobile transmission over medium to short distances and Bluetooth is used for very short distance transmissions. In terrestrial mobile telephony, the transmission occurs between the mobile phone and a network of antennas (cell stations). In recent years, bandwidth and access in remote areas have constantly improved with decreasing costs of the services.

The standardized Global System for Mobile Communication (GSM), a 'second generation' (2G) mobile telephone technology, was introduced in the 1990s and is to date the most widespread mobile telephony standard. It enables Short Message Service (SMS) the exchange of short text messages, which is in ubiquitous use nowadays. With SMS technology, text messages up to 160 characters can be interchanged between mobile phone users [4]. The low rate of data transmission (9.6 kbit/s) with GSM technology limits image transmission considerably. Consequently, GPRS was introduced. General Packet Radio Service (GPRS) has a transmission capacity of about 50–100 kbit/s and enables Multimedia Messaging Service (MMS). MMS technology enables sending of text, images, audio files and video files [4]. GPRS allows for Internet access through WAP (Wireless Access Protocol). The third generation (3G) cellular systems that enable wideband mobile telecommunication, are based on Universal Mobile Telecommunication System (UMTS) that has a transmission capacity of 384 kbit/s. The further development HSDPA (High-Speed Downlink Packet Access) with maximum transmission rate of 14 megabytes per second (Mbit/s) and beyond is approaching the quality of a landline. The fourth generation of mobile telephony aims at providing broadband wireless telecommunication and comprises WIMAX (Worldwide Interoperability for Microwave Access), that provides mobile Internet access with up to 40 Mbit/s [7] (Table 10.2).

The Success Story of Mobile Phone Technology

Mobile phone technology is well integrated in our daily lives and already utilized by a substantial proportion of the global population. Thus, the entry barrier to adopt the technology for use in health care is low. There is no necessity to purchase yet another new device. Furthermore, it is the one device that most people will constantly carry with them.

Compared to computer technology accessibility of mobile phone technology is higher in populations with a low socioeconomic status [3]. The United Nations agency for information and communication technology issues (ITU) reported in 2008 a growth of global mobile phone subscribers averaging 24% per year since 2000, with mobile penetration estimated to reach more than 60% or four billion by the end of 2008, and 4.6 billion by the end of 2009. Increased mobile phone usage especially in Russia, India and China were reported to spur the growth of subscriptions [12]. Costs of installation of fixed line connections are higher than the cost of installing a mobile communication system. Reports conducted in Africa and Asia reported life changing developments through integration of mobile telephony in previously unconnected areas of developing countries in commercial but also health care perspectives. The number of mobile Internet subscribers was estimated to increase from 577 million in 2008 to 1.7 billion in 2013 due to the growth of web 2.0 applications. It was estimated that Internet access by mobile phones will account for around 50% of Internet usage [13].

Spurred by the increasingly ubiquitous availability of mobile technology in developing countries, the teledermatology enterprise ClickDiagnostics has been founded in 2008 (http://clickdiagnostics.com). It has implemented mobile-phone based tele-consultation services in underserved areas in Africa, South Asia, North America, and South America, enabling individuals with limited possibilities to see a doctor in a face-to-face visit, access to health care.

Table 10.2 Mobile technologies and data transmission rates. Transmission rates have substantially improved throughout the last years. Transfer rates given are an approximation and are subject to change as the real-world configuration of cellular networks does often not reach the theoretical full potential of transmission rates and technology is constantly changing

Type	Generation	Acronym	Full name	Data transmission rate
Mobile Internet access	–	WLAN	Wireless local area network	11–120 Mbit/s
Mobile telephone standards	2G	GSM	Global System for Mobile Communication	9.6 kbit/s [8]
	2.5G	GPRS	General Packet Radio Service	56–114 kbit/s [9]
	3G	UMTS	Universal Mobile Telecommunication System	384 kbit/s–2 Mbit/s [8, 10]
	3.5	HSDPA	High Speed Downlink Packet Access	>14 Mbit/s [11]
	4G	WIMAX	Worldwide Interoperability for Microwave Access	10–100 Mbit/s [11]

Overview of Scientific Publications and Examples for Applications of Mobile Telemedicine

Telediagnosis

The earliest investigations focusing on diagnostic power of teledermatology using mobile devices of the first generation in general were performed by Massone and colleagues. Skin lesions, excluding melanoma, of 95 subjects were photographed with the integrated camera of a commercially available cell phone [14]. Images of the skin lesions were consequently sent to three teledermatologists in store-and-forward mode, using the web application www.telederm.org. Teledermatologists made a diagnosis blinded to the face-to-face diagnosis and the diagnoses of the other teledermatologists. Diagnostic agreement with the face-to-face diagnosis in the mobile phone study ranged from 68% to 73%, with an average of 70%.

The group then went on to investigate the feasibility of teleconsultation using personal digital assistants (PDAs). 87 subjects were photographed with the integrated camera of a personal digital assistant (PDA) by a medical student [15]. The three teledermatologists assessing the PDA photos (which had considerably higher image quality) had an agreement with the face-to-face dermatologist of 66–90%, averaging 80%. A limitation of these pilot projects conducted in 2005 were limited resolution and image quality by the images acquired with the first generation of mobile devices with integrated cameras. However, principal feasibility was proved.

A recent study by Tran et al. [16] explored the applicability of mobile teledermatology in Egypt, Africa. 30 patients with various skin diseases were given a face-to-face diagnosis by a junior dermatologists and these were compared to diagnoses of two senior dermatologists made by means of a mobile-based teleconsultation using a software-enabled mobile telephone. Diagnostic agreement between the observers was achieved in overall 75% of cases. A limitation to this study was the lack of a gold standard (such as histopathology) to formulate a "final" diagnosis, which is a common problem to telemedicine studies.

Homecare

An important focus of mobile teledermatology is homecare of subjects affected with chronic diseases such as leg ulcers and psoriasis. Chronic wounds and leg ulcers require long-term treatment with several follow-up visits and thus are a burden for the health care system to which transportation contributes significantly. In many countries, visiting nurses provide home care but often need feedback from the physician in charge. In a preliminary feasibility study in 2005 by Braun and colleagues, face-to-face examination of in total 61 chronic leg ulcers in 52 patients were compared to examination of two teledermatologists [6]. On the images of the ulcer surface taken by visiting nurses with a mobile phone under routine conditions, teledermatologists estimated the proportion of granulation tissue, epithelization, fibrin, and necrosis of the ulcer surface as well as erythema, cyanosis, eczema and hyperpigmentation at the periphery. The same evaluation was done by the dermatologist performing the face-to-face examination. The reported kappa value for the diagnostic agreement among the three physicians of ranged between 0.69 for extent of granulation tissue and 0.94 for the assessment of epithelialization. (in Cohen's kappa statistics, a value of 1 represents complete agreement, 0 indicates a level of agreement corresponding to statistical chance).

Monitoring of patients with psoriasis, one of the most common chronic skin disease, is another potential application of telemedicine. Individuals affected equipped with mobile phones with integrated cameras can take images of their lesions and forward them to a dermatologist together with health parameters who can monitor potential side effects of treatment and determine a PASI (Psoriasis Area and Severity Index) score. These applications are discussed in detail in Chaps. 13 and 14.

Screening and Triage

A subsequently performed study by Massone et al. [17] focused on teledermoscopy of pigmented skin tumors performed with mobile phones as a tool for melanoma screening. Images of melanocytic skin lesions were taken with the built-in camera of a mobile phone and included both clinical and dermoscopic views. The dermoscopic images were acquired by applying the integrated camera of the mobile phone on a hand-held dermoscopic device. The two teleconsultants that evaluated the images obtained a correct telediagnosis when compared to the face-to-face diagnosis in 89% and 91.5% of cases, respectively. This study revealed the feasibility of store-and-forward teledermoscopy as a triage tool in the future. An individual concerned about a changing mole or new mole can capture the image of a given lesion and send it via MMS (Multi Media Message) to a specialized telemedicine centre for triage. In the future, an icon on the screen of a mobile phone could directly lead to a telemedical consultation including advice for new and suspicious moles.

Previously, image quality has been identified as being a major limiting factor in mobile teledermatology. However, recent technical advances led to such significant improvement in the specifications of the small built-in cameras of mobile devices and in the transmission capability that image quality should no longer be considered as an obstacle.

However, the sample sizes in previous studies such as these described above have been limited and may therefore conceal the true values of the method. For an advanced model of practice in mobile teledermatology to be developed and implemented, a systematic clinical examination is required.

Seven billion text messages month are sent vial cell phone in the United States of America every month [18]. The idea to use this ubiquitous technology for health care has been explored in various studies. A recent review by Krishna et al. [3] identified 25 studies of which 20 were controlled randomized trials and five controlled trials conducted in America, Europe, Asia and Australia, that reported the use of mobile phones for health management via voice feature or SMS. Applications ranged from delivery of healthcare (notification of diagnosis, appointment reminders), outcome of care (medication reminder, smoking cessation advice) to clinical improvement (diabetes management, hypertension). One study reported the reduction of stress levels in patients receiving narratives on exploring a tropical beach or new age music via mobile phone. Significant differences between control and intervention groups with mobile phone or SMS interventions was reported in 20 of the 25 studies.

In California, an Internet based platform designed for the prevention of sexually transmitted diseases – Internet Sexuality Information Services (see URL: Internet: http://www.isis-inc.org/sexinfo.php) offers young people the possibility obtain advice about sexually transmitted diseases with direct links to specialized clinics using text messages.

One randomized controlled trial applied mobile teledermatology as a reminder strategy to improve adherence to sunscreen as means of prevention from skin cancer [19]. Sunscreen use was measured by an electronic measuring device attached to the sunscreen tube, that send a SMS to a data storage unit each time the cap was removed during a 6 week study period. Mobile phone text messages were sent to remind 35 individuals in the intervention group of daily sunscreen use and gave general weather information. The daily sunscreen use of the individuals who received text messages was significantly higher than in the control group who did not receive reminders. In the intervention group, 69% ($n=24$) reported to be willing to continue the reminder system, and 89% ($n=31$) said that they would recommend it to others.

Data suggests that text messaging as a reminder tool could promote preventive behavior. It can help to overcome non-adherence to medical advice due to simple forgetfulness [4]. Text messages are seen immediately wherever the patient is at a given time without delay.

The studies mentioned above only covered a relatively short periods and long term effects need to be assessed. However the potential for the future holds great promise. For example, "intelligent" drug tubes might send reminders directly to the phone of an individual when used too infrequently. In conclusion these applications go far beyond the "normal" established medical face-to-face care and enable empowerment of the individual to take care of their own health status.

Application Programs

Mobility is not only an advantage for the patients but also for physicians that are often also constantly moving, on ward rounds or house calls. Little books to carry around in the pocket are thus very popular, but the amount of information is limited and there is need to be up-to date in the ever changing world of medicine. Smartphones with computer-like functionalities and PDAs allow for installation of so-called Apps (short form of Application software), i.e. specialized software programs with various features, comprising medical databases for example [20]. As with every health-related Internet content, the quality of these applications vary significantly and features underlie a constant change.

One of the best-known medical application programs, for use by physicians is ePocrates (www.epocrates.com). It started as a drug database that allows the user to search for a special medication or substance class and to check dosing, contraindications, drug interactions and adverse effects for example. Nowadays it also offers information on laboratory values, diagnoses and infectious diseases [21, 22], the basic application being free with possible pay-for use upgrades. Other applications comprise online tools to find the right diagnosis with possible download on PDAs/smartphones (Diagnosaurus http://www.accessmedicine.com/diag.aspx), or mobile platforms to learn to distinguish key heart sounds (iMurmur http://www.appstorehq.com/imurmur-iphone-53982/app) [20].

Applications for dermatology comprise tools for self monitoring of skin lesions accompanied with educational background for the patient (http://www.iappfun.com/item/368835200.html) and dermatology learning platforms. (http://appshopper.com/medical/dermatology-and-the-skin) Many applications, will have to stand the test of time regarding their true value.

Conclusion

Currently, telemedicine research in many medical specialities is focusing on developing and testing new ways to utilize mobile telecommunication technology that exceeds the traditional health care services. The main advantage is that can make use of devices that are already ubiquitous used as mobile phones are nowadays a normal part of many people's lives. They are increasingly distributed in remote areas and developing countries that have formerly been traditionally been underserved, allowing personal empowerment in access to healthcare and disease self-management.

The opportunities of potential application seem endless but there are considerable challenges to bring them to successful implementation. Data security and privacy are special restraints arising in mobile teledermatology. Wireless applications could become susceptible targets to intrusion (to assess private information) and even interference. Commercial mobile network operators use different modes of data encryption features and MMS settings which renders standardization of service difficult. Furthermore, data encryption features are often disabled – without the knowledge of the user – to improve network performance [23]. Implementation requires to overcome other obstacles such as lacking standardization, inadequate telemedicine resources and staff as well as lack of funding in the health care system. In the end, the success of mobile telemedicine, will be determined by how well medicine can solve these problems and integrate the vast variety of advanced telecommunication and information technology as mobile technical equipment, such as mobile devices and connected telemedicine technologies are undergoing a rapid development. The challenge is to adapt the end devices and software for medical purposes. Mobile telemedicine holds great potential for revolutionizing the delivery of health care if applied with consideration. It could equalize access of healthcare for everyone independent of geographic location and social background, all with a little device the size of a shirt pocket.

References

1. Waegemann CP (2010) mHealth: the next generation of telemedicine? Telemed J E Health 16:23–25
2. Smith AC, Gray LC (2009) Telemedicine across the ages. Med J Aust 190:15–19
3. Krishna S, Boren SA, Balas EA (2009) Healthcare via cell phones: a systematic review. Telemed J E Health 15:231–240
4. Terry M (2008) Text messaging in healthcare: the elephant knocking at the door. Telemed J E Health 14:520–524
5. McCullagh PJ, Zheng H, Black ND, Davies R, Mawson S, McGlade K (2008) Section 1: medical informatics and eHealth. Technol Health Care 16:381–397
6. Braun RP, Vecchietti JL, Thomas L, Prins C, French LE, Gewirtzman AJ et al (2005) Telemedical wound care using a new generation of mobile telephones: a feasibility study. Arch Dermatol 141:254–258
7. Istepanian RH, Philip NY (2009) Provisioning of medical quality of services for HSDPA and mobile WiMAX in healthcare applications. Conf Proc IEEE Eng Med Biol Soc 2009:717–720
8. Richardson K (2000) UMTS overview. Electron Commun Eng J 12:93–100
9. Granbohm H, Wiklund J (1999) GPRS-General packet radio service. Ericsson Review 2:82–88
10. Larsen SB, Clemensen J, Ejskjaer N (2006) A feasibility study of UMTS mobile phones for supporting nurses doing home visits to patients with diabetic foot ulcers. J Telemed Telecare 12:358–362

11. Ko YF, Sim ML, Nekovee M (2006) Wi-Fi based broadband wireless access for users on the road. BT Technol J 24(2):123–129
12. ITU (International Telecommunication Union). [cited 2010 December]; Available from: http://www.itu.int/newsroom/press_releases/2008/29.html
13. ITU (International Telecommunications Union) Newslog. (2010) [cited 2010 November]; Available from: http://www.itu.int/ITU-D/ict/newslog/Mobile+InternetInternet+Users+To+Top+17+Billion+By+2013.aspx
14. Massone C, Lozzi GP, Wurm E, Hofmann-Wellenhof R, Schoellnast R, Zalaudek I et al (2005) Cellular phones in clinical teledermatology. Arch Dermatol 141:1319–1320
15. Massone C, Lozzi GP, Wurm E, Hofmann-Wellenhof R, Schoellnast R, Zalaudek I et al (2006) Personal digital assistants in teledermatology. Br J Dermatol 154:801–802
16. Tran K, Ayad M, Weinberg J, Cherng A, Chowdhury M, Monir S et al (2010) Mobile teledermatology in the developing world: implications of a feasibility study on 30 Egyptian patients with common skin diseases. J Am Acad Dermatol 64(2):302–309
17. Massone C, Hofmann-Wellenhof R, Ahlgrimm-Siess V, Gabler G, Ebner C, Soyer HP (2007) Melanoma screening with cellular phones. PLoS One 2:e483
18. Boland P (2007) The emerging role of cell phone technology in ambulatory care. J Ambul Care Manage 30:126–133
19. Armstrong AW, Watson AJ, Makredes M, Frangos JE, Kimball AB, Kvedar JC (2009) Text-message reminders to improve sunscreen use: a randomized, controlled trial using electronic monitoring. Arch Dermatol 145:1230–1236
20. Terry M (2010) Medical apps for smartphones. Telemed J E Health 16(1):17–22
21. Fox GN, Gill KU, Music RE (2005) Epocrates essentials: is the expanded product an improvement? J Fam Pract 54:57–63
22. Hyler SE (2002) ePocrates 4.0. J Psychiatr Pract 8:57–58
23. M-Health News. [cited 2010 December]; Available from: http://www.m-healthconference.com/393/413/articles/195.php

Skin Emergency Telemedicine

11

James Muir, Cathy Xu, and H. Peter Soyer

Core Messages

- Rapidly delivered and reliable specialist dermatology advice is needed by accident and emergency departments.
- Most patients with skin disease can be well managed by non-specialist medical staff who have ready access to specialist dermatologist advice.
- Teledermatology routinely achieves diagnostic and management outcomes comparable with face to face consultations.
- A Skin Emergency Telemedicine Service (SETS) can provide a consultation service which is reliable and sufficiently rapid to be clinically useful. This is currently not possible with traditional methods in most centers.
- A SETS can provide dermatology advice far more cheaply, quickly, efficiently and with many fewer staff then traditional face to face consultation.

  The equipment and technical expertise to utilize a SETS is already present within the vast majority of modern accident and emergency units.

Introduction

Teledermatology has been well shown to provide comparable diagnostic accuracy to face to face consultation in the management of skin disease [1–3]. Combine this with the fact that almost all dermatological treatment and procedures can be adequately carried out by non-specialist medical staff, it has long been used for the delivery of specialist dermatology services around the world. In general these are delivered via store and forward technology [4–8].

Longer response times when managing skin disease are usually acceptable. This is because the majority of dermatological disorders are not acutely life threatening. Often the condition has been present for many months before a teledermatology consult is sought. In many parts of the world due to a shortage of specialist dermatologists there is a considerable delay before patients with skin disease can access face-to-face consultation with a dermatologist. It can be argued that a teledermatology service does not have to be as good as a traditional face to face consultation service, just better then the services available to the patient otherwise. Thus a teledermatology service in areas where specialist face to face consultation is not readily available for reasons of geographic isolation or long waiting times for appointments may be a very good option for delivery of dermatological care. This would be true even if response times to requests for advice were prolonged provided they were significantly shorter than the time needed for the same patient to access a traditional appointment with a dermatologist. In practice, turnaround times between submission of a request for advice and response from a teledermatologist vary. One of the

J. Muir (✉) • C. Xu • H.P. Soyer
Dermatology Research Centre, The University of Queensland, School of Medicine, Princess Alexandra Hospital, Brisbane, QLD, Australia
e-mail: arnoldmuir@optusnet.com.au; c.xu@uq.edu.au; p.soyer@uq.edu.au

H.P. Soyer et al. (eds.), *Telemedicine in Dermatology*,
DOI 10.1007/978-3-642-20801-0_11, © Springer-Verlag Berlin Heidelberg 2012

authors (JM) has been able to respond to 96% of all submitted teledermatology cases within 24 h. This may not be quick enough in all situations.

Dermatological Emergencies

There are circumstances where a close to immediate response is needed. The obvious example being severe drug reactions such as toxic epidermal necrolysis where early diagnosis and withdrawal of the offending agent is associated with better patient outcomes [9–12]. The same can be said for life threatening systemic illnesses which present with or at least manifest dermatological features. Many of these conditions are readily diagnosed on visual features alone by an experienced dermatologist but can present an insurmountable diagnostic challenge to practitioners untrained in skin disease. Examples include erysipelas, septicaemia, HIV seroconversion reactions, secondary syphilis, leucocytoclastic vasculitis, calciphylaxis, disseminated intravascular coagulation and so on. Then there are skin problems presenting in the setting of an acute and possibly related illness where the treating doctor needs immediate advice on their diagnosis and management. A recent case from the authors practice was one of severe pyoderma gangrenosum occurring in the setting of a flare of long standing ulcerative colitis. The treating doctors were about to debride and graft the ulcerated lesions when they sought an urgent teledermatology opinion. The surgery was cancelled and the condition responded rapidly to appropriate medical therapy.

For logistic reasons specialist advice may also be needed rapidly. Factors such as geographic isolation, unit workload and resources may mean it is not practical or indeed possible for a patient to return to a treating doctor on another day to receive the answer to a submitted teledermatology consultation.

The most likely setting where an urgent dermatology opinion will be needed is in a busy accident and emergency unit. Patients need to be assessed, diagnosed, managed and discharged from these units in a timely manner otherwise new patients cannot be accommodated. This is true regardless of the severity of the presenting complaint. Ideally the patients should be discharged appropriately and with an optimal management plan in place. If specialist advice is needed, it must be rapid even if the condition is not life threatening or particularly severe. These units cannot afford to have patients waiting long periods of time whilst specialist review is awaited.

Far from being a rare event skin disease represents between 4% and 12% of all presentations to an accident and emergency unit [13, 14]. Teledermatology is an obvious way to meet this need. Even in a large hospital with specialist dermatologists on site it may be difficult to get a face to face dermatology consultation in a suitable time frame. This is not solely because the conditions seen are 'dermatological emergencies'. Patients with more mundane and even chronic skin disease present to accident and emergency units. Medical staff need to manage these patients in an appropriate, timely and efficient way. This is for reasons of logistical efficiency in the running of the unit as well as for purely medical reasons. Rapid access to specialist dermatology advice allows accident and emergency staff to discharge these patients either to the wards, home, dermatology outpatients or the care of their local doctor as appropriate.

Incorporating Teledermatology into Accident and Emergency

Is it possible to provide accident and emergency units with accurate and rapid dermatology advice via telemedicine? There is plenty of published literature documenting the accuracy of teledermatology [1–5]. It has been well shown to be as accurate as a face to face consultation in the great majority of cases [14–17]. The challenge therefore is not so much in providing accurate advice but rather in timely service delivery. Clearly in the rare instances of a true dermatological emergency a diagnosis is needed as quickly as possible. However due to the dynamic of an accident and emergency unit a rapid response allowing patients presenting with skin disease to be managed and discharged as quickly as possible is essential. If not these patients typically end up waiting for long periods of time before a decision is made as to their management. This can be because junior doctors who conducted the initial assessment are awaiting the opinion of more senior staff members. In hospitals with a dermatology department an opinion may be sought from a dermatologist. This can still require a wait of hours. These patients, even if not unwell place an avoidable logistical burden on the accident and emergency unit. Usual teledermatology services utilizing store and forward technology have a response time measured in hours or days which is inappropriate to the needs of an accident and emergency unit seeking dermatological advice.

The crucial difference between a teledermatology service to an accident and emergency department and one providing advice to a primary care physician is rapidity of response. A patient in accident and emergency needs to be managed in a timely fashion which ensures optimal patient outcome and promotes the efficient working of the unit. We felt that a suitably designed telemedicine service providing dermatology advice to an accident and emergency service could fulfil these aims.

Skin Emergency Telemedicine Service

The model adopted is called 'Skin Emergency Telemedicine Service' or SETS for short. In common with teledermatology services worldwide it utilizes store and forward methodology. The crucial difference is that concurrent with submission of a case the teledermatologist is notified via a phone call or text message that there is a case needing their immediate attention. The teledermatologist can then immediately view the e-mail bearing the case history and digital images and respond with advice. The reply from the teledermatologist can be via a telephone call, e-mail or text message. After discussion with accident and emergency staff it was felt that an acceptable delay between submission of a case and response would be up to 1 h. Provided they received immediate notification of a submitted case the teledermatologists involved [Prof HP Soyer and Dr J Muir] felt this was a readily achievable goal.

Thus a typical SETS consultation would run as follows:

- Patient presents to accident and emergency with a dermatological problem.
- Medical staff asses the patient and decide that advice from a dermatologist is needed.
- An electronic proforma (Table 11.1) giving details of the patients presenting complaint and history is filled out by accident and emergency department staff. This does not have to be physically done by medical staff but needs to be confirmed as being complete and accurate.
- Digital images illustrating the extent and character of the skin problem are taken.

Table 11.1 SETS proforma

Patient ID number:	DOB:	Sex: □Male □Female
History of presenting complaint:		
Duration:		
Progression:		
Associated symptoms (e.g. itch, fever, arthralgia, malaise):		
Results of any investigations (e.g. blood/urine tests, biopsies, x-rays):		
Treatment to date:		
General medical history:		
Surgical:		
Medication: (including prescribed, non-prescribed, over the counter drug, natural, intermittent and regular, also alcohol/ tobacco/ illicit drugs) and chronology		
Allergies:		
Occupation/Pastimes:		
Exposure to animals:		
Overseas travel:		
Examination:		
Diagnoses:		
1. Emergency Department:		
2. Teledermatology:		
Differential diagnosis:		
3. Biopsy performed:	□ No □ Yes Results:	
4. Face-to-Face consultation:		

Please attach images showing the extent of the eruption i.e. we need to know where it isn't as well as where it is. Good quality close ups are essential. If any pathology present please send images. They need to be clearly labeled as to site and patient. If possible send images that do not allow patient identification

- The completed proforma and images are e-mailed to the SETS web site and the on call SETS dermatologist.
- The dermatologist is notified by a telephone or text message that there is a case needing urgent attention.
- The on call dermatologist immediately views the case and contacts the referring doctor with diagnostic and management advice. This contact can be via telephone, text or e-mail.

The possible sources of delay in this model are; recognition that a particular patient needs a SETS consultation, collecting, documenting and forwarding the information and images to the on call dermatologist, notification of the teledermatologist that there is a case submitted and finally the time taken for the on-call dermatologist to assess the submitted material and then formulate and deliver a response.

To test this model we set up a year long study in the accident and emergency unit of the Princess Alexandra Hospital, Brisbane, Australia. This is a 750 bed major tertiary hospital providing a full range of medical services except for obstetrics. The accident and emergency unit is a busy one seeing about 46,000 patients per year [18, 19]. Earlier discussions between senior dermatology and accident and emergency staff had revealed that getting a timely dermatology opinion was difficult when only face to face consultation was available. Emergency staff felt that there was a need for ready access to dermatology advice. This was because dermatological issues were not uncommon as either the primary reason for presentation or as part of a more complex problem. It was felt that many staff found dermatological disease difficult to diagnose and manage. This reflects the low priority given to dermatology education in under- and post- graduate medical training. Although this hospital has a dermatology unit the staff in accident and emergency felt that often they could not get an opinion quickly enough to be of practical use to them. As with all busy units around the world there is considerable pressure on staff, resources and space resulting in the need for patients to be managed as quickly as possible.

The pilot SETS study was designed to test the theory that telemedicine could provide rapid, accurate and clinically relevant advice to accident and emergency staff managing patients with dermatological problems without in anyway compromising patient safety. We hoped to show that by using telemedicine this outcome could be achieved significantly more quickly than with the current practice of managing patients within the unit or awaiting face to face dermatologist consultation.

To this end we only recruited patients presenting with skin problems who were over the age of 18 who gave informed consent to participating in the study. All patients not admitted to hospital were given appointments to be reviewed in dermatology outpatients within 2 weeks of their initial presentation. This was to confirm the accuracy of the teledermatology diagnosis and management as well as ensuring optimal patient care. It should be noted that waiting times for dermatologist appointments are often considerably longer than 2 weeks. The dermatologists who reviewed the patients face to face were not involved in providing teledermatology advice in this study. Their diagnoses and management were later compared with that of the teledermatologists. Any pathology tests taken were also used to help determine the accuracy of the teledermatologists.

Table 11.2 Conditions seen in SETS

Conditions	No. of cases	Conditions	No. of cases
Vasculitis	2	Dermatitis/eczema	10
Drug eruptions	8	Urticaria	9
Scabies	3	Psoriasis	6
Tinea	2	Erysipelas/cellulitis	3
Darier disease	2	Photo drug/contact	4
Others	9	Acute varicella/zoster	2
Total			$N=60$

In the course of this year long study a total of 60 patients were referred to the SETS. In 82% or 49 of the submitted cases a response was received by the referring medical staff in less than 1 h. In fact almost two thirds of cases were answered within 30 min.

Conditions seen were many (Table 11.2) and 20 of the 60 patients were actually admitted for inpatient care. As expected not all patients returned for review. Of the 50 who did return diagnostic concordance between the face to face and teledermatology consultation was seen in 80% and the remaining cases all showed relative diagnostic agreement. This of course reflects the results of numerous studies of diagnostic accuracy of store and forward dermatology and was thus expected. It should be remembered that diagnostic concordance between face to face dermatologists is no better than this [17].

Perhaps more importantly from a practical standpoint is the concordance rate for clinical management. This was measured at a 96% rate of complete agreement by the face to face dermatologist with the management advice given by the teledermatologist.

In short it is possible to provide accurate dermatological advice to an accident and emergency department within a time frame that makes such a service clinically relevant and useful to treating medical staff. In fact such a service could be provided to any practitioner able to take and send digital images, e-mail and who has a reliable telephone service. Thus a SETS service could also provide accurate and reliable dermatological advice to small hospitals, remote clinics, flying doctors or even ships at sea. This service would provide a far more rapid response then that possible with face to face consultation. Importantly this can be done without in anyway compromising patient care. In fact patient outcomes can be expected to be improved as in most of these situations no dermatological advice is currently available.

A SETS service can provide diagnostic and management advice equal to that of a face to face service but far more quickly and to patients who currently cannot access any form of specialist dermatology advice.

Discussion

As expected we did discover areas where such a service can be improved. Surprisingly one obstacle to an efficient service was availability of staff sufficiently familiar with digital photography and e-mail who were able to take and send adequate photographic images. It was not uncommon to be sent images that were poorly focused or too large a file size to be sent over the internet. This difficulty with simple technical issues can be easily overcome with a brief familiarization course with digital photography and use of e-mail. As the new generations of 'techno savvy' medical staff take over this issue should cease to be a concern.

Our data revealed that patients often spent many hours in accident and emergency before a SETS case was submitted. There are many possible reasons for this. As this was a new initiative not all staff would have been aware of the service or comfortable using it. This may have created delays in initiating a request for a SETS consultation. Cases presenting to accident and emergency are triaged according to degree of urgency. Only one of our 60 cases was felt to be imminently life threatening. Thus other patients would have been given priority. To reduce this delay it should be possible once a patient has been triaged to recognize that a SETS consultation will likely be needed. Non medical staff would be able to fill in the profroma and take and send the necessary digital images. The teledermatologists response would then be available to medical staff when they saw the patient thus expediting management and reducing the period of time patients spend within the accident and emergency unit.

In the few instances where there was a prolonged delay in response from the teledermatologist it was usually because there had been no completed notifying call. In this circumstance the teledermatologist was unaware that there was a case waiting assessment. It should be noted that this service ran 24 h a day, 7 days a week. The dermatologists providing the advice were able to respond promptly in almost all instances even when involved in their usual professional duties. A major reason for this is that the time consuming aspects of a medical consultation (collection of data, examination, explanation

Table 11.3 Rates of diagnostic agreement

Assessments	Diagnostic agreement (ED vs Tele) (N=60)	Diagnostic agreement (Tele vs Final) (N=50)
Complete agreement	26 (43%)	40 (80%)
Relative agreement	23 (38%)	10 (20%)
No agreement	3 (5%)	0
Not applicable	8 (13%) [No ED diagnoses]	10 [No FTF]

and initiation of management, performance of biopsies, writing prescriptions etc.) were all performed by others. All the teledermatologists had to do was form a differential diagnosis and communicate their management plan. This can be done in minutes provided the history is complete and the images adequate. It does mean that the referring medical staff need to have the skills to carry out the teledermatology advice. The only procedure that needed to be performed was punch biopsy which should be within the capabilities of any medical graduate [20].

Improving Medical Education

Not to be forgotten is the educational benefit a SETS service has. With a traditional referral to a dermatologist medical staff may remain unaware of the eventual diagnosis and management and how this was arrived at. By using SETS referring doctors receive almost instantaneous feedback as to the diagnosis, investigation and treatment of the problem referred. Although not specifically assessed in our study informal feedback from referring doctors supports the concept that this service offered considerable educational benefit.

Furthermore ready access to specialist opinion at any time of day can instill clinical confidence in medical staff when they are called on to deal with issues for which they feel themselves ill equipped. This is especially so for junior doctors working alone in the more remote areas of Australia. It is common for referrals to dermatologists to be made even when the diagnosis is known to the referring doctor. These patients are referred for advice on management. This was reflected in our study where quite often the emergency department staff had made a correct provisional diagnosis. The SETS dermatologist was able to confirm their diagnostic assessment and offer advice on further investigation and management (Table 11.3).

One reason telemedicine is ideally suited for management of skin disease in accident and emergency is that all management can be performed by clinicians without specialist skills. There is no need for specialized procedural skills requiring advanced training as would be the case for surgical presentations. There are few specialized clinical skills needed to make a diagnosis other then the ability to recognize the clinical signs of a given skin disease. This can almost always be done as readily from a clinical image as from a face to face examination. With the aid of a SETS dermatologist clinicians in the emergency department can be guided to historical and clinical clues which may help make a diagnosis.

For a SETS to give optimal results referring doctors have to be able to perform a skin biopsy. This is of course well within the skill set of any doctor. Ideally a SETS case biopsy sample should be reviewed by a specialist dermatopathologist. The SETS dermatologist can guide the referring clinician on optimal biopsy site and whether investigations such as direct immunofluoresence, biopsy for culture or skin swabs etc. are needed. The ability for a SETS to direct appropriate collection of pathology samples also means that treatment can be initiated without the concern that confirmatory pathology testing has not been ordered. This avoids the all too common problem of patients presenting to a dermatologist for assessment of a resolved or significantly altered skin eruption after the referring doctor has commenced treatment. In this situation diagnosis is often impossible as clinical features and pathology results have been altered so much that they bear little relationship to the original eruption.

Improving Clinical Outcomes

As can be seen in the list of cases submitted (Table 11.2) in our study almost all can be diagnosed on clinical features alone. Simple pathology testing would have confirmed the diagnoses. In the cases of vasculitis, triggers and involvement of organs other then the skin would need to be sought by history, examination and appropriate investigation. This can be guided by the SETS dermatologist but readily performed by the referring medical staff. This avoids delays in identifying and removing triggers. Systemic involvement if present will be found and addressed earlier than would otherwise have been the case.

Drug eruptions were common and often identified as such by the referring doctors. A SETS can give advice on the need for biopsy and most importantly which, of often multiple medications is the likely cause. Early recognition of infectious illnesses such as varicella, eczema herpeticum and scabies has clear health benefit to both the affected patients and others they may come in contact with.

It is interesting to note that many of the conditions seen were not examples of dermatological emergencies. However these patients did present to accident and emergency and thus needed assessment and management. Although familiar to dermatologists conditions such as Darier's disease, psoriasis, scabies or even tinea can represent a management challenge to accident and emergency staff even if the diagnosis is obvious. From the point of view of the doctor consulted it would be professionally, ethically and medicolegally unsatisfactory to turn away patients presenting with non urgent skin conditions without at least an attempt to address their problem. Clearly these patients considered their skin problems serious enough to attend a busy unit knowing that there would likely be a long wait. With the aid of immediate and accurate advice from a teledermatologist the needs of both the patients with skin disease and their treating doctors can be addressed.

Cost Effectiveness

An important issue with any medical service is cost effectiveness. A SETS is clearly a cheaper and far more efficient approach to the delivery of dermatological care to patients then any that could be delivered by traditional face to face consultation.

The equipment and staff needed are already available in accident and emergency departments throughout Australia. From a technical perspective all that is needed is a basic digital camera capable of taking macro images and the ability to send and receive e-mails and images. The actual work of taking the images, filling in the proforma and sending these to the teledermatologist could be done by suitably supervised non-medical staff. Thus any modern accident and emergency department wishing to utilize a SETS would not incur extra equipment or labor costs.

A major determinant of the cost of specialist consultation is time. A dermatologist staffing a SETS can offer management advice on a submitted case in a far shorter time then is possible face to face. Using electronic communication the on-call dermatologist has no need to travel. This means that any time spent by the dermatologist is used solely for addressing the case submitted and formulating and transmitting a management plan. The other time consuming aspects of a dermatology consultation (history taking, biopsies, explaining the diagnosis and management, writing prescriptions etc.) are all performed by the referring staff.

A single dermatologist could easily provide a SETS to multiple accident and emergency departments. Cost savings in on call allowances would be very large. As there are no geographical or indeed time zone restrictions to locations that can be serviced by a SETS far fewer dermatologists would be needed then with any equivalent level of service delivery by traditional means.

A further cost saving would be in the increased ability for patients to be managed within their own communities with no need to travel for specialist assessment and care.

Improving Access to Dermatology Care

A SETS also addresses the issue of equity in the delivery of medical care. Many areas of the world have no access to specialist dermatological advice. This is true even in wealthy nations such as Australia. Patients with skin disease often have to rely for help on medical staff with no advanced or often even basic training in skin disease. This is especially true with acute presentations. A SETS allows access to reliable management advice for skin disease in a timely, efficient and cost effective manner. This advice can be available virtually immediately and at any time. There is no reason why a SETS cannot be delivered to multiple centers in geographically disparate areas.

A dermatologist providing consultations for a SETS can offer advice from any area of the world which has adequate coverage by telecommunication services. As e-mails and digital images can be received and responded to on a variety of hand held mobile communication devices the dermatologist is free to undertake any other activities whilst awaiting a consultation request. They can travel away from their home base and still provide the same service. This has profound implications for recruitment of specialist staff to provide this service. Unlike traditional 'on call rosters' which meant the doctor would have to be in close physical proximity to any center requesting advice, a SETS dermatologist is completely free of any restrictions on movement or activity other than being contactable electronically and immediately. Thus a single dermatologist can provide continuous coverage to multiple centers with minimal impact on other activities.

In the study recently completed by the authors requests for assistance were answered 7 days a week and at any hour of the day. At the time of addressing a SETS consultation the dermatologists were often away from their work place or home. Consultations were even answered when the dermatologist was in another hemisphere. As each case could usually be assessed and answered in a few minutes the study dermatologists could provide SETS advice whilst working in their usual capacity. This means that a dermatologist providing emergency advice via a SETS will be far less inconvenienced and thus more likely to take on and continue in such a role.

Conclusion

The time has come to start providing more medical services via innovative use of technology. It is important that this should not compromise patient care. A SETS has the capacity to efficiently, cheaply and readily provide comprehensive dermatological advice for patients in any area that has modern telecommunications services. Such a service would make specialist dermatology care available to patients previously denied this service by reason of geographical isolation or work force issues.

References

1. Lim AC, Egerton IB, See A, Shumack SP (2001) Accuracy and reliability of store-and-forward teledermatology: preliminary results from the St George teledermatology project. Australas J Dermatol 42:247–251
2. Levin YS, Warshaw EM (2009) Teledermatology: a review of reliability and accuracy of diagnosis and management. Dermatol Clin 27(2):163–176
3. Whited JD, Hall RP, Simel DL, Foy ME, Stechuchak KM, Drugge RJ (1999) Reliability and accuracy of dermatologists' and clinic-based and digital image consultations. J Am Acad Dermatol 41(5 pt 1):693–702
4. Heffner VA, Lyon VB, Brousseau DC, Holland KE, Yen K (2009) Store-and-forward teledermatology versus in-person visits: a comparison in pediatric teledermatology clinic. J Am Acad Dermatol 60(6):956–961

5. van der Heijden JP, Spuls PI, Voorbraak FP, de Keizer NF, Witkamp L, Bos JD (2010) Tertiary teledermatology: a systematic review. Telemed J E-Health 16:1–7
6. Wurm EM, Campbell TM, Soyer HP (2008) Teledermatology: how to start a new teaching and diagnostic era in medicine. Dermatol Clin 26(2):295–300, vii. Review
7. Burg G, Hasse U, Cipolat C, Kropf R, Djamei V, Soyer HP, Chimenti S (2005) Teledermatology: just cool or a real tool? Dermatology 210:169–173
8. Eedy DJ, Wootton R (2001) Teledermatology: a review. Br J Dermatol 144:696–707
9. Abrahamian FM, Talan DA, Moran GJ (2008) Management of skin and soft-tissue infections in the emergency department. Infect Dis Clin North Am 22(1):89–116
10. Browne BJ, Edwards B, Rogers RL (2006) Dermatologic emergencies. Prim Care 33(3):685–695
11. Freiman A, Borsuk D, Sasseville D (2005) Dermatologic emergencies. CMAJ 173(11):1317–1319
12. Brady WJ, DeBehnke D, Crosby DL (1994) Dermatological emergencies. Am J Emerg Med 12(2):217–237
13. Wootton R, Oakley A (eds) (2002) Teledermatology. London, The Royal Society of Medicine Press, pp 13–14
14. Scheinfeld N, Fisher M, Genis P, Long H (2003) Evaluating patient acceptance of a teledermatology link of an urban urgent-care dermatology clinic run by residents with board certified dermatologists. Skinmed 2(3):159–162
15. Muir J, Campbell TM, Soyer HP (2009) Telemedicine in skin emergencies. In: Revuz J et al (eds) Life-threatening dermatoses and emergencies in dermatology. Springer, Berlin, Heidelberg, pp 247–253
16. Lim AC, See AC, Shumack SP (2001) Progress in Australian teledermatology. J Telemed Telecare 7(Suppl 2):55–59
17. Burdick AE (2007) Teledermatology: extending specialty care beyond borders. Arch Dermatol 143(12):1581–1582
18. Princess Alexandra Hospital Health Service District (2008) Annual Report 2007–2008. Queensland Government, Brisbane
19. Princess Alexandra Hospital Health Service District (2009) Annual Report 2008–2009. Queensland Government, Brisbane
20. Muir J, Xu C, Paul S, Staib A, McNeill I, Singh P, Davidson S, Soyer HP, Sinnott M (2011) Incorporating teledermatology into emergency medicine. Emerg Med Australas 23(5):562–568

Telewoundcare

12

Barbara Binder and Rainer Hofmann-Wellenhof

Core Messages

- Chronic wounds are a significant problem for patients and the health care system.
- Ulcers are dynamic and regular assessment of the wound status and the surrounding skin is mandatory and adjustments of therapy are required.
- Telewoundcare offers patients in rural and remote areas expert medical consultation without loss of quality medical care while maintaining their independence and mobility.
- Several studies and trials have proven that with e-consultations the classification and assessment of a wound can be made reliably. Treatment suggestions and treatment adjustments, as well as wound healing monitoring, are feasible.
- Teledermatology is an evolving technology especially in the field of telewoundcare and holds great potential for the future.

B. Binder (✉) • R. Hofmann-Wellenhof
Department of Dermatology, Medical University of Graz, Graz, Austria
e-mail: barbara.binder@klinikum-graz.at; rainer.hofmann@medunigraz.at

Main Part

Chronic wounds are a significant problem for patients and the health care system. About 2.5% of the community suffer from chronic wounds of various origins, and an even higher portion is seen with increasing age [22]. The causes of wounds include vascular diseases (venous or arterial ulcers), neuropathic or hematological disorders, trauma, pressure and others [8, 17]. Vascular diseases are responsible for the majority of leg ulcers, 70% due to venous insufficiency, 20% due to peripheral arterial occlusive disease and only 10% caused by underlying diseases such as vasculitis, metabolic imbalances, medications or neuropathy. In patients suffering from diabetes mellitus, the leg ulcers are often due to a combination of causes, e.g. venous and arterial vessel impairment and neuropathy [18, 19]. Pressure ulcers, caused by various forms of immobility, are a major problem for the community. According to the literature, the prevalence data range between 0.4% and 38% [15, 20].

Ulcers are dynamic and therefore regular assessment of the wound and surrounding skin is required to facilitate necessary adjustments to therapy. These examinations should be performed by physicians trained in wound care; however, in many cases such specialists are not always available locally to the patient and therefore they have to travel to a specialized wound care center. Many of these patients are older with various comorbidities and traveling long distances can be exhausting for them. For another group of patients it may be very difficult to organize the transportation because of total immobility caused by spinal injury. The visits can be time consuming because of the long travel distance and prolonged waiting time

H.P. Soyer et al. (eds.), *Telemedicine in Dermatology*,
DOI 10.1007/978-3-642-20801-0_12,

in the outpatient departments. The inconveniences related to these regular visits at a specialist in wound care cause major discomfort to the patient therefore further reducing the patient's quality of life. Patient transportation also imposes additional economic strain on the health care system. In Styria, a province of Austria, the transportation costs for the ambulance range between 0.65 and 1.26 EUR/km [21, 23]. To avoid travel and additional waiting times in an outpatient wound care center for assessment and treatment, patients are often admitted to a hospital for inpatient care associated with great costs for the community [11]. Furthermore, the patients lose some of their independence and may acquire additional complications associated with bed rest [25]. During hospital stay the wounds are effectively treated according to wound management standards however the wound often worsens when the patient returns home due to the lack of wound care professionals in remote areas. This leads to a discomfort for the patient, hinders the wound healing process and once again impacts on the patient's quality of life.

Another fact that should not be neglected is the aging population and therefore increasing prevalence of chronic wounds among society. Indeed, the prospective number of patients with chronic wounds would overwhelm hospital services and offices of professionals making the provision of good wound care to all affected, a challenge for the community [17].

Telemedicine, especially teledermatology, holds great potential to solve the above mentioned problems. Since the first employment of telemedicine by NASA in the early 1960s, the technical advances led to different possibilities of applied telemedicine. Reasonably priced photographic equipment or the possibility of taking photographs with the mobile phone, coupled with the quick electronic transfer of high-quality digital images make it possible to get expert opinion for diagnosis or recommendations for wound management without delay [5, 6]. As such, patients in rural and remote areas could potentially receive expert medical consultation whilst maintaining their independence and mobility. As chronic wounds are disabilities of the older population and these patients often suffer from numerous comorbidities, telemedicine also offers great advantage for the underlying diseases. Various trials have been published on this issue. Neurological disorders are common in older patients and Dorsey et al. reported about a positive effect of using telemedicine in Parkinson's disease [7]. They showed, relative to baseline, that nursing home patients experienced trends toward improvement in quality of life and patient satisfaction and demonstrated the feasibility of providing subspecialty care via telemedicine for individuals with Parkinson's disease living remotely. Different studies are investigating the potential for telemedicine supported home care in Alzheimer's disease and dementia [27]. An interesting multicentre study investigated the feasibility of a telerehabilitation intervention in home care setting in patients after stroke, traumatic brain injury and multiple sclerosis [9]. They found that the Home Care Activity Desk Training was as effective as standard care in terms of clinical outcomes with both therapists and patients were satisfied with this kind of intervention. Chronic heart failure and chronic obstructive pulmonary disease are common among the elderly and studies of telemonitoring have proven to be effective, leading to improved self-care skills among these patient groups [14, 16, 24]. Bernstein et al. published an interesting model comparing the outcome for patients treated in hemodialysis units with onsite nephrologist and without onsite nephrologist in a remote area [2]. They concluded that chronic hemodialysis patients receiving remotely delivered care in specialized facility attain comparable, if not better, survival outcomes than their urban counterparts with direct onsite nephrology care. Telemedicine promises to become a novel twenty-first-century tool for diabetes mellitus health care providers to communicate with patients to improve the quality and lower the costs of health care [13]. Looking at these data, telemedicine in the elderly population could become important among many specialist fields, including effective wound management.

Numerous studies have been published on telemedical wound care, investigating accuracy and feasibility in addition to acceptance by patients and professionals. Kim et al. performed a prospective study including 70 patients with pressure ulcers stage II–IV, diabetic foot ulcers and venous stasis ulcers to compare the diagnostic evaluation of a wound by the treating physician (in-person assessment – considered as gold standard) with the diagnostic evaluation by remote physician using a telemedicine system [12]. A nurse took digital photos and collected other data of the patient and of the wound and sent the information via Internet to a database where they were posted for access by the telemedicine physician. The wounds were assessed during in-person visit and from the telemedicine physician. Percentage agreement for all visits ranged from 67.1 for "not healing" to 88.8 for "cellulitis present." The authors conclude that telemedicine has the potential to improve access to speciality care for patients who are not currently receiving routine monitoring by specialized nurses or physicians.

Braun et al. investigated the feasibility of telemedical wound care using mobile phones with built-in digital cameras [4]. Three physicians assessed nine variables of the wound status – one performed the face-to-face consultation and the other two the remote evaluation –. A total of 61 leg ulcers were included. Images were taken and sent by e-mail to the remote physician. The image quality was judged to be good in 59% and very good in 20% and the participants felt comfortable making a diagnosis based on the pictures in 82% of cases. Therefore this method offers the possibility of a direct interaction between visiting nurse or physician and the specialists with immediate access to the image and the consequence of improved wound care.

In 2007, Rees RS and Bashshur N published a study investigating the effects of a telewound program on the use of service and financial outcome among homebound patients with chronic wounds [23]. Nineteen patients with chronic pressure ulcers were included in this prospective study and followed up for 2 years. This sample was matched to a historical control group from hospital records. Once a week a digital photograph was taken by the nurse and sent, together with a clinical protocol, to the plastic surgeon experienced in wound care. The telemedicine group had 50% fewer emergency visits, 50% fewer hospitalization associated with shorter lengths of stay. In this study, the telewound program led to lower costs in the management of pressure ulcers and possibly to better health outcomes.

From Veracruz, Mexico, the experience of using telemedicine in the successful assessment and treatment of patients with hard-to-heal leg ulcers was reported [5, 6]. Three patients were included: one 53-year-old man had ulcers on both lower legs and hypertension, morbid obesity, chronic venous insufficiency, recurrent erysipelas and lymphoedema; a 73-year old very obese woman with ulcers on her right leg after surgical debridement of bullous erysipelas and a 51-year old female suffering from rheumatoid arthritis with one ulcer on each lower leg. Images were sent via e-mail to a wound care specialist weekly. The remote specialist was confident to give diagnosis and therapeutic recommendations. This method offers high quality wound care at low cost. In countries with few wound care specialists telemedicine provides a useful tool to obtain expert input remotely.

The experience of our research group with teledermatology and wound management began in 2001. A study was conducted with the aim to examine the feasibility of teledermatology in wound assessment and therapeutic recommendations for patients with chronic leg ulcers [23]. One hundred and ten leg ulcers of different origin were included. We compared the assessment of the wounds by two young physicians doing their internship at our department and a teledermatologist who was an expert in wound care. The two physicians took 1–4 digital images of each ulcer. The images together with selected clinical data (e.g. recent treatment, response to therapy, additional underlying disease) were transmitted to the expert via web application for independent teledermatological assessment. The teledermatologist was blinded to the results of the assessment of the face-to-face visit. A high accordance was found between direct consultations and e-consultation, especially for slough (98.2%) and granulation tissue (76.4%). The teledermatologist assessed the ulcer edges more often than the physicians in the face-to-face consultation (100% vs. 94.5%). The surrounding skin also was more often assessed by the teledermatologist than by the young physicians (99.1% vs. 60%). The last results could be explained by the fact that the younger physicians were less experienced in wound care and therefore they underestimated the impact of surrounding skin changes for the wound healing success. In summary, the results of this study showed that the correct classification of leg ulcers can be made by clinical examination or based on a digital image. For assessment by e-consultation additional data from the patient's history and results of certain previous investigations are recommended; for treatment suggestions, information of previous therapeutic modalities and therapeutic response in addition to known allergic reactions should be transmitted to the teledermatologist. In those cases in which sufficient clinical information was transmitted, the teledermatologist felt confident in recommending further treatment strategies and in planning further e-consultations. Therefore a standardized data sheet – transmitted with the photographs – would be helpful in providing adequate assessment of the wounds and treatment suggestions to increase the medical care of patients with chronic wounds in remote areas.

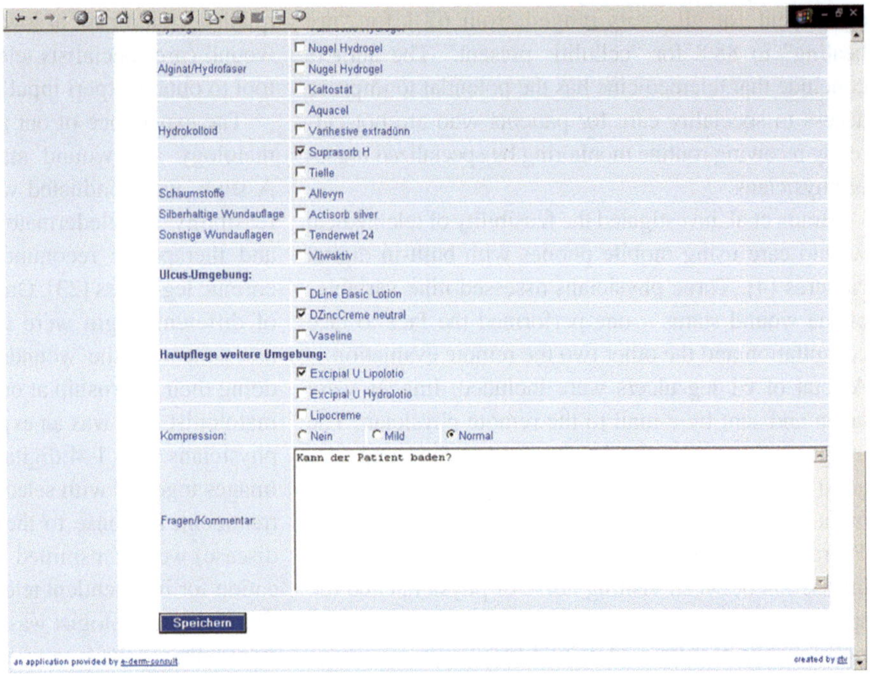

Fig. 12.1 Standardized data sheet for the teledermatologist

Based on this experience, a further study was conducted. We investigated the efficacy of telemedicine for managing leg ulcers in a setting with home care nurses [3]. The reduction of costs and the acceptance of teledermatology by patients and home care nurses were also evaluated. Sixteen patients with a sum total of 45 leg ulcers were enrolled. The treatment regime was determined following an initial outpatient visit at our outpatient department for assessment and classification of the ulcers. Teledermatological follow up was performed by home care nurses once a week for 3 months. A standardized data sheet with relevant clinical information completed by the nurses and 1–4 images were transmitted to the experts in the wound care center via a secure web site specifically designed for this study (Figs. 12.1 and 12.2). The quality of the images was excellent or sufficient in 89% and the experts were confident in giving therapeutic recommendations. The combination of teledermatological expert monitoring and treatment performance by home care nurses led to a good healing rate. More than 70% of the ulcers decreased in size, and approximately one third completely healed. During the treatment phase, patients with leg ulcers visited their general physician or a wound care center every 1–3 weeks for treatment adjustment. A marked decrease in outpatient visits was noted in our study and transportation costs were reduced about 46%. The acceptance of teledermatological monitoring by home care nurses was very good and they believed that the quality of their treatment had improved. Twelve patients were satisfied with the telemedicine wound care and they thought that teledermatology was able to replace a face-to-face visit with the general physician or a wound expert. Teledermatological monitoring of leg ulcers could increase the quality of medical care by enabling general practitioners and home care nurses to receive support from wound care experts from any location. Reduction of the need for travel also lead to lowering the costs of the insurance companies and to improving the quality of life for the 16 almost elderly patients.

An ongoing pilot trial (named "TeleUlcus") concerning teledermatology and wound healing was commenced in March 2009 and includes three provinces of Styria, Austria. The aim is to reduce in-patient care and outpatient visits for patients with chronic wounds, to improve the wound management in home care settings, to reduce the economic burden to the health care system by reducing the transportation costs and enhance the healing rate of chronic wounds. Before starting the pilot trial, general physicians, home care nurses and the stuff of the included hospitals were trained in using teledermatology and specialized in wound care. Standards for diagnostic and therapeutic procedures, and standards for wound care were

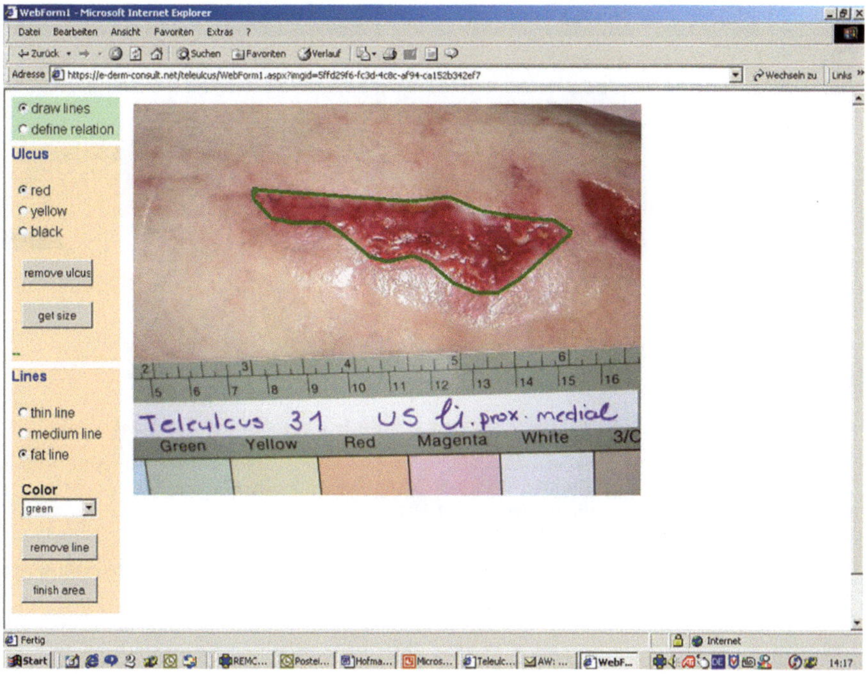

Fig. 12.2 Digital image sent to the teledermatologist. A color scale was photographed together with each lesion. The centimeter scale enables the teledermatologist to measure the area of the ulcus

introduced before starting the trial. The experts of wound care are located at the Department of Dermatology, Medical University of Graz and give support in diagnosis and procedure to all healthcare professionals by teledermatology (Fig. 12.3). The acceptance of teledermatology is very high in this trial and the members welcome the possibility of consulting the experts on each occasion.

To date, teledermatology has not been introduced into the general Austrian health care system. One difficulty met during the trial is the lacking reimbursement of devices and wound dressings for the physicians by the insurance companies. In Styria only patients treated by home care nurses have free access to the required wound dressings therefore patients treated by general physicians often don't get the appropriate wound dressing. In the pilot trial we had special offers from the insurance company to overcome this barrier. This is not only true for Austria, Barret et al. also reported about such set of problems in Western Australia [1]. After evaluation of our data we hope that teledermatology in woundcare will become an appealing field for the health care system and the insurance companies in Austria.

In the Netherlands, KSYOS TeleMedical Centre has been introduced as a state-certified institution for specialized telemedical care, e.g. teledermatology. Cameras, software, training and help service are provided by the telemedicine institution. The teledermatological consultation is fully reimbursed by the Dutch healthcare insurance system. Telewoundcare is also a field of this institution and patients receive proper care, in good time, at the best location and from the proper actor [26].

In Soenderjylland, Denmark, telemedicine was introduced as an interdisciplinary tool to remit patients with chronic wounds to the specialists in the hospitals, with the aim to avoid visits to the outpatient clinic, to control the quality of treatment given and to support the district nurses in wound care of patients with chronic wounds. The concept is named "Saar-I-Syd" (Wounds in the South). Patients are registered in the web base database, and digital images taken by mobile phone and clinical data are sent by the district nurse to this database. The expert gets a sms that new information has been submitted to the database. After 12 months, they found that the set-up based on electronic web-based wound care record works very well, is simple to use and reliable. Specialist support is rapidly available for healthcare professionals far away from the hospital with the outcome of shortening the wound treatment period and of fewer visits to the outpatient's clinic [10].

In conclusion, several studies and trials have proven that with e-consultations the classification and assessment of a wound can be made reliably. Treatment

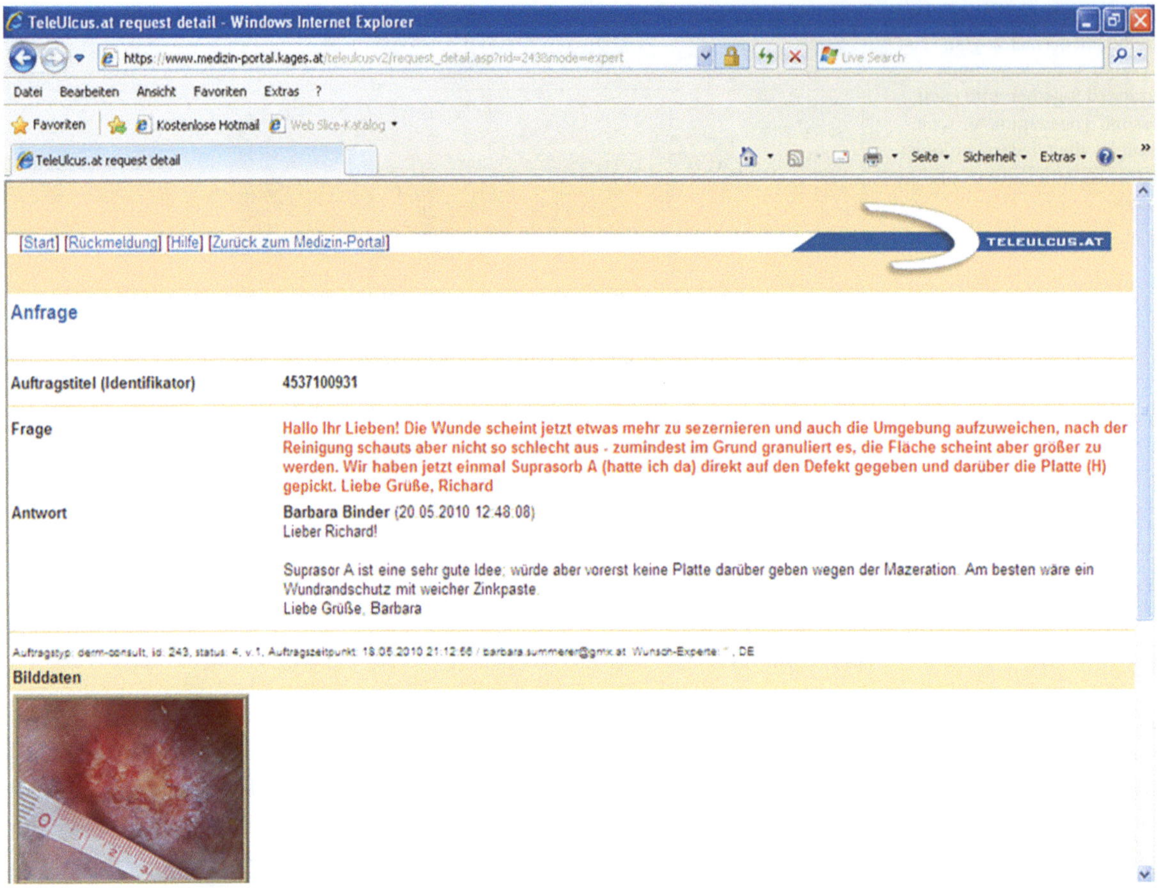

Fig. 12.3 Question of a general physician (*red*) to the expert including the digital image – answer (*black*) of the expert

suggestions and treatment adjustments as well as wound healing monitoring are feasible; only digital images – taken by digital camera or mobile phone – and additional information of the patients underlying diseases and previous treatment modalities are required. Such an approach could potentially increase the quality of medical care in patients with chronic wounds by enabling health care professionals in any location to receive diagnostic and treatment support from experts in wound care. Reduction in the need to travel to an expert or a wound care center leads to lower costs for the health care systems. The quality of life for these almost elderly patients improves by avoiding inconveniences such as long waiting times for appointments at speciality clinics, often located some distance away, and repeated visits to those clinics. The patients maintain their independency and mobility. Because of the regular contact between experts in wound healing and the health care professionals high standard in wound care for all patients with chronic wounds could be achieved. By this improvement of wound care the period of treatment time could be shortened with reduction of costs for wound dressings. Teledermatology is an evolving technology especially in the field of telewoundcare and holds great potential for the future.

References

1. Barrett M, Larson A, Carville K, Ellis I (2009) Challenges faced in implementation of a telehealth enabled chronic wound care system. Rural Remote Health 9:1154
2. Bernstein K, Zacharias J, Blanchard JF et al (2010) Model for equitable care and outcomes for remote full care hemodialysis units. Clin J Am Soc Nephrol 5:645–651
3. Binder B, Hofmann-Wellenhof R, Salmhofer W et al (2007) Teledermatological monitoring of leg ulcers in cooperation with home care nurses. Arch Dermatol 143:1511–1514
4. Braun RP, Vecchetti JL, Luc T et al (2005) Telemedical wound care using a new generation of mobile phones. Arch Dermatol 141:254–258
5. Burg G, Soyer HP, Chimenti S (2009) Skin diseases in Europe – teledermatology. Eur J Dermatol 19:656–662

6. Chanussot-Debrez C, Contreras-Ruiz J (2008) Telemedicine in wound care. Int Wound J 5:651–654
7. Dorsey ER, Deuel LM, Voss TS et al (2010) Increasing access to speciality care: a pilot randomized controlled trial of telemedicine for Parkinson's disease. Mov Disord 25(11):1652–1659
8. Hafner J, Läuchli S, French LE (2010) Phlebology and wound healing. Ther Umsch 67:200–205
9. Huijgen BC, Vollenbroeck-Hutten MM, Zampolini M et al (2008) Feasibility of a home-based telerehabilitation system compared to usual care: arm/hand function in patients with stroke, traumatic brain injury and multiple sclerosis. J Telemed Telecare 14:249–256
10. Jelnes R, Ejskaer N (2007) The use of telemedicine in wound care. EWMA J 7:35–36
11. Jones SM, Banwell PE, Shakespeare PG (2004) Telemedicine in wound healing. Int Woud J 1:225–230
12. Kim HM, Lowery JC, Hamill JB, Wilkens EG (2003) Accuracy of web-based systems for monitoring chronic wounds. Telemed J E Health 9:129–140
13. Klonoff DC (2009) Using telemedicine to improve outcomes in diabetes – an emerging technology. J Diabetes Sci Technol 3:624–628
14. Lewis KE, Annandale JA, Dl W et al (2010) Does home telemonitoring after pulmonary rehabilitation reduce healthcare use in optimized COPD? A pilot randomized trial. COPD 7:44–50
15. Lyder HC (2003) Pressure ulcer and management. JAMA 289:223–226
16. Maric B, Kaan A, Araki Y et al (2010) The use of the internet to remotely monitor patients with heart failure. Telemed J E Health 16:26–33
17. Nelzen O, Bergqvist D, Lindhagen A, Hallböök T (1991) Chronic leg ulcers: an underestimated problem in primary health care among elderly patients. J Epidemiol Community Health 45:184–187
18. Nelzen O, Bergqvist D, Lindhagen A (1991) Led ulcers etiology – a cross sectional population study. J Vasc Surg 14(4):557–564
19. Phillips TJ, Dover JS (1991) Leg ulcers. J Am Acad Dermatol 25:965–987
20. Reddy M, Gill SS, Rochon PA (2006) Preventing pressure ulcer: a systemic review. JAMA 296:974–984
21. Rees RS, Bashshur N (2007) The effects of telewound management on use of service and financial outcome. Telemed J E Health 13:663–674
22. Riedel K, Ryssel H, Koellensperger E et al (2008) Pathogenesis of chronic wounds. Chirurg 79:526–534
23. Salmhofer W, Hofmann-Wellenhof R, Gabler G et al (2005) Wound teleconsultation in patients with chronic leg ulcers. Dermatology 210:211–217
24. Schmidt S, Schuchert A, Krieg T, Oeff M (2010) Home telemonitoring in patients with chronic heart failure. Dtsch Arztebl Int 107:131–138
25. Simon DA, Dix FP, McCollum CN (2004) Management of venous leg ulcers. BMJ 328:1358–1362
26. Van der Heijden J (2010) Teledermatology integrated in the Dutch national healthcare system. J Eur Acad Dermatol Venereol 24:615–616
27. Williams R (2010) Neurology at distance. Lancet Neurol 9:346–347

Telepsoriasis

13

Julia Frühauf and Rainer Hofmann-Wellenhof

Core Messages

- Psoriasis mainly manifests with chronic inflammation of the skin that may cause significant physical and psychological burden.
- It is essential for healthcare professionals to work together with patients suffering from psoriasis planning treatment regimens, as active participation may improve patient compliance.
- Teledermatology, and in particular mobile teledermatology, might prove to be the preferable tool empowering the chronic-ill to effectively take control of their life with psoriasis.
- The feasibility of teledermatology services in the management of psoriasis patients has already been proven.
- Further effectiveness studies are needed to widely adopt this mode of care.

Introduction

Psoriasis is a chronic, immune-mediated, multisystem disease with predominantly skin and joint manifestations that affects approximately 2% of the general population [1]. It is characterized by scaly, erythematous patches, papules, plaques and occasionally, pustules that may be pruritic or even painful. It is associated with high morbidity and its impact on patient's social life and emotional and physical wellbeing is dramatic [2, 3]. Conditions that may be associated with psoriasis, psoriasis arthritis, or both include autoimmune diseases, such as inflammatory bowel disease, components of the metabolic syndrome such as diabetes and cardiovascular disease, lymphoma, and depression [1]. Psoriasis waxes and wanes during a patient lifetime, is often modified by treatment initiation and cessation and has few spontaneous remissions [1]. Although clearance of the physical presence of psoriasis may enhance an individual well being in the short term, the notion of relapse once therapy is withdrawn is a constant psychological burden. Patient support groups are one source of psychological assistance, designed to develop and reinforce positive coping styles. Results of a recent online survey about the role of psoriasis online support communities confirmed that these platforms offer both, a valuable educational resource and a source of psychological and social support [4]. Despite initial concerns that online activity might lead people to withdraw from social interaction [5], a number of recent reports have noted that use of the Internet can empower people [6], thus improving social support and self-esteem [7]. In addition, it allows individuals to access information at a time and place of their choice [5].

As physicians who care for the large majority of patients with psoriasis, dermatologists play an important role in identifying the morbidity of all aspects of psoriatic disease.

In this respect, telemedicine, and in particular teledermatology, which combines telecommunication and information technologies, offers new possibilities for patients and doctors to interact with each other. When

J. Frühauf (✉) • R. Hofmann-Wellenhof
Department of Dermatology, Medical University of Graz, Graz, Austria
e-mail: julia.fruehauf@medunigraz.at; rainer.hofmann@medunigraz.at

H.P. Soyer et al. (eds.), *Telemedicine in Dermatology*,
DOI 10.1007/978-3-642-20801-0_13, © Springer-Verlag Berlin Heidelberg 2012

the practice of teledermatology first began, most communication was between physicians (generally specialist to generalist) [8]. For this purpose, digital cameras were used to produce high-quality images of a dermatologic condition and then to forward them via E-mail or other communication networks for referral. Teledermatology has since evolved to allow direct communication between patients and dermatologists. This advancement was partially fueled by the rapid progress in computer and information technologies incorporating expensive digital cameras into low-cost mobile phones, as well as patients becoming increasingly comfortable using this technology. With mobile teledermatology [9, 10] a ubiquitous and easy-to-use solution for data acquisition was gained in the management of the chronic-ill. Teledermatology has revolutionized some aspects of health care delivery by transforming relationships between patients and physicians shifting the power of consultation so that patients may become more informed and assertive [11]. Even for patients with chronic skin diseases such as psoriasis, loss of body control is one of the most bothersome aspects [12]. Therefore, teledermatology may have the potential to strengthen patient confidence and motivation to use their own skills and knowledge to take effective control over their life, even with this chronic illness. Even simple strategies including telephoning the patient 2–3 weeks after consultations [13] and involving patients in the selection of their treatment [14] might enhance patients' motivation and adherence to treatment plans, and even led to improved health outcomes [15–19]. Due to remote and immediate medical access, also waiting time and travel expenses might be effectively reduced for the patients. Many therapeutic options are available for the treatment of psoriasis [1]. Limitations of traditional therapies and the improved understanding of psoriasis have led to the recent introduction of new bioactive agents, also called biologics. These agents have been effective even in high-need psoriasis patients, for whom at least two other systemic therapies were unsuitable [20]. Most of these medications can be self-administered subcutaneously at home, making possible a more flexible lifestyle for the patients. However, even there are limitations, as close monitoring is needed e.g. to adjust treatment plans when psoriasis flares or adverse effects from medications occur. Teledermatology seems a valuable tool to effectively monitor such patients, and moreover to reduce health care costs related to psoriasis exacerbations, as it makes timely interventions possible. American studies demonstrated that treatment costs are a notable portion of psoriasis-related expenditures [21] and that total and out-of-pocket expenditures rise with increasing disease severity [22]. Hospitalizations accounted for one third of the expenditures arising for outpatient visits. To date, there is little information available about the economic impact of psoriasis in European countries [23, 24] In a cost-of-illness study from Italy [23], the mean costs for psoriasis with moderate disease amounted less than half of those for patients with more severe disease. In another study from Germany [24] the annual total costs were highest in high-need patients, who also showed the highest PASI score.

Technical Infrastructure

Image quality is an essential component in assuring the optimal communication of patient image data to the dermatologist for teleconsultation [25]. Therefore, there are minimum requirements for digital images such as resolution, contrast and color discrimination, and guidelines for technical specifications of image acquisition have been recently proposed by the American Telemedicine Association [26]. It is remarkable that color discrimination seems less important in the evaluation of psoriasis than in other skin diseases. Despite basic requirements for image standardization, such as constant room lighting and the use of a non-reflective, white backdrop behind the region of interest, the ability to overview the whole body area involved mainly impacts the reliability of remote diagnosis. This might be due to the fact that psoriasis severity scores are an area-weighted measure, where the final score is determined more by the Body Surface Area (BSA) and less by the morphological characteristics of the disease [27, 28]. This finding is also reflected by previous research that found the BSA component to be mainly responsible for substantial inter-rater variability in psoriasis severity scorings [29–32]. Till date, the current gold standard methods, PASI (Psoriasis Area and Severity Index) and Palmoplantar PASI (PPPASI), are used to measure psoriasis severity by evaluating the average redness, scaling and thickness (PASI), and average number of erythema, pustules and scaling (PPPASI) of the plaques, respectively, weighted by the area of involvement [33]. For calculating the scores, each area is given a numeri-

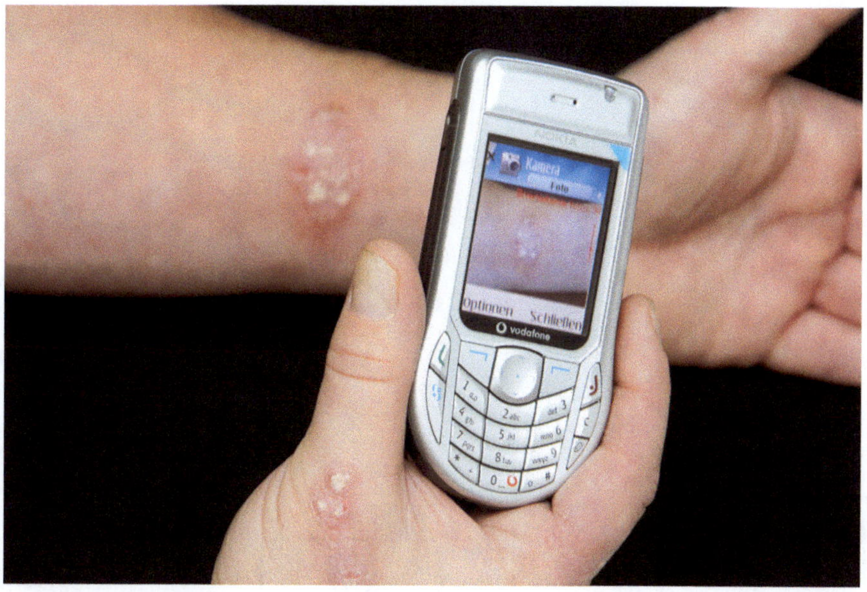

Fig. 13.1 Data capture using mobile phones. Photographs of lesions are made using a common mobile phone with a built-in camera (Image published Frühauf [39])

cal score representing the proportion involved. The two scores vary from 0 to 72 with higher scores indicating severer conditions. Therefore, overview-images of each anatomical region and detailed views of some defined target lesions should be conveyed for teleconsultation to adequately display the area of involvement and the composition of the plaques. However, when using the Self-Administered PASI (SAPASI) [34] for disease severity scorings, which is a patient-rated PASI with equivalent value [35], image acquisition of some target lesions might be sufficient. It is understandably uncomfortable for patients to expose sensible body regions (e.g. the genitals) in front of a camera. Furthermore, some body regions (e.g. the scalp) are inaccessible to the camera. To assess disease severity at these sites, the use of respective questionnaires might be useful. Furthermore, assistance e.g. by family members could be necessary in case of very widespread disease or locations, which are inaccessible by the patients themselves (e.g. lesions on the back). Taking into account the morphologic characteristics of the disease, teledermatology may have some diagnostic limitations; due to the inability to palpate the lesions and the danger to put too much emphasis on minute details, induration and scaling, might be misdiagnosed [36]. However, these limitations may only marginally impact psoriasis severity scorings, as diagnostic accuracy of remote PASI/PPPASI assessments has been shown to be adequate and comparable to that of in-person clinical encounters [37]. Regarding image resolution, pictures of 720×500 pixels have been demonstrated to be adequate for dermatological diagnosis [38]. Thus, any standard digital camera and even any built-in camera with a, e.g., 1.3 mega-pixels capability and an image resolution of 1,280×960 pixels is more than sufficient for decision-making. To date, the technical architecture mainly used in the management of psoriasis patients consists of a conventional mobile phone equipped with a built-in camera and an implemented application. The software integrates both a section for image capturing (Fig. 13.1) and one for the input of patients' medical history via questionnaire. The captured pictures are stored and sent as JPEG (joint photographic experts group, a compression algorithm for digital images) files. In the last years, various mobile transmission technologies with improved transmission rates have been developed. The technology commonly used is a packet-based wireless data transfer via General Packet Radio Service (GPRS) or Universal Mobile Telecommunication System (UMTS) to a central web-server. The simplest method for remote analysis of incoming patient data is the use of a Hypertext Preprocessor (PHP), a server-side scripting language, and a relational database engine, which are both implemented on a web-server to create a database driven webpage. PHP processes the page request and converts the data from the database into a web-interface with login-protected user access. Although reducing the flexibility of mobile care, data might be also transferred to

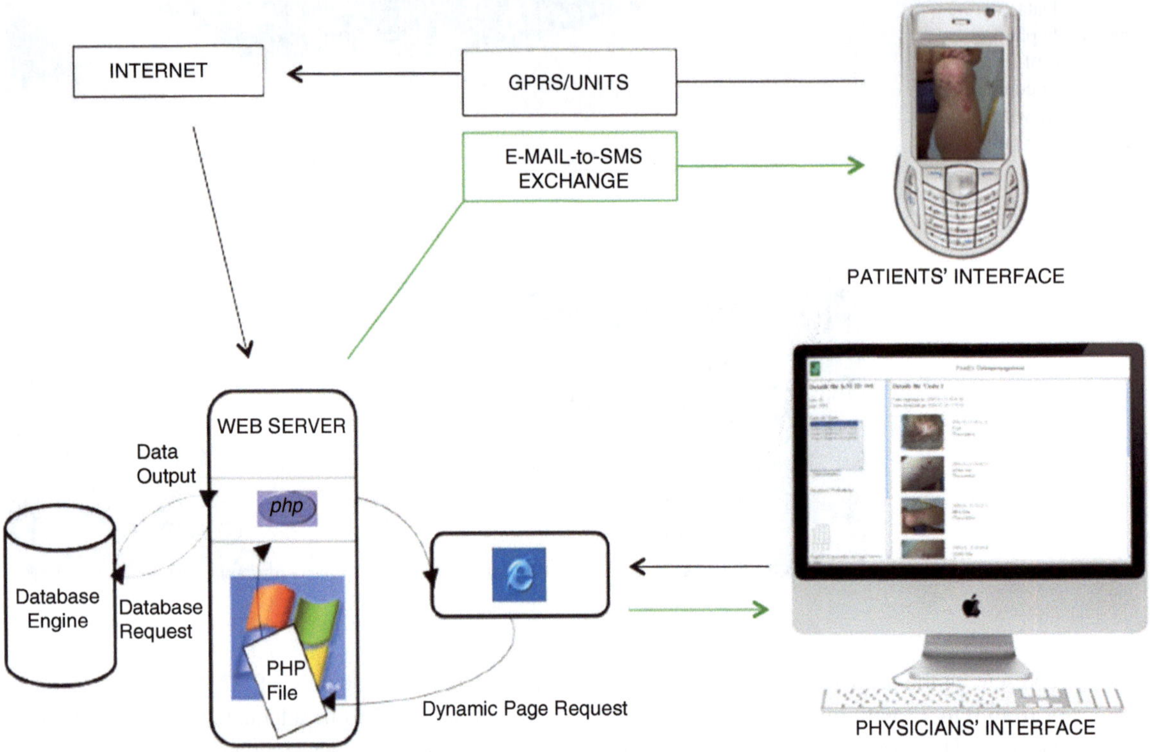

Fig. 13.2 Technical architecture of a mobile teledermatology system: Patient data stored on a mobile phone are then transmitted to a central web-server, using a packet-based wireless data transfer via General Packet Radio Service (*GPRS*) or Universal Mobile Telecommunication System (*UMTS*). For analysis of incoming patient data by the teledermatologists, Hypertext Preprocessor (*PHP*), a server-side scripting language, and a relational database engine using the scripting language Structured Query Language (*SQL*) are implemented on the web-server to create a database driven webpage. PHP processes the page request and converts the data from the database into a web-interface with login-protected user access (Modified Version of artwork published Frühauf [39])

the computer via Universal Series Bus (USB), and then stored and uploaded to a Web-application. To directly send treatment instructions from the remote examiner to the correspondent mobile phones of the patients, an additional mobile phone-based feedback system that converts email messages into short text messages (Email-to-SMS) seems very useful (Fig. 13.2).

Status of Research and Application

A long time, generalized skin eruptions were thought to be more difficult to diagnose by remote than by in-person examinations, even if presenting with indurated lesions varying over time in intensity, extent and distribution [40]. As an adjunct to visual inspections, dermatologists routinely palpate the skin during clinical examination. This sensory modality is lacking, when using teledermatology for skin examination. This might explain some of the concerns dermatologists have had about the accuracy of teledermatology diagnoses in psoriasis patients, as induration seems an important clinical sign of the disease [41]. In other fields of application, however, teledermatology has already been intensely utilized. It has been applied to melanoma screenings, in the surveillance of long-term therapy of leg ulcers, or in medical attendance in rural and remote areas [42]. Since 2005, increasing emphasis was also put on the evaluation of teledermatology services for patients with inflammatory skin diseases. It has been found that teledermatology techniques could be reliably applied to diagnosis of atopic skin eruptions [43], and the additive value of second opinion teleconsultations in patients with challenging inflammatory, neoplastic skin diseases among experts was confirmed [44]. In the latter case, it is remarkable that up to 30% of the patients were correctly diagnosed by teleconsultation only. The authors assumed that this finding was not related to the diagnostic teledermatology method itself, but could be a result of selection of diagnostic criteria or qualification of the submitting physician and of the expert consultants. Recently, good accuracy and sensitivity of teledermatological examination could be also demonstrated in the area of occupational medicine, where minimal skin changes, such as erythema, vesicles, papules or lichenification, need to be assessed [36].

Till date, only three studies have been performed using teledermatology particularly in the management of psoriasis patients [37, 39, 45, 46]. Klotz et al. [45] investigated the value of second opinion teleconsulting in the monitoring of phototherapy of psoriasis patients living in areas devoid of dermatologists. Two groups of patients were instituted. One group, received phototherapy by their local physician, the other received the same treatment, but was additionally supervised by a dermatologist via telemedicine services. In the monitored group, 40% more patients were clear of psoriasis at time of discharge and treatment time decreased from 140 to 37 days. The number of patients with side effects decreased. The number of self-and family practice-referred patients dropped; the clinic became a valuable referral center for dermatologists. At that time, when the settings of the two other telepsoriasis studies were instituted, teledermatology has already evolved to allow direct communication between patients and physicians, spotlighting mobile phones as the preferable tool for flexible and patient-centered data transfer. Self-imaging e.g. via mobile phones is thought to empower patients to participate in their care actively, therefore resulting in improved clinical outcomes [12], and reduced numbers of return visits to the dermatological clinic [47]. The ability of patients in taking and submitting high-quality images for dermatological evaluation has been shown before [38, 48, 49]. In contrast to previous studies evaluating mobile teledermatology services [48, 50–52], Hayn et al. [46] and Frühauf et al. [37, 39] independently developed mobile monitoring systems for psoriasis patients outside hypothetical in-office scenarios, without any intermediary (e.g. research assistant) between patients and dermatologists. Data transmission was not computer-based; instead, mobile communication networks were used, enhancing the flexibility of mobile care. The software (Java 2 Micro Edition or C++ application), which was implemented on the mobile phones (Sony Ericsson K770i or K800i, both with a built-in 3.2 megapixel camera [Sony Ericsson, London, UK], and Nokia 6630 with a built-in 1.3 megapixel camera [Nokia, Helsinki, Finland], respectively), consisted of a section for image capturing, and a section for the input of historical information (e.g. occurrence of undesirable side effects or skin lesions in regions inaccessible to the camera, and body temperature) and information on quality of life via questionnaires. Of note, both systems were implemented as an adjunct to routine follow-up consultations. The system of Hayn et al. [46] was used in the course of a medical case series, in which 19 psoriasis patients (age 46.3 ± 12.3 years) requiring biologic therapy were included. Together, 70 consultations were performed and more than 1000 pictures were conveyed from the patients. Severity measurements were performed using the SAPASI. In addition, digital images of up to five target lesions were specifically evaluated regarding plaque-composition. Preliminary results indicate that the mobile phone-based image acquisition by psoriasis patients themselves is feasible with sufficient quality for therapy assessment. A detailed statistical analysis is on the way and results will be soon available. In the 12-week pilot-study by Frühauf et al. [37, 39], 10 high-need psoriasis patients (median age: 40 years, range: 25–67 years) with generalized or palmoplantar psoriasis were enclosed. Instead of the SAPASI, herein PASI/PPPASI calculations were used to assess disease severity. Therefore, patients photographed their skin lesions according to the anatomical areas of PASI or PPPASI [34]. 80 mobile visits and 486 images were conveyed from the patients. Both remote examiners rated quality and resolution of the images submitted by the patients very similarly. On average, 86% of each patient images (min-max, 66–95%) were judged as very good, 12% (5–28%) as satisfactory, and 2% (0–6%) as poor. Data from routine outpatient consultations, were compared with those obtained by two teledermatologists with particular attention to accuracy of PASI/PPPASI and therapeutic outcome assessments (≥50% reduction from baseline PASI/PPPASI scores (PASI/PPPASI 50) at week 12) [53]. PASI/PPPASI assessments correlated significantly between the face-to-face consultant and the two teledermatologists (Table 13.1), as well as between the two teledermatologists. The remote examiners assessed the therapeutic outcome in agreement with the face-to-face consultant in 8 of 10 and 9 of 10 cases, respectively. Together, therapeutic outcome assessments marginally differed in two patients, which is also a common finding during regular clinical consultations [54]. Even with experienced in-person examiners, an inter-rater variability of up to 8.1 PASI scores has been described [54]. In this study, however,

Table 13.1 Comparison and correlation of disease severity measurements obtained by the face-to-face consultant (*FTF*) and two teledermatologists (*TD1*, *TD2*) in 10 high-need psoriasis patients receiving etanercept

	FTF	TD1				TD2			
Visits	PASI/PPPASI[a], median (range)	Correlation[b] with FTF	*P* value[c]	Inter-rater variability[d]	PASI/PPPASI[a], median (range)	Correlation[b] with FTF	*P* value[c]	Inter-rater variability[d]	PASI/PPPASI[a], median (range)
Week 0	18.65 (5.2–34.8)	0.90	<0.001	3.39	15.85 (5.7–29.6)	0.95	<0.001	2.97	16.50 (5.0–29.6)
Week 1	13.70 (5.2–29.4)	0.96	<0.001	2.11	14.50 (5.6–23.4)	0.98	<0.001	2.57	12.95 (4.4–27.2)
Week 6	5.05 (2.2–23.2)	0.88	0.001	1.50	6.55 (3.3–20.0)	0.78	0.008	1.27	5.85 (3.2–23.9)
Week 12	3.55 (1.3–20.0)	0.71	0.02	1.11	3.75 (2.1–19.0)	0.80	0.005	0.86	4.75 (1.5–20.1)

[a]Disease severity measurements: *PASI* Psoriasis Area and Severity Index, *PPPASI* Palmoplantar PASI. Shown as combined scores established from eight patients with plaque psoriasis and two patients with palmoplantar psoriasis
[b]Spearman's rank correlation coefficient
[c]*P* value for correlation coefficient
[d]Mean PASI/PPPASI deviation from FTF (Table published in *Archives of Dermatology* [37])

the inter-rater variability was very low (Table 13.1) indicating that mobile teledermatology is a feasible method for monitoring disease severity in psoriasis patients. Together, it has been demonstrated that both approaches, either using patient-rated (SAPASI) or physician-rated (PASI or PPPASI) measures for severity scoring, could be reliably applied to remote diagnosis of psoriatic skin eruptions.

Patient and Physician Acceptance

The willingness to be educated is one of the highest among patients with psoriasis [55]. Therefore, a collaborative model of management whereby both patients and dermatologists take responsibility for the process and outcome of consultation would appear to be essential in enhancing patient satisfaction in this challenging condition. Validated instruments to assess user satisfaction with or acceptance of store-and-forward teledermatology do not currently exist [56]. Particular emphasis should be put on the understanding how patients and physicians perceive the interaction resulting from this new mode of care. Using specifically developed questionnaires (Fig. 13.3), it could be recently demonstrated that mobile teledermatology is highly accepted by psoriasis patients [39]. All ten patients were satisfied with the remote treatment instructions, and the possibility offered to discuss their health-related problems. In addition, 80% of the patients believed the mobile monitoring system to be an adequate alternative to in-person consultation, and 90% felt to be in good hands. As expected, the system exerted great influence on patient daily life. All patients perceived savings of time and expenses, and moreover, they believed to have gained a more flexible and empowered lifestyle (Fig. 13.3). Contrary to a recent report that found patient acceptance and satisfaction with telemedicine services to be complicated by patients' perceived health status [57], in the above-mentioned study no significant correlations were observed. One may speculate whether this finding was due to the fact that this care model had greatly diminished the flaws of store-and-forward teledermatology, including insufficient privacy [57–59] embarrassment being photographed [57, 59], limitations to expression of problems and concerns [57], completeness of information transmitted [60, 61], anxiety about the unfamiliar technology [60], frustration with technical problems [60], delayed or absent follow-up [62], and concerns about never having been evaluated directly by a dermatologist [58]. With regard to consultant dermatologists' acceptance of store-and-forward teledermatology, there is little information available [62], but dermatologists have commonly reported greater confidence when making the diagnosis by in-person examinations [62]. Remarkably, image quality has not been reported as major source of dissatisfaction among consultants [62]. To date, only two studies have been performed also evaluating consultants' acceptance of telepsoriasis services. In the study by Hayn et al. [46], the teledermatologists felt that this method simplified patient-physician interaction, shortened the mean duration of a regular outpatient-follow-up visit, and facilitated individual therapy adjustment based on the

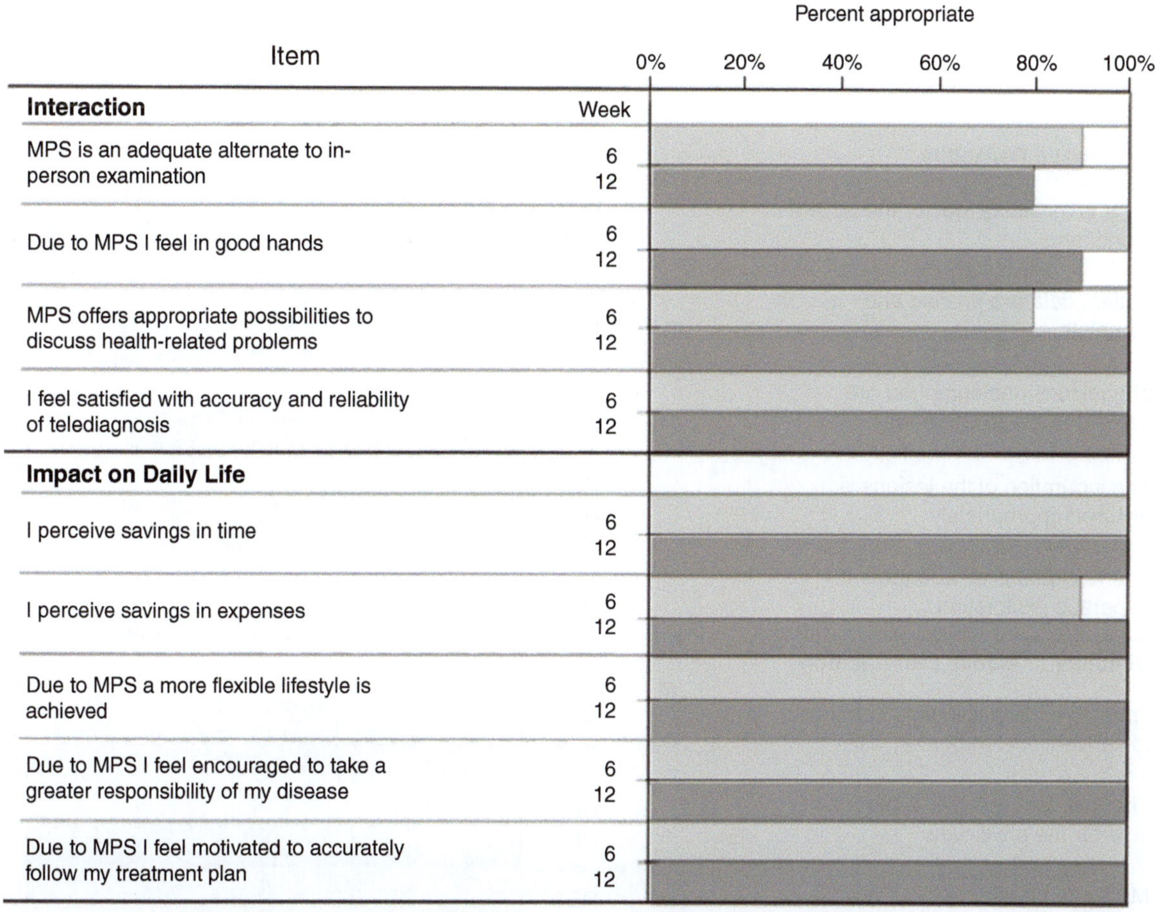

Fig. 13.3 Patient responses (in percentages) to the 9-item acceptance questionnaire about the mobile patient-support (*MPS*) system at weeks 6 and 12, grouped by the two subscales 'interaction' and 'impact on daily life' (Modified Version of artwork published Frühauf [39])

availability of photos from lesions in regular intervals. In the study by Frühauf et al. [39], the two remote examiners believed the text information to be adequate in comparison to a directly obtained history, and the remote consultation service to be a reliable tool for the patient-driven home monitoring in all of the cases. Some concerns, however, were expressed with comparability of photographed lesions and the inability to appreciate dermal swelling and induration (Fig. 13.4).

Conclusion

Patient empowerment has been found to be a key factor for achieving improved health outcomes in psoriasis. Thus, providing a patient-driven follow-up care to those patients seems an area of considerable potential. Furthermore, dermatologists are in short supply and are geographically maldistributed, creating a lack of access to care even of the chronic-ill. Teledermatology has the potential to bridge this gap in access because the rapid advancement of technologies has made close and less time-consuming support and even coaching in the home possible. Supporting ongoing management of existing patients as an adjunct to conventional care may prove to be its most valuable application in the care of psoriasis patients. So far, prerequisite conditions for the successful application, such as very good image quality and high concordance of diagnostic and therapeutic decisions between remote and in-person consultations have been demonstrated. Although the sample size was very small in previous studies, it seems likely that both patients and physicians would also adopt this method for routine usage. In the future,

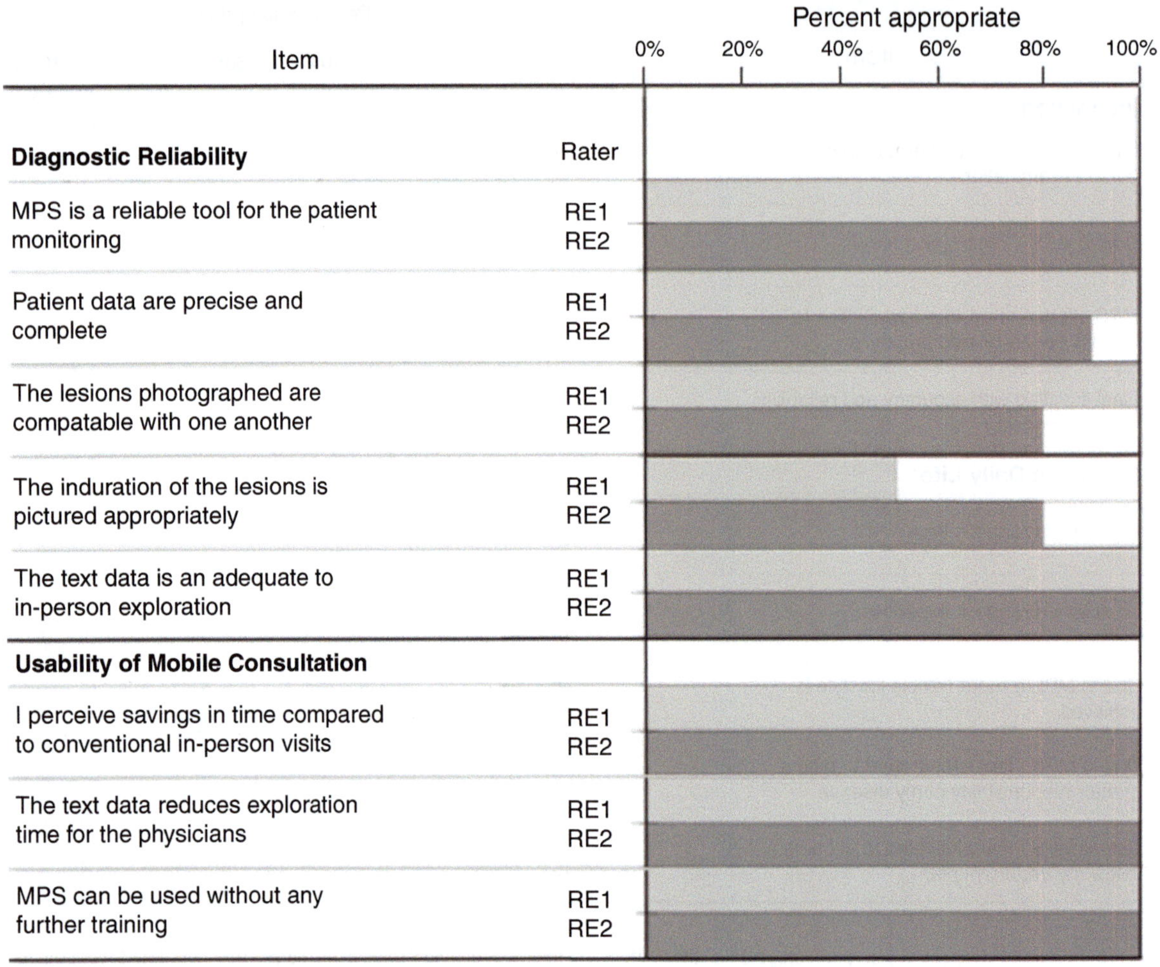

Fig. 13.4 Remote examiner (*RE1*, *RE2*) responses to the 8-item acceptance questionnaire about the mobile patient-support (*MPS*) system at week 12, grouped by the two subscales 'diagnostic reliability' and 'usability of mobile consultation' (Modified Version of artwork published Frühauf [39])

larger controlled studies are required to evaluate the impact of remote follow-up care on consultants' satisfaction, patient empowerment and its influence on the therapeutic outcome, and furthermore to demonstrate its economic viability in order to be widely adopted.

References

1. Menter A, Gottlieb A, Feldman SR et al (2008) Guidelines of care for the management of psoriasis and psoriatic arthritis: section 1. Overview of psoriasis and guidelines of care for the treatment of psoriasis with biologics. J Am Acad Dermatol 58:826–850
2. Peters BP, Weissman FG, Gill MA (2000) Pathophysiology and treatment of psoriasis. Am J Health Syst Pharm 57:645–662
3. Idriss SZ, Kvedar JC, Watson AJ (2009) The role of online support communities. Benefits of expanded social networks to patients with psoriasis. Arch Dermatol 145:46–51
4. Kraut R, Patterson M, Lundmark V et al (1998) Internet paradox: a social technology that reduces social involvement and psychological wellbeing? Am Psychol 53:1017–1031
5. Van Uden-Kraan CF, Drossaert CH, Taal E et al (2008) Empowering processes and outcomes of participation in online support groups for patients with breast cancer, arthritis, or fibromyalgia. Qual Health Res 18:405–417
6. Shaw LH, Gant LM (2002) In defense of the internet: the relationship between internet communication and depression, loneliness, self-esteem, and perceived social support. Cyberpsychol Behav 5:157–171

7. Whited JD (2001) Teledermatology. Current status and future directions. Am J Clin Dermatol 2:59–64
8. Massone C, Lozzi GP, Wurm E et al (2005) Cellular phones in clinical teledermatology. Arch Dermatol 141:1319–1320
9. Massone C, Lozzi GP, Wurm E et al (2006) Personal digital assistants in teledermatology. Br J Dermatol 154:801–802
10. Finch TL, Mort M, Mair FS et al (2008) Future patients? Telehealthcare, roles and responsibilities. Health Soc Care Community 16:86–95
11. Lamb CA, Fried RG, Feldman SR (2004) Giving patients 'perceived control' over psoriasis: advice for optimizing the physician-patient relationship. J Dermatolog Treat 15: 182–184
12. Harris DR (1999) The art of treating psoriasis: practical suggestions for improved treatment. Cutis 64:335–336
13. Van de Kerkhof PC, de Hoop D, de Korte J et al (2000) Patient compliance and disease management in the treatment of psoriasis in the Netherlands. Dermatology 200: 292–298
14. DiMatteo RM (1994) Enhancing patient adherence to medical recommendations. JAMA 271:79, 83
15. Von Korff M, Gruman J, Schaefer J et al (1997) Collaborative management of chronic illness. Ann Intern Med 127:1097–1102
16. Prochaska JO, Velicer WF, Rossi JS et al (1994) Stages of change and decisional balance for 12 problem behaviours. Health Psychol 13:39–46
17. Seeman M, Seeman TE (1983) Health behavior and personal autonomy: a longitudinal study of the sense of control in illness. J Health Soc Behav 24:144–160
18. Brody DS (1980) The patient's role in clinical decision-making. Ann Intern Med 93:718–722
19. Rich SJ, Bello-Quintero CE (2004) Advancements in the treatment of psoriasis: role of biologic agents. J Manag Care Pharm 10:318–325
20. Galadari I, Rigcl E, Lebwohl M (2001) The cost of psoriasis treatment. J Eur Acad Dermatol Venereol 15:290–291
21. Feldman SR, Fleischer AB Jr, Reboussin DM et al (1997) The economic impact of psoriasis increases with psoriasis severity. J Am Acad Dermatol 37:564–569
22. Colombo G, Altomare GF, Peris K (2008) Moderate and severe plaque psoriasis: cost-of-illness study in Italy. Ther Clin Risk Manag 4:559–568
23. Sohn S, Schoeffski O, Prinz J et al (2006) Cost of moderate to severe plaque psoriasis in Germany: a multicenter cost-of-illness study. Dermatology 212:137–144
24. Kanthraj GR (2009) Classification and design of teledermatology practice: what dermatoses? Which technology to apply? J Eur Acad Dermatol Venereol 23:865–875
25. Krupinski E, Burdick A, Pak H et al (2008) American telemedicine association's practice guidelines for teledermatology. Telemed J E Health 14:289–302
26. Ashcroft DM, Li Wan Po A, Williams HC (1999) Clinical measures of disease severity and outcome in psoriasis: a critical appraisal of their quality. Br J Dermatol 141:185–191
27. Feldman SR (2004) A quantitative definition of severe psoriasis for use in clinical trials. J Dermatolog Treat 15:27–29
28. Exum ML, Rapp SR, Feldman SR et al (1996) Measuring severity in psoriasis: methodological issues. J Dermatolog Treat 7:119–124
29. Ginsburg IH (1995) Psychological and psychophysiological aspects of psoriasis. Dermatol Clin 13:793–804
30. Marks D, Barton SP, Shuttleworth D et al (1989) Assessment of disease progress in psoriasis. Arch Dermatol 125:235–240
31. Ramsey B, Lawrence CM (1991) Measurement of involved surface area in patients with psoriasis. Br J Dermatol 124:565–570
32. Tiling-Grosse S, Rees J (1993) Assessment of area involvement in skin disease: a study using schematic figure outlines. Br J Dermatol 128:69–74
33. Fredriksson T, Pettersson U (1978) Severe psoriasis – oral therapy with a new retinoid. Dermatologica 157:238–244
34. Feldman SR, Fleischer AB Jr, Reboussin DM et al (1996) The self-administered psoriasis area and severity index is valid and reliable. J Invest Dermatol 106:183–186
35. Henseler T, Schmitt-Rau K (2008) A comparison between BSA, PASI, PLASI and SAPASI as measures of disease severity and improvement by therapy in patients with psoriasis. Int J Dermatol 47:1019–1023
36. Baumeister T, Weistenhöfer W, Drexler H et al (2009) Prevention of work-related skin diseases: teledermatology as an alternative approach in occupational screenings. Contact Dermatitis 61:224–230
37. Frühauf J, Schwantzer G, Ambros-Rudolph CM et al (2010) Pilot study using teledermatology to manage high-need patients with psoriasis. Arch Dermatol 146(2):200–201
38. Qureshi AA, Brandling-Bennett HA, Giberti S et al (2006) Evaluation of digital skin images submitted by patients who received practical training or an online tutorial. J Telemed Telecare 12:79–82
39. Frühauf J, Schwantzer G, Ambros-Rudolph CM et al (2009) Acceptance of a mobile patient-support system for the home monitoring of high-need psoriasis patients. In: G. Schreier, D. Hayn, E. Ammenwerth eHealth 2009. Books@ocg.at 250:107-114
40. Lewis K, Gilmour E, Harrison PV et al (1999) Digital teledermatology for skin tumours: a preliminary assessment using a receiver operating characteristics (ROC) analysis. J Telemed Telecare 5(Suppl 1):S57–S58
41. Cox NH (2007) A literally blinded trial of palpation in dermatologic diagnosis. J Am Acad Dermatol 56:949–951
42. Baumeister T, Drexler H, Küttnig B (2007) Teledermatology – a hitherto underestimated tool in occupational medicine – indications and limitations. J Occup Health 49:504–508
43. Wallach D, Coste J, Tilles G (2005) The first images of atopic dermatitis: an attempt at retrospective diagnosis in dermatology. J Am Acad Dermatol 53:684–689
44. Lozzi GP, Soyer HP, Massone C (2007) The additive value of second opinion teleconsulting in the management of patients with challenging inflammatory, neoplastic skin diseases: a best practice model in dermatology? J Eur Acad Dermatol Venereol 21:30–34
45. Klotz J, Muir L, Cameron C et al (2005) Monitoring a remote phototherapy unit via telemedicine. J Cutan Med Surg 9:47–53
46. Hayn D, Koller S, Hofmann-Wellenhof R et al (2009) Mobile phone-based teledermatologic compliance management – preliminary results of the TELECOMP study. Stud Health Technol Inform 150:468–472

47. Baldwin L, Clarke M, Hands L et al (2003) The effect of telemedicine on consultation time. J Telemed Telecare 9(suppl 1):71–73
48. Ebner C, Wurm EM, Binder B et al (2008) Mobile teledermatology: a feasibility study of 58 subjects using mobile phones. J Telemed Telecare 14:2–7
49. Eminovic N, Witkamp L, Ravelli AC et al (2003) Potential effect of patient-assisted teledermatology on outpatient referral rates. J Telemed Telecare 9:321–327
50. Braun RP, Vecchietti JL, Thomas L et al (2005) Telemedical wound care using a new generation of mobile telephones: a feasibility study. Arch Dermatol 141:254–258
51. Massone C, Hofmann-Wellenhof R, Ahlgrimm-Siess V et al (2007) Melanoma screening with cellular phones. PLoS One 2:e483
52. Hsieh CH, Jeng SF, Chen CY et al (2005) Teleconsultation with the mobile camera-phone in remote evaluation of replantation potential. J Trauma 58:1208–1212
53. Nast A, Kopp IB, Augustin M et al (2007) Evidence-based (S3) guidelines for the treatment of psoriasis vulgaris. J Dtsch Dermatol Ges 5(Suppl 3):1–119
54. Langley RG, Ellis CN (2004) Evaluating psoriasis with psoriasis area and severity index, psoriasis global assessment, and lattice system physician's global assessment. J Am Acad Dermatol 51:563–569
55. Arican O (2007) E-dermatology: emails about dermatological disease on the internet. J Dermatol 34:375–380
56. Demiris G, Speedie SM, Hicks LL (2004) Assessment of patients' acceptance of and satisfaction with teledermatology. J Med Syst 28:575–579
57. Williams TL, Esmail A, May CR et al (2001) Patient satisfaction with teledermatology is related to perceived quality of life. Br J Dermatol 145:911–917
58. Weinstock MA, Nguyen FQ, Risica PM (2002) Patient and referring provider satisfaction with teledermatology. J Am Acad Dermatol 47:68–72
59. Williams T, May C, Esmail A et al (2001) Patient satisfaction with store-and-forward teledermatology. J Telemed Telecare 7(Suppl 1):45–46
60. Van den Akker TW, Reker CH, Knol A et al (2001) Teledermatology as a tool for communication between general practitioners and dermatologists. J Telemed Telecare 7: 193–198
61. Oakley AM, Duffill MB, Reeve P (1998) Practicing dermatology via telemedicine. N Z Med J 111:296–299
62. Whited JD (2006) Teledermatology research review. Int J Dermatol 45:220–229

Skin Cancer Telemedicine

14

David Moreno-Ramirez and Lara Ferrandiz

Core Messages

- The special characteristics of dermatology have turned telemedicine into a feasible methodology to deliver dermatologic care in areas where in-person specialized consultations are difficult or in those clinical settings in which transmitted pictures and clinical information allow a remote dermatologist to make management decisions.
- Skin cancer offers additional advantages for telemedicine management (lower clinical information needed to make decisions, high quality pictures from single lesions, possibility to make decision on the referral to the skin cancer clinic, etc.).
- The triage of skin cancer patients through telemedicine has been evaluated with excellent results in terms of diagnostic accuracy, effectiveness, and efficiency.
- The preoperative management of skin cancer patients through telemedicine has been also implemented and tested with favorable results.
- Telemedicine may also be of help in managing skin cancer patients not suitable for surgical treatment (i.e. topical immunomodifiers).
- The use of telemedicine in skin cancer clinics is supported by levels of evidence Ib-IIa, with strength of recommendations of A-B.

Introduction

Telemedicine can be defined as the use of telecommunication technologies to provide medical information and services [1]. Non-melanoma skin cancer (NMSC) is the most common group of neoplastic conditions in humans whose incidence has been rising worldwide over the last several decades. According to recent reports, the incidence rates of NMSC are 2,074 cases of basal cell carcinoma per 100,000 inhabitants/year in Australian males and 65 cases of squamous cell carcinoma per 100,000 Americans/year [2]. In Spain, the incidence of non-melanoma skin cancer ranges from 71.4 to 158.5 patients/100,000 inhabitants/year, the highest incidence rates corresponding to male patients living in rural areas.

Pigmented lesion and skin cancer clinics (PLC and SCC) have been set up at reference hospitals over the last decades in an attempt to provide general practitioners (GPs) with a direct referral system for patients with skin growths suspicious of cancer. Theoretically, this approach would improve the early diagnosis and treatment of malignant melanoma and NMSC, which is of utmost importance for patients' prognosis. In that

D. Moreno-Ramirez (✉) • L. Ferrandiz
Skin Cancer and Teledermatology Clinic, Dermatology Department, Hospital Universitario Virgen Macarena, Seville, Spain
e-mail: dmoreno@e-derma.org; lferrandiz@e-derma.org

H.P. Soyer et al. (eds.), *Telemedicine in Dermatology*,
DOI 10.1007/978-3-642-20801-0_14, © Springer-Verlag Berlin Heidelberg 2012

sense, these specialized clinics have demonstrated an increased diagnostic accuracy when compared with general dermatology clinics or non-dermatology specialists [3, 4]. However PLCs, and in many cases SCCs, are busy clinics. Public health campaigns on skin cancer and sun protection have led to a general concern about moles resulting in an increased attendance at dermatology departments. As a consequence of this public interest, the evaluation of patients having benign lesions actually represents an important burden of the workload of those clinics with no established filtering or triage systems.

The special characteristics of dermatology, a morphological discipline based on visual diagnosis, along with the advances on digital imaging and internet transmission have turned teledermatology (TD) into a rather feasible, accurate and reliable methodology to make remote decisions on patients. Moreover, different studies have demonstrated that TD is more suitable for the diagnosis and management of circumscribed lesions than for generalized dermatoses, with sensitivities ranging from 0.82 to 1.00, and specificities between 0.62 and 1.00 for the remote diagnosis of skin cancer [5–9]. Thus, the transmission of digital pictures and clinical information between the primary care center (PCC) and the PLC or SCC would provide the dermatologists with enough information to manage patients with suspicious skin growths.

Teledermatology for Skin Cancer Patients Methodologies and Applications

Teledermatology applications for skin cancer patients may be based on two different methodologies, the asynchronous or store-and-forward teledermatology (SFTD), and the synchronous or real-time teledermatology. In **SFTD**, digital pictures of skin tumors or pigmented lesions together with clinical data from the patients are transmitted to a remote dermatologist via internet or intranet; the participants, the GP and the dermatologist, are separated by time and space, which means one of the main advantage of this methodology. In contrast, **real-time TD** uses videoconferencing equipment to permit a live and direct interaction between the remote dermatologist, the patient and the GP; thus, the in vivo interaction between the participant allows the dermatologist a more comprehensive collection of clinical information which indeed means the main advantages of this methodology (Table 14.1) [2, 3].

Table 14.1 Advantages and disadvantages of store-and-forward and real-time telemedicine for skin cancer

Store-and-forward	Real time
Less time-consuming	More time-consuming
High quality pictures (digital photography)	Video quality
High quality dermoscopic pictures possible	High quality dermoscopy not possible
Clinical information limited to standard forms	Possibility to get additional clinical information directly from the patient
Dermatologist, GP and patient do not need to communicate at the same time	Dermatologist, GP and patient do need to communicate at the same time
More appropriate as a triage tool	Probably more appropriate as a diagnose-and-treat facility
Lower cost of the equipments and time	Difficult to organize

Store-and-Forward Teledermatology for Skin Cancer Triage

A specific application of TD, which has been repeatedly tested, involves the use of store-and-forward systems for the management of patients' referral in skin cancer clinics. The fact that less clinical information is needed to make decisions about skin growths (compared to generalized dermatoses), the high quality that digital transmitted pictures may provide in tumoral lesions, and the diagnostic advantage of dermatologists against non-dermatologist physicians when dealing with skin cancer, have been argued in favor of the implementation of such dermatologist-directed triage systems [1, 3, 4]. For a better understanding of these systems it must be emphasized that the main goal of TD triage applications is not to reach clear-cut diagnosis but to make decisions on the need for a patient to be referred to a face-to-face skin cancer clinic. After the evaluation of teleconsultations, those patients having suspicious or already malignant lesions would be immediately referred to the face-to-face clinic whereas patients having clear-cut benign lesions would directly discharged by the GP without unnecessary travels to the hospital.

The University Hospital Virgen Macarena (UHVM) TD Network Experience

A SFTD system aimed at the triage of patients with suspicious skin growths was implemented at the UHVM skin cancer clinic in 2003 [6, 10]. The TD facility is available for 31 PCCs which cover a total population of 550,000 inhabitants of a southern Spain province with living distances from 5 to 100 km to the hospital. The technical basis of the facility was rather straightforward; digital pictures (1600×1200 pixels, Nikon Coolpix® 4300), and clinical information taken by the GP at the PCC are uploaded to a web framework supported by the intranet of the regional public health system (ATM, ISDR-B and Frame Relay/ADSL networks) using standardized forms (Fig. 14.1a, b); after the evaluation of the pictures and clinical information by a remote dermatologist at the skin cancer clinic, a decision and management report is written to be downloaded by the GP. Since the application is aimed at the triage of skin cancer patients, the management decision always involves the referral or not-referral of the patient to an in-person visit at the Skin Cancer Clinic of the UHVM. Those patients having suspicious or malignant lesions are directly referred to the SCC, whereas patients presenting clear-cut benign lesions are directly managed by the GP with no need of hospital visits (Figs. 14.2 and 14.3). Seven years after the setting up of the system, TD has turned into an essential complementary tool for the daily practice at the skin cancer clinic with an average number of 450 teleconsultations evaluated per month.

TD for Skin Cancer Triage: Outcomes

Teledermatology as a tool for the triage of skin cancer patients' has undergone a deep evaluation in terms of effectiveness as a referral system, diagnostic performance of transmitted pictures of skin cancer, and also from an economic point of view.

Regarding the effectiveness of TD triage systems for skin cancer, the lack of quantifiable clinical endpoints that may be applied to this clinical setting (i.e. mortality and quality of life) has led to the consideration of intermediate clinical outcomes (i.e. consultations avoided, time to intervention, and consultation time requirements) as the most descriptive outcome indicators [11]. Thus, the studies that have evaluated TD triage of skin cancer have reported mean waiting intervals between 2 and 50 days for against the 88–137 waiting days for the conventional letter referral [12–14]. In the UHVM network, the patients referred to the in-person clinic were attended within the following 2 weeks (mean time = 12.31 days) since they first visited the general practitioner [6, 10].

Another secondary endpoint evaluated in TD triage systems has been the capability of the teleconsultation to avoid unnecessary face-to-face hospital visits. In previous studies, in-person evaluations avoided have ranged between 44% and 82% for real-time TD systems. At the UHVM network, the store-and-forward teleconsultation has demonstrated a filtering rate of 51%, with 49% of patients being referred to the face-to-face hospital visit.

A pre-requisite for TD to be effective in triaging skin cancer patients is an acceptable reliability and diagnostic performance of internet transmitted clinical pictures. In this regard, simple agreement percentages ranging from 55% to 100% have been reported for biopsy decisions in SFTD-based skin cancer triage systems [10, 15, 16]. TD has also disclosed excellent agreement, or diagnostic concordance, as compared to face-to-face consultations, with kappa statistic of 0.81 in one prospective series [6]. Regarding validity of TD as a triage tool for skin cancer, the few studies available have also yielded sensitivities between 0.90 and 1, and specificities between 0.62 and 1.00 [6, 10, 15, 16].

For a better performance of this type of TD based triage systems the application of stringent inclusion criteria is mandatory. In the case of the UHVM network, the GPs were trained in a set of criteria that yielded the best results for the decision making process (Table 14.2). Other clinical situations were proven not suitable for teleconsultation as clinical pictures and information transmitted were not enough to make decisions. This is the case of patients having multiple melanocytic lesions, or congenital nevi, who need a comprehensive anamnesis and physical and dermoscopic examination, or even digital mapping or counseling which makes them not suitable for an effective teleconsultation.

Skin cancer triage through TD has also been demonstrated as an efficient approach to deal with patients' referrals in skin cancer clinics, also yielding a clear economical advantage against the conventional letter referral. In the cost-effectiveness analysis conducted at the HUVM TD network the unit cost for patients attended through TD was 79.78€ per patient against 129.37€ per patient managed through the conventional circuit ($p < 0.005$). The cost ratio between SFTD and conventional care was of 1.62. The Spearman correlation test also yielded an inverse relation between the unit cost in each participating center and the number of teleconsultations transmitted from each primary care center ($p < 0.001$) [17]. TD resulted in a more cost-effective, or dominant, methodology. Thus, from an economic point of view, it may be concluded that in a public health system equipped with intranet or

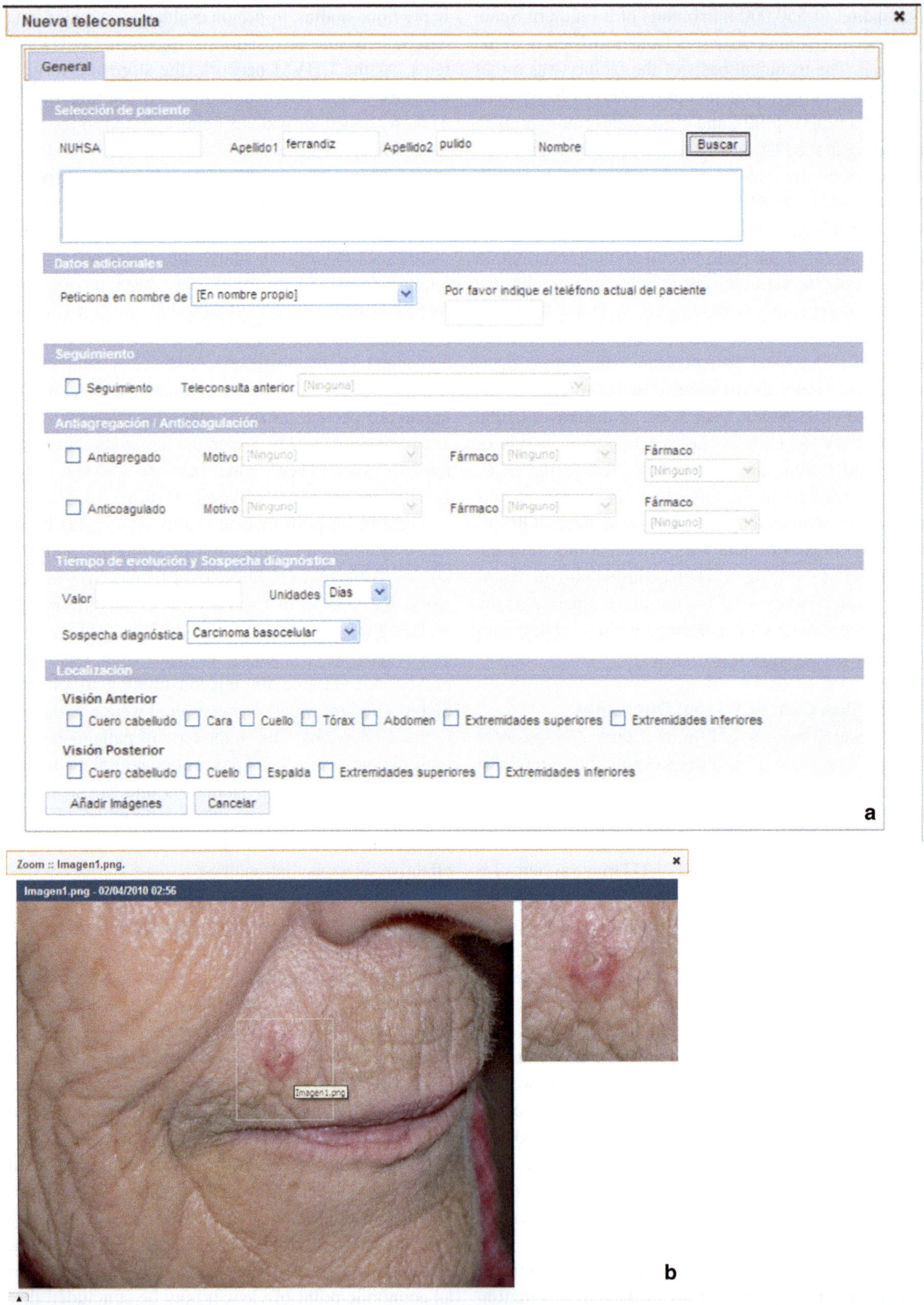

Fig. 14.1 Standardized web form for teleconsultation. (**a**) Clinical items to be fulfilled by the GP. (**b**) Picture inserted in the form to be evaluated by the remote dermatologist

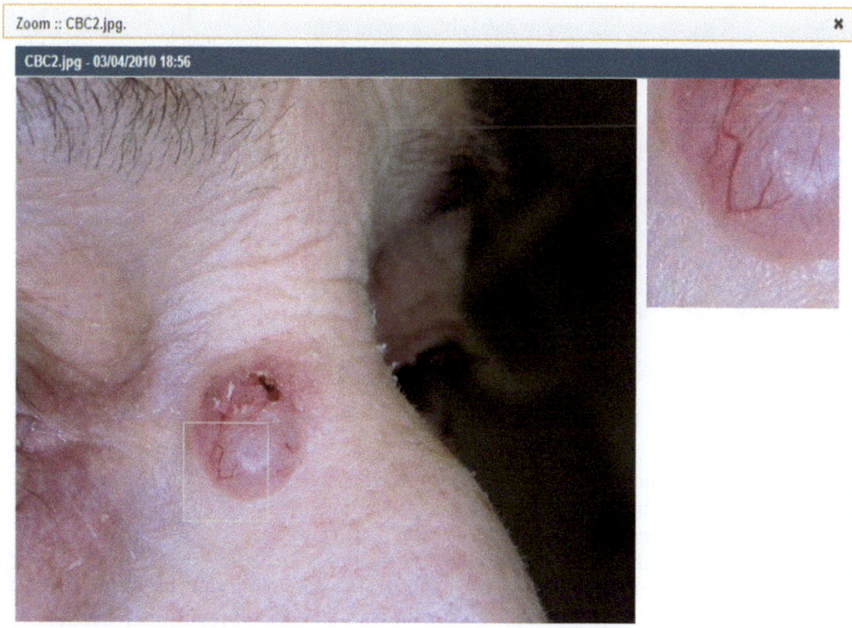

Fig. 14.2 Teleconsultation of a 77-year-old woman with a 3-year history lesion on the nose. Teleconsultation diagnosis: basal cell carcinoma. Management: referred to the skin cancer clinic, or presurgical teledermatology

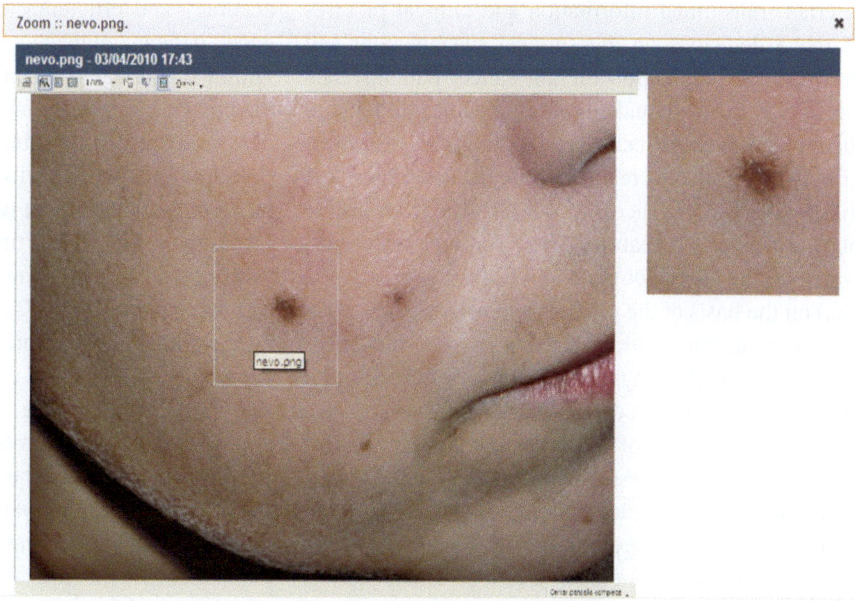

Fig. 14.3 Teleconsultation of a 26-year-old woman with a 10-year history pigmented lesion on the cheek. Teleconsultation diagnosis: common acquired melanocytic nevus. Management: not referred to the skin cancer clinic

Table 14.2 Inclusion and exclusion criteria for triage of skin cancer through teledermatology

Inclusion criteria	Exclusion criteria[a]
• Circumscribed cutaneous lesion suspicious of skin cancer	• Congenital nevus
	• Multiple melanocytic lesions
	• Lesions on hairy areas
• Changing or recent evolution cutaneous lesion	• Ungueal lesions
	• Mucosal lesions

University Hospital Virgen Macarena Teledermatology Network

[a]Exclusion criteria does not mean that the patient is not suitable for in-person dermatology consultation

internet networks the routine use of SFTD in skin cancer clinics is a cost-effective methodology to manage with patients' referrals.

Presurgical Teledermatology for Skin Cancer Patients

Store-and-forward TD may represent a suitable tool for the routine practice in dermatologic surgery units. Presurgical teledermatology involves the use of

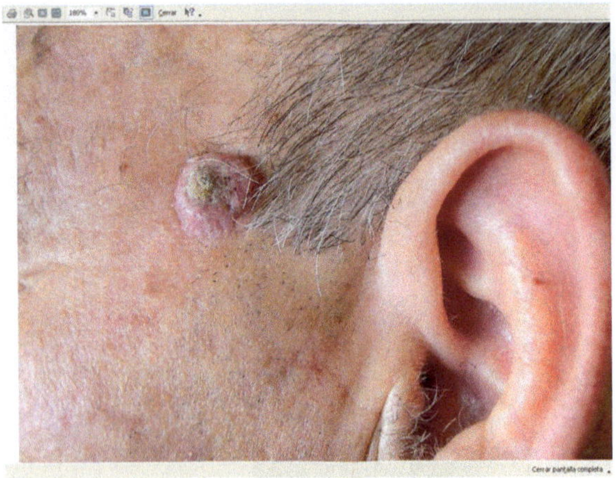

Fig. 14.4 Teleconsultation of a 63 year-old man with a 6-month history lesion on the temple. Teleconsultation diagnosis: keratoacanthoma. Management: presurgical teledermatology. This teleconsultation is enough to decide the need for surgical excision under local anesthesia and to plan a possible closure through a Limberg flap

Table 14.3 Inclusion and exclusion criteria for presurgical teledermatology skin cancer management

Inclusion criteria	Exclusion criteria
• Clear-cut diagnosis of skin cancer through teleconsultation	• No clear-cut diagnosis of skin cancer • Benign lesions
• Skin cancer suitable to be excised under local anesthesia	• Tumor or patient suitable for surgery under general anesthesia or under anesthesiologist support
• Special consideration for patients with physical limitations, confined to bed, resident in institutions or from remote areas	• Severe comorbidity that merits a careful evaluation

internet transmitted information and clinical pictures to make decisions on the surgical management and preoperative preparation of skin cancer patients. The capability of store-and-forward teleconsultations to distinguish between benign and malignant cutaneous growths, and also to reach in many cases a clear-cut diagnosis of skin cancer allows the dermatologist to plan the surgical treatment (i.e. surgical technique, type of anesthesia, outpatient vs. inpatient surgery, etc.) on the basis of the pictures and information transmitted via intranet with no need of pre-operative hospital visits [18–20] (Figs. 14.2 and 14.4). With this aim presurgical TD does specially work for patients with a clear-cut diagnosis of non-melanoma skin cancer (basal cell carcinoma, squamous cell carcinoma, etc.), or a fast-growth vascular tumor (i.e. pyogenic granuloma), suitable for surgery under local anesthesia after the evaluation of the teleconsultation. Those lesions expected to need a major reconstruction (i.e. large grafts or flaps), or to be operated on under general anesthesia after the telemedical evaluation represented formal contraindications for the remote presurgical management (Table 14.3). However, despite these apparently self-limiting inclusion criteria 80% of patients with skin cancer are eligible to be managed through presurgical teledermatology. Finally, it should be taken into consideration that a presurgical TD program necessarily relies on the facilities available at the primary care centers like the anticoagulation monitoring program, domiciliary nursing, blood test extraction and web-based platform for blood test results, etc.

Presurgical teledermatology has undergone a comprehensive evaluation as for clinical effectiveness, accuracy and efficiency [20]. In the UHVM experience, patients managed through TD were operated within an average interval of 26.10 days since the first visit to the GP, and with only one visit to the hospital. The average waiting interval of patients managed through the conventional referral system was 60.57 days, with at least two visits to the Dermatology Department before the final intervention. On-the-day surgery cancellations were significantly lower for the TD-managed patients (2.99%) than for patients managed through the conventional referral system (8.85%). Moreover, the accuracy of the teleconsultation to plan the surgical technique was of kappa=0.75 [20]. An economic evaluation of this presurgical teledermatology system has also been completed, and compared with the conventional system. The unit cost of patients managed through TD was of 156.40€, against 278.42€ per patient in the conventional system. The conventional methodology resulted 1.78-fold more expensive than TD. Teledermatology resulted in a more cost-effective intervention, with an incremental cost-effectiveness ratio of 3.10€ saved per patient and waiting day avoided in patients without physical limitations, and of 4.87€ in patients with physical limitations to visit the hospital [21].

As the results of this experience suggest, one of the most remarkable advantages of presurgical TD is the avoidance of unnecessary visits to the hospital, which specially applies to patients with physical limitations,

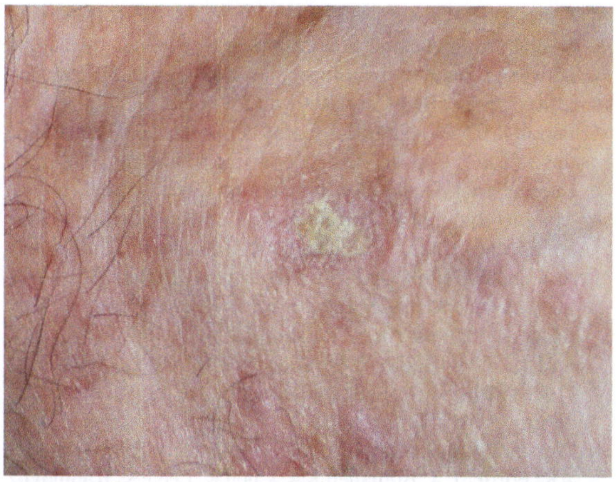

Fig. 14.5 Clinical picture transmitted showing a clear-cut actinic keratosis

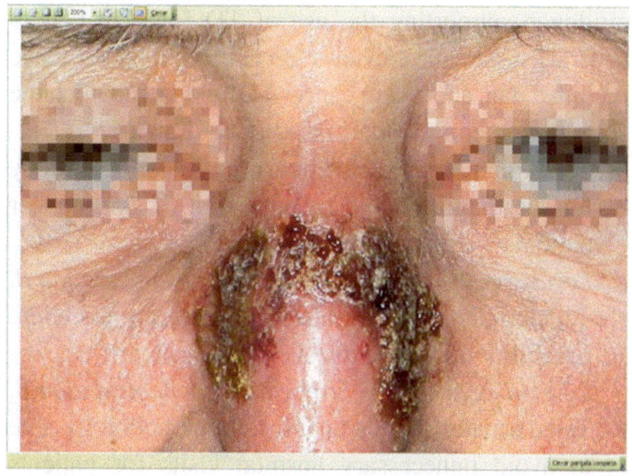

Fig. 14.6 Teleconsultation showing severe local irritation by topical imiquimod

confined to bed or resident in institutions. Presurgical TD has also demonstrated to be a more cost-effective intervention than the conventional presurgical management in health services equipped with communication networks. However, the success of this multidisciplinary approach relies on a close collaboration with the GP and nurses working at primary care centers. If this pre-requisite is fulfilled, SFTD may also be considered a suitable tool for the routine practice in dermatologic surgery units aimed at the improvement of the standards of care of skin cancer patients.

Teledermatology for the Non-Surgical Treatment of Skin Cancer Patients

The frequency of actinic keratoses (AK) is directly related to cumulative sun exposure, mainly in patients older than 50 years with outdoor occupations. These factors come together in patients living in rural areas, which makes AK a prevalent condition in these settings, with rates from 11% to 26% in the United States [22].

The prescription and monitoring of topical immune response modifiers (imiquimod) in patients having AK may also be readily carried out through SFTD (Fig. 14.5). In these patients, once a clear-cut diagnosis of actinic keratosis is made, and the suitability of topical treatment established, a teleconsultation report with the diagnosis and detailed instructions about how to apply imiquimod is uploaded or sent via intranet to the GP to be explained to the patient. Two-four weeks after the completion of the treatment the patient is attended at the face-to-face clinic to evaluate the clinical response.

The main aim of this approach is to avoid a first visit to the dermatologist in those cases of clear-cut AK suitable for treatment with 5% imiquimod cream, an approach specially beneficial for patients with physical limitations or living in remote areas. A close monitoring of side effects of imiquimod is also possible through teleconsultation since digital pictures from patients presenting irritation are readily evaluated (Fig. 14.6).

However, this interesting application of TD does not lack limitations. Clinical response after the completion of the topical therapy is not properly evaluated through teleconsultation. Thus, despite TD may avoid the first visit, and further visits related to side effect of the imiquimod cream, all the patients on imiquimod will finally visit the skin cancer clinic. Another controversial issue of TD for AK patients is the difficult management of cancerization field through TD. These limitations have led us to restrict this use of TD to patients with special difficulties to visit the hospital.

Evidence About Teledermatology for Skin Cancer

Despite the many studies published in recent years about teledermatology, the wide variety of TD methodologies, clinical applications, and outcome measures analyzed hinder the interpretation of the results available. In an attempt to find out the real evidence supporting the use of TD for skin cancer several systematic reviews recently published have included data about skin cancer TD, and from which the following recommendations may be drawn [23–26]:

- Teledermatology has demonstrated a good accuracy for the diagnosis and management of skin cancer patients
  Level of evidence IIa. Strength of recommendation B.
- Teledermatology has demonstrated an excellent reliability for the diagnosis of skin cancer
  Level of evidence IIa. Strength of recommendation B.
- Teledermatology is a health care methodology able to avoid unnecessary hospital visits for patients with cutaneous growths
  Level of evidence Ib. Strength of recommendation A.
- Teledermatology is a health care methodology able to shorten waiting periods to final intervention for skin cancer patients
  Level of evidence Ib. Strength of recommendation A.
- Teledermatology is an accurate methodology for the preoperative management of skin cancer patients
  Level of evidence IIa. Strength of recommendation B.
- Presurgical teledermatology is effective in avoiding unnecessary pre-operative visits for skin cancer patients
  Level of evidence IIa. Strength of recommendation B.
- In health services equipped with communication networks, teledermatology is a cost-effective approach for the management of patients' referral in skin cancer clinics
  Level of evidence Ib. Strength of recommendation A.
- In health services equipped with communication networks, teledermatology is a cost-effective approach for the preoperative management of skin cancer patients
  Level of evidence IIa. Strength of recommendation B.

Conflict of Interest None declared.

References

1. Eedy DJ, Wootton R (2001) Teledermatology: a review. Br J Dermatol 144:696–707
2. Rigel DS, Cockerell CJ, Carucci J, Wharton J (2008) Actinic keratosis, basal cell carcinoma and squamous cell carcinoma. In: Bolognia JL, Jorizzo JL, Rapini RP (eds) Dermatology. Mosby Elsevier, St. Louis
3. Jorizzo JL, Phillips CM, Balch DC, Schanz SJ, Branigan AE (2002) Teledermatology: issues in remote diagnosis and management of cutaneous disease. Curr Probl Dermatol 14:5–38
4. Osborne JE, Chave TA, Hutchinson PE (2003) Comparison of diagnostic accuracy for cutaneous malignant melanoma between general dermatology, plastic surgery and pigmented lesion clinics. Br J Dermatol 148:252–258
5. Parkin MD, Whelan SL, Ferlay J, Teppo L, Thomas DB (eds) (2002) Cancer incidence in five continents, IIIth edn. International Agency for Research on Cancer, Lyon
6. Moreno-Ramirez D, Ferrandiz L, Nieto-Garcia A, Carrasco R, Moreno-Alvarez P, Galdeano R, Bidegain E, Rios-Martin JJ, Camacho FM (2007) Store-and-forward teledermatology in skin cancer triage. Experience and evaluation of 2009 teleconsultations. Arch Dermatol 143:479–484
7. Phillips CM, Burke WA, Allen MH, Stone D, Wilson JL (1998) Reliability of telemedicine in evaluating skin tumors. Telemed J 4:5–7
8. Warshaw EM, Lederle FA, Grill JP, Gravely AA, Bangerter AK, Fortier LA, Bohjanen KA, Chen K, Lee PK, Rabinovitz HS, Johr RH, Kaye VN, Bowers S, Wenner R, Askari SK, Kedrowski DA, Nelson DB (2009) Accuracy of teledermatology for nonpigmented neoplasms. J Am Acad Dermatol 60:579–588
9. Shapiro M, James WD, Kessler R, Lazorik FC, Katz KA, Tam J et al (2004) Comparison of skin biopsy triage decisions in 49 patients with pigmented lesions and skin neoplasms: store-and-forward teledermatology versus face-to-face dermatology. Arch Dermatol 140:525–528
10. Moreno-Ramirez D, Ferrandiz L, Perez-Bernal AM, Carrasco R, Rios JJ, Camacho F (2005) Teledermatology as a filtering system in pigmented lesion clinics. J Telemed Telecare 11:298–303
11. Whited JD (2007) Summary of the Status of Teledermatology Research. Center for Health Services Research in Primary Care, VA Medical Center, Durham, NC
12. Whited JD, Hall RP, Foy ME et al (2002) Teledermatology's impact on time to intervention among referrals to a dermatology consult service. Telemed J E Health 8:313–321
13. Krupinski E, Barker G, Rodriguez G et al (2002) Telemedicine versus in-person dermatology referrals: an analysis of case complexity. Telemed J 8:143–147
14. Taylor P, Goldsmith P, Murray K, Harris D, Barkley A (2001) Evaluating a telemedicine system to assist in the management of teledermatology referrals. Br J Dermatol 144:328–333
15. Lewis K, Gilmour E, Harrison PV, Patefield S, Dickinson Y, Manning D et al (1999) Digital teledermatology for skin tumors: a preliminary assessment using a receiver operating characteristics (ROC) analysis. J Telemed Telecare 5(Suppl 1):57–58
16. Ohran Oztas M, Calikoglu E, Baz K, Birol A, Onder M, Calikoglu T et al (2004) Reliability of web-based teledermatology consultations. J Telemed Telecare 10:25–28
17. Moreno-Ramirez D, Ferrandiz L, Ruiz-de-Casas A, Nieto-Garcia A, Moreno P, Galdeano R, Camacho FM (2009) Economic evaluation of a store-and-forward teledermatology system for skin cancer patients. J Telemed Telecare 15(1):40–45
18. Eadie LH, Seifalian AM, Davidson BR (2003) Telemedicine in surgery. Br J Surg 90:647–658
19. Board of Governors of the Society of American Gastrointestinal Endoscopic Surgeons (1997) Guidelines for the surgical practice of telemedicine. Surg Endosc 11: 789–792

20. Ferrandiz L, Moreno-Ramirez D, Nieto-Garcia A, Carrasco R, Moreno-Alvarez P, Galdeano R, Bidegain E, Rios-Martin JJ, Camacho F (2007) Teledermatology-based presurgical management for non-melanoma skin cancer: a pilot study. Dermatol Surg 33:1092–1098
21. Ferrandiz L, Moreno-Ramirez D, Ruiz-de-Casas A, Nieto-Garcia A, Moreno P, Galdeano R, Camacho FM (2008) An economic analysis of presurgical teledermatology in patients with nonmelanoma skin cancer. Actas Dermosifiliogr 99:795–802
22. Salasche SJ (2000) Epidemiology of actinic keratoses and squamous cell carcinoma. J Am Acad Dermatol 42(1 Pt 2):4–7
23. Massone C, Wurm EM, Hofmann-Wellenhof R, Soyer HP (2008) Teledermatology: an update. Semin Cutan Med Surg 27:101–105
24. Moreno-Ramirez D, Ferrandiz L, Nieto-Garcia A, Villegas-Portero R (2008) Teledermatology. Med Clin (Barc) 130:496–503
25. Romero G, Cortina P, Vera E (2008) Telemedicine and teledermatology (II): current state of research on dermatology teleconsultations. Actas Dermosifiliogr 99:586–597
26. Whited JD (2006) Teledermatology research review. Int J Dermatol 45:220–229

Real-Life Teledermatology Cases

15

Eshini Perera, Cathy Xu, and Shobhan Manoharan

Core Messages

- Junior doctors and non specialist practitioners often have difficulties diagnosing and managing skin conditions.
- The discrepancy in the distribution of dermatology specialists has resulted in significant waiting times for outpatient appointments.
- Teledermatology is an accurate and reliable way to diagnosis dermatological conditions.
- A field trial of a telederm proforma demonstrates five successful cases of teledermatology.

Introduction

Dermatological complaints make up roughly 25% of medical visits [1]. This often presents as a problem as there is a large discrepancy between the number of dermatologists in most metropolitan hospitals compared to both private and public non metropolitan hospitals [2]. The discrepancy in distribution of specialists has resulted in a significant waiting time for dermatology outpatient appointments, which moreover are related often with immense travel costs given the particular geographic situation in Australia. Concurrently, in undergraduate medical courses there is a lack of dermatology training in Australia, with less than 40 hours being taught [1]. This has resulted in junior doctors and non-specialist practitioners having every so often difficulties in diagnosis and management of dermatologic conditions. Many primary care providers often find it difficult to determine the nature of skin complaints and as a consequence skin ailments are often not efficiently managed.

Given the highly visual nature of skin diseases teledermatology has become an extremely accurate and reliable resource in diagnosis skin diseases [3, 4]. A recent analysis has shown that accuracy rates ranged from 30% to 92% for clinical dermatologists and from 19% to 95% for teledermatologists [5]. The diagnostic agreement rate between teledermatologists and clinic-based dermatologists is in the range of 41–94% in complete agreement and 50–100% in partial agreement [6]. Clinical management agreement rates between teledermatologists and clinic dermatologists have revealed similar high agreement rates.

Process

A field trial is currently ongoing at the Dermatology Department of the Princess Alexandra Hospital (PAH) in Brisbane based on the protocol of a recent study carried out in collaboration with the Emergency and Dermatology Department at the PAH [7]. A primary care physician completes our Telederm proforma (Table 15.1) which requires a brief history about the

E. Perera (✉) • C. Xu
Princess Alexandra Hospital, Queensland Health, Brisbane, QLD, Australia
e-mail: eshini_perera@health.qld.gov.au; c.xu@uq.edu.au

S. Manoharan
Westside Dermatologist, Brisbane, QLD, Australia

Department of Dermatology, Princess Alexandra Hospital, Brisbane, QLD, Australia
e-mail: info@westderm.com.au

H.P. Soyer et al. (eds.), *Telemedicine in Dermatology*,
DOI 10.1007/978-3-642-20801-0_15, © Springer-Verlag Berlin Heidelberg 2012

Table 15.1 Telederm proforma

		Place Patient Label Here
Patient ID number:	**DOB:**	**Sex:** ☐ Male ☐ Female
History of presenting complaint:		
Duration:		
Progression:		
Associated symptoms (e.g. Itch, fever, arthralgia, malaise):		
Results of any investigations (e.g. blood/urine tests, biopsies, x-rays):		
Treatment to date:		
General medical history:		
Surgical:		
Medications: (including prescribed, non-prescribed, over the counter drug, natural, intermittent and regular, also alcohol/ taobacco/ illicit drugs) and chronology		
Allergies:		
Occupation/Pastimes:		
Exposure to animals:		
Overseas travel:		
Examination:		
Diagnoses:		
1. Emergency Department:		
2. Teledermatology:		
Differential diagnosis:		
3. Biopsy performed:	☐ No ☐ Yes	
	Results:	
4. Face-to-Face consultation:		

Please attach images showing the extent of the eruption i.e. we need to know where it isn't as well as where it is. Good quality close ups are essential. If any pathology present please send images. They need to be clearly labelled as to site and patient. If possible send images that do not allow patient identification.

presenting complaint, the examination, results of any investigations performed, current treatments and general medical history. The patient's skin lesions are then photographed with a variety of digital cameras including Sony Cybershot DSC-P73, a Canon PowerShot G9, a Canon Digital IXUS 85 IS and a Panasonic Lumix DMC-TZ3. This information is then send to a secure mail server and automatically forwarded to a dermatologist who is notified via mobile phone or email alert. The dermatologist suggests a provisional diagnosis and a differential diagnosis if appropriate and provides management recommendation via telephone or email. In case it is necessary follow-up consultations are performed within 1–2 weeks at a public dermatology department.

The five cases presented below are examples of patients managed successfully using this protocol.

Teledermatology Cases

Case 1: Morbus Darier with Superimposed Generalised Herpes Simplex Infection (Kapoi's Varicelliform Eruption)

Clinical Scenario

A 47-year-old female with a known history of Darier's disease presented to the Emergency Department with an eruption on her chest and back which was becoming increasingly painful (Fig. 15.1a, b). The patient was taking 50 mg of Acitiretin for her Darier's disease and she had been recently reviewed at another hospital 1 month ago and had subsequently commenced flucloxacillin with no improvement. The patient reported having fevers at home but was afebrile on presentation. The treating doctor was concerned that the patient had an acute flare of Darier's disease with a superimposed bacterial infection resistant to the antibiotic treatment. Investigations initially undertaken in the Emergency Department included a FBE (WCC 11.2 and CRP 7.1) and bacterial/viral swabs which were pending.

Teledermatology Report

The reply was sent by a consultant dermatologist (who was in Italy at the time) within 1 h. The provisional diagnosis of generalized Herpes simplex infection commonly referred to as Kaposi's varicelliform eruption was made and admission of the patient for intravenous antivirals, antibiotics and topical therapy was recommended.

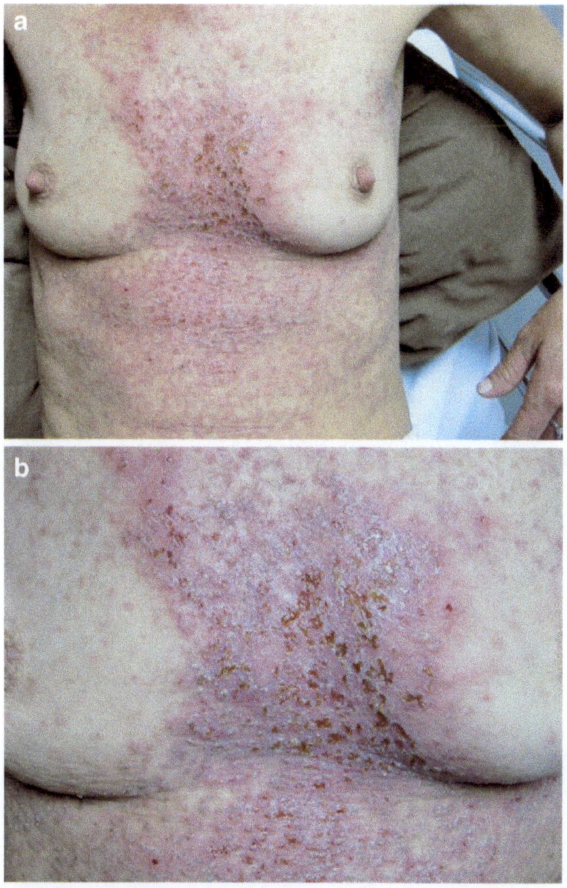

Fig. 15.1 (**a**) Images submitted for diagnosis. Note the crusted erosions present over the sternum. (**b**) Close up of sternum

Further Management and Outcome

The viral swab, PCR and bacterial swab were positive for HSV type I and staphylococcus aureus. The patient was admitted to the ward and treated with intravenous acyclovir and flucloxacillin as well as adequate topical treatment. Outpatient follow-up revealed that the rash has settled down with residual signs of Darier's. She was advised to continue taking Acitretin and return for a review in 3 months.

Comment

This case highlights how dermatological emergencies can be diagnosed and managed rapidly and efficiently by non-dermatologic medical staff through an online consultation process.

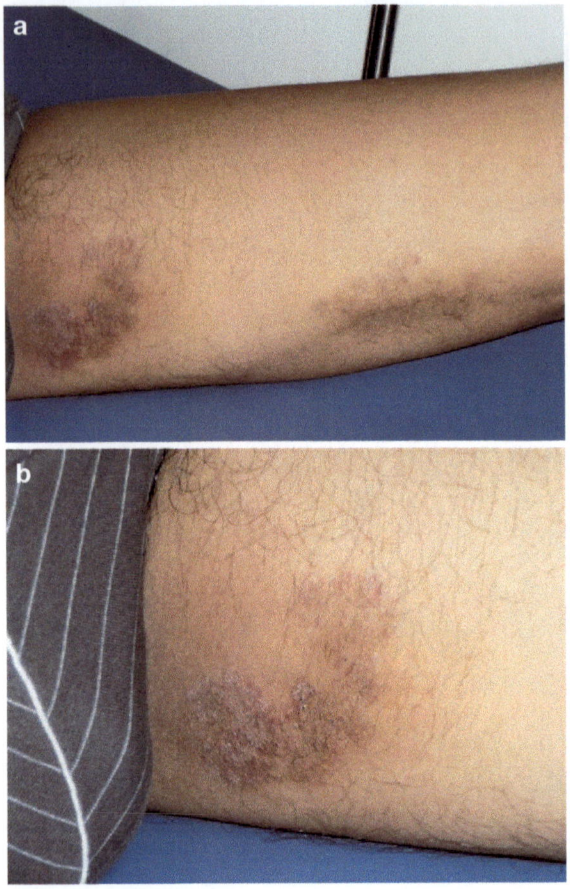

Fig. 15.2 (a) Rather well demarcated erythrosquamous plaques on thigh with evidence of postinflammatory hyperpigmentation. (b) Close-up of brown colored plaque on the left thigh. Note the scale and definite border

Case 2: Tinea Corporis and Pedis

Clinical Scenario

A 22 year old Nepalese male presented to the Emergency Department with a 2 month history of a progressively worsening pruritic rash on the dorsum of his right foot, thigh and groin (Fig. 15.2a, b). A diagnosis was not provided.

Teledermatology Report

The consultant diagnosed tinea corporis as provisional diagnosis and subacute eczema and lichen simplex chronicus as the differential diagnoses. He suggested performing skin scrapings in search for fungal elements by microscopy and culture. The patient, however, had already been discharged from the Emergency Department without any treatment and a Dermatology outpatient follow-up appointment.

Further Management and Outcome

The follow-up examination revealed a well circumscribed scaly plaque on the groin, thighs and right foot. Skin scrapings of both the right foot and groin were performed. Trichophyton rubrum was cultured in both areas. The patient was prescribed terbinafine cream twice daily and advised to visit his GP for further follow-up. The patient was contacted per telephone 1 month after the outpatient appointment and he reported that the rash on his foot and groin had cleared following the terbinafine cream.

Comment

This case underlines the relevance of a teledermatology service for Emergency and non-specialist Outpatient Departments for subacute/chronic skin conditions.

Case 3: Amoxicillin-Induced Drug Eruption

Clinical Scenario

A 55-year-old female presented to the emergency department with a 2 week history of a pruritic widespread erythematous rash over the forearms, legs, abdomen, thighs and back (Fig. 15.3a, b). She had no lip swelling or airway compromise. The patient had been treated with prednisolone 50 mg for the last 3 days, celestone M cream and phenergan which had minimal effect on the rash. The patient was treated 4 weeks prior with amoxicillin for an ear infection and had developed a rash around her face after completing the first course. She ceased amoxicillin 1 week prior to presentation. Her other regular medications included: Olmesartan and perindopril. No investigations were undertaken in the emergency department and the treating doctor was concerned that the patient had developed a drug reaction to penicillin.

Teledermatology Report

Despite relatively poor image quality the diagnosis of amoxicillin-induced drug eruption was considered as the most likely diagnosis by the virtual consultant. On the advice of the dermatologist the patient was discharged home with oral Keflex and oral prednisolone, promethazine and a potent topical steroid cream.

Further Management and Outcome

She was reviewed in Dermatology Outpatient clinic 3 days later. By this time her rash was nearly completely gone and her pruritis had resolved. She was weaned of her course of prednisolone.

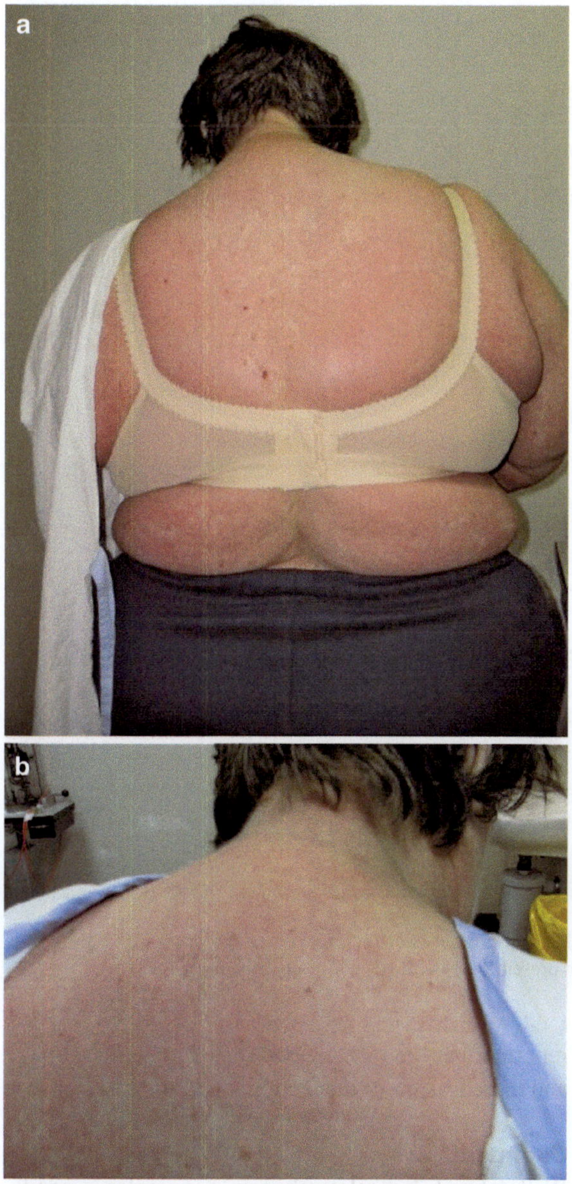

Fig. 15.3 (**a**) A 55-year-old female with an extensive erythematous rash with indistinct borders on her back. (**b**) Close up of rash on the back

Comment

Teledermatology supports emergency doctors with the diagnosis of the many faces of drug eruptions, some of which are potential life-threatening.

Case 4: Varicella

Clinical Scenario

A 24-year-old male on a background of poorly controlled type 1 diabetes mellitus, presented with a 2-day history of a rash, which began over his scalp and face and progressed to his trunk and mucosa (Fig. 15.4a–d). The patient was vague on the history of his prior immunizations but reported that he had not previously had varicella/zoster. He had not travelled overseas and not been exposed to anyone with a similar rash. On presentation he was afebrile. Bacterial and viral swabs as well as viral serology were undertaken in the Emergency Department. The diagnosis of varicella, however, was not raised. The patient blood results were as follows: FBE: Hb 143, WCC 5.7. Blood glucose level 11.8.

Teledermatology Report

A reply by the teledermatology consultant was sent 20 min later (from Singapore) and the provisional diagnosis of a varicella infection with other viral exanthemas as a differential diagnosis was made. The consultant recommended admission with antiviral treatment consisting of acyclovir or famvir. He also suggested ruling out varicella associated complications including pneumonia and meningitis.

Further Management and Outcome

Varicella DNA was detected on swab PCR and a chest x ray showed scattered reticulo-nodular shadowing suggestive of pneumonitis. The patient was admitted under the endocrine team for diabetic ketoacidosis secondary to a varicella infection. He was commenced on intravenous antivirals, insulin infusion and fluids.

The patient self-discharged against medical advice after 2 days of treatment and no follow-up appointments were made.

Comment

Teledermatology supports emergency doctors with the diagnosis of the many faces of viral exanthemas as exhibited here with the example of varicella infection.

Case 5: Palmoplantar Pustulosis

Clinical Scenario

A 75-year-old female, on a background of Chronic Obstructive Pulmonary Disease and peripheral vascular disease presented to a metropolitan Emergency Department with a 1 month history of a scaly pustular rash on the soles of her feet (Fig. 15.5a, b). The treating doctor was concerned that she had pyoderma. The patient had been treated with Betnovate cream with no resolution of the rash. A swab of the lesion was sent with results pending.

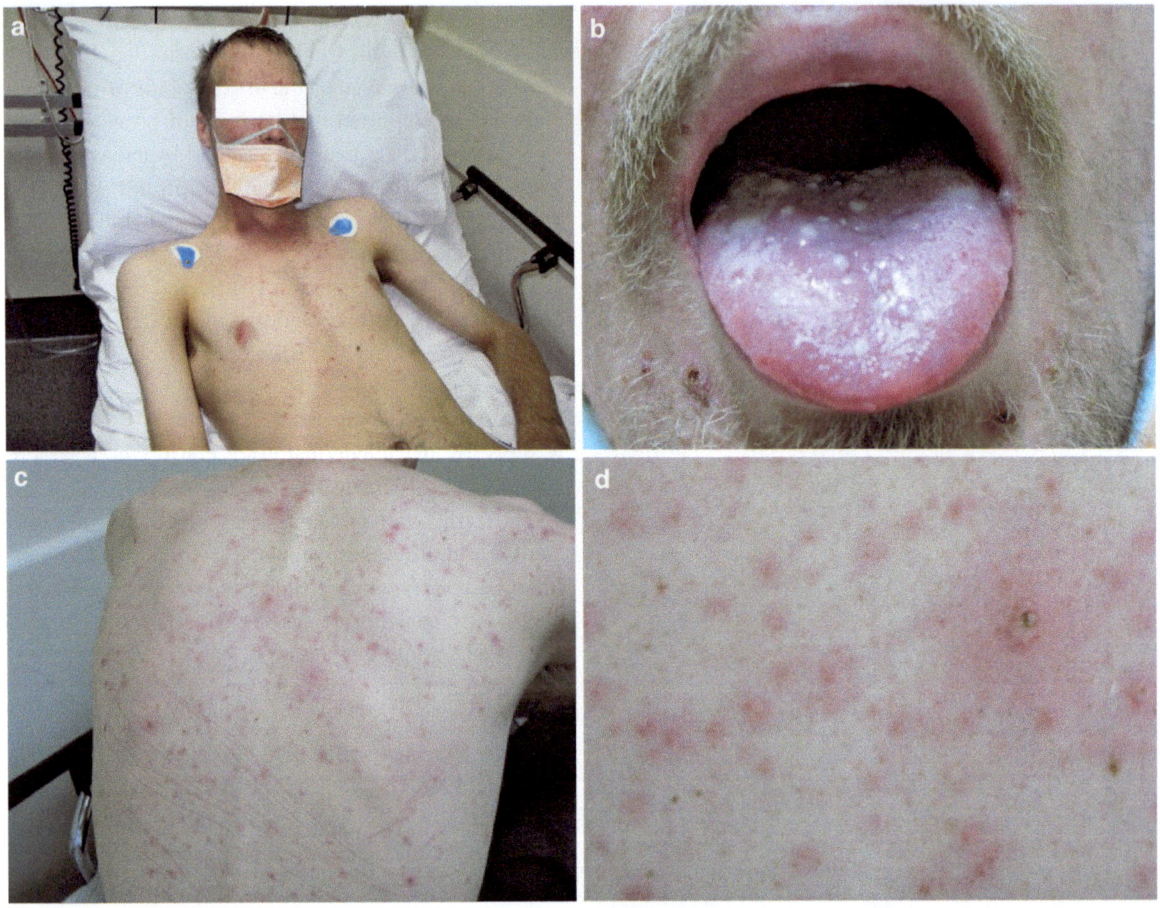

Fig. 15.4 (a) A 24-year-old male with widespread papulovesicular rash present over the face, chest and arms. (b) Close-up of vesicles present on the tongue. (c) Widespread papulovesicular rash present over back. (d) Close-up of back

Teledermatology Report

The reply from the Dermatological registrar was sent several hours later with palmoplantar pustolosis as the provisional diagnosis. She suggested potassium permanganate soaks with topical application of diprosone ointment and paraffin cream to the area. The consultant replied soon after concurring with this diagnosis and management plan.

Further Management and Outcome

Viral and bacterial swabs yielded no growth and a scraping for fungi was negative. The treating doctor reported that the rash cleared completely after 3 days and there was no further follow-up of the rash.

Comment

Well-defined, but relatively rare dermatologic conditions can be diagnosed well by telederm consultations and help to increase the quality of care for patients affected with these specific dermatologic diseases as demonstrated on this example of palmoplantar pustulosis.

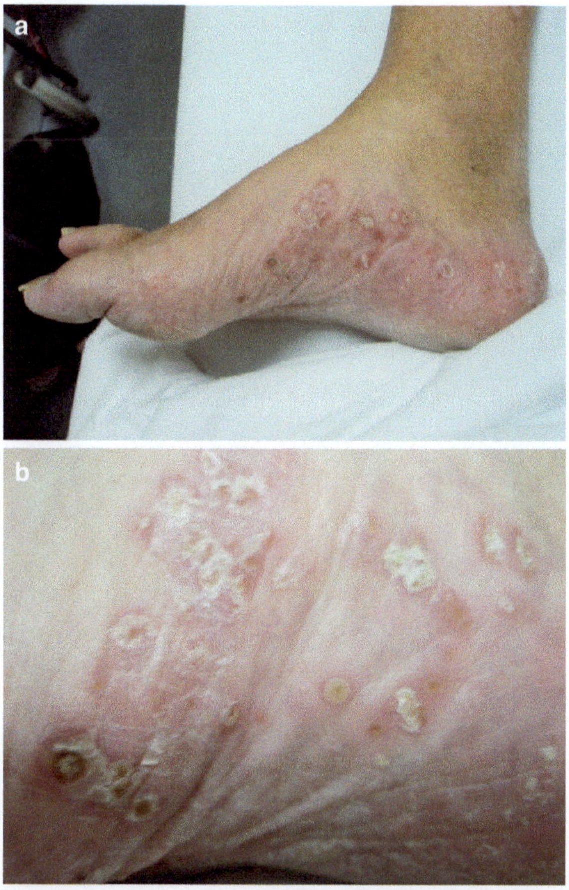

Fig. 15.5 (**a**) A 75-year-old female with well demarcated erythrosquamous pustular eruption on plantar aspect of the left foot. (**b**) Note the pustules and sharp border

References

1. Wootton R, Oakley A (eds) (2002) Teledermatology. The Royal Society of Medicine Press, London, p xiii–4
2. The Australasian College of Dermatologists, Annual Report 2009–2010. http://www.dermcoll.asn.au/downloads/ACD_AReport2010_web.pdf. Accessed May 2011
3. Burg G, Hasse U, Cipolat C, Kropf R, Djamei V, Soyer HP, Chimenti S (2005) Teledermatology: just cool or a real tool? Dermatology 210:169–173
4. Oztas MO, Calikoglu E, Baz K, Birol A, Onder M, Calikoglu T, Kitapci MT (2004) Reliability of Web-based teledermatology consultations. J Telemed Telecare 10:25–28
5. Whited JD, Hall RP, Simel DL, Foy ME, Stechuchak KM, Drugge RJ (1999) Reliability and accuracy of dermatologists' and clinic-based and digital image consultations. J Am Acad Dermatol 41(5 pt1):693–702
6. Levin YS, Warshaw EM (2009) Teledermatology: a review of reliability and accuracy of diagnosis and management. Dermatol Clin 27(2):163–176
7. Muir J, Xu C, Paul S, Staib A, McNeill I, Singh P, Davidson S, Peter Soyer H, Sinnott M (2011) Incorporating teledermatology into emergency medicine. Emerg Med Australas (in press)

Part III

Practical Guidelines

Teledermatology PACS

16

Liam J. Caffery

Core Messages

- Digital Image Communication in Medicine (DICOM) is a global information technology standard that facilitates the transfer of medical images from one biomedical device to another.
- DICOM has significantly contributed to the success of teleradiology and picture archiving and communication systems (PACS).
- PACS is a computer system – both the hardware and software – used for the acquisition, storage, and distribution of biomedical images.
- Store-and-forward teledermatology can be implemented using the DICOM standard.
- DICOM defines a file format, various transmission and retrieval protocols – all of which can be used for acquisition, transmission, storage and review of dermatological images.
- DICOM provides a standards-based method for dermatology to contribute to an electronic health record.
- DICOM also provides mechanism for the consistent display of images and leverages security protocols that ensure patient confidentiality during a teledermatology consultation.

Introduction

Store-and-forward teledermatology is used for the transmission of dermatological and dermascopic images together with supplementary information (e.g. patient history) from a referral site to a remote dermatologist. A number of technological solutions can be used to implement a store-and-forward teledermatology service such as ordinary email or web-based applications.

In addition to facilitating dermatology consultations, specific requirements of a store-and-forward teledermatology application include the ability to:

- Securely transmit patient identifiable information that uses the Internet as a communication medium;
- Interoperate with other information systems used within an organisation – for example, an electronic health record (EHR); and
- Meet legislative requirement for the archive of medical records.

Ordinary email and web-applications may be deficient in providing teledermatology services due to their inability to support these ancillary requirements of teledermatology in a consistent, non-proprietary manner. Hence, interest in using the digital imaging and communication in medicine (DICOM) standard for teledermatology is increasing. In 2008, the American telemedicine medicine association (ATA) published *Practice Guidelines for Teledermatology* [1]. In this policy document the ATA identified "the DICOM standard is likely to impact the practice of teledermatology in the very near future".

In the radiology domain, the DICOM standard has been essential to the success of teleradiology and picture archiving and communication systems (PACS).

L.J Caffery
Centre for Online Health, Level 3, Foundation Building, Royal Children's Hospital, The University of Queensland, Herston, QLD, Australia
e-mail: l.caffery@uq.edu.au

H.P. Soyer et al. (eds.), *Telemedicine in Dermatology*,
DOI 10.1007/978-3-642-20801-0_16, © Springer-Verlag Berlin Heidelberg 2012

There is potential DICOM can contribute to successful store-and-forward teledermatology and form the building blocks of teledermatology and dermatology PACS.

This chapter will examine DICOM and PACS and how these concepts relate to teledermatology. Software requirements for DICOM-enabled teledermatology are discussed. Example workflows are presented to demonstrate numerous ways DICOM can contribute to teledermatology. Further, the standards-based contribution of teledermatology to an electronic health record (EHR) is explored.

Background

Picture Archiving and Communication Systems (PACS)

A PACS is a computer system – both the hardware and software – used for the acquisition, storage, distribution and review of biomedical images. A PACS is made up of many components – including a database, an image archive, one or more client or web-based review stations, DICOM gateways and a web-server.

The concept of PACS arose with the need to manipulate digital medical images following the invention of the computed tomography (CT) scanner – the first modality to produce images in a digital format. The development of the CT was also the catalyst for the development of the DICOM standard.

Most modern hospitals use a PACS to manage their radiographic services allowing the hospital to operate a filmless and paperless imaging service. In these instances, all radiographic images are acquired in a digital format, stored digitally in an archive and retrieved and viewed on a review station. An *image archive* is a repository of medical images whose function is to not only store images but allow retrieval for clinical use. A secondary function of an image archive is to permanently store images for the period of time mandated by legislation. Under legislation medical images (and all medical records) need to be retained for a minimum period of time – for example, the *Queensland Health (Clinical Records) Retention and Disposal Schedule* of the state's health department requires images to be stored for at least it 5 years [2]. An image archive is usually is made up of number of tiers allowing the storage of multiple copies of images. This architecture obviates loss of data due to hardware failures. To a clinical user, a *review station* is often the only part of a PACS they will interact with. A review stations is typically a personal computer (PC) which runs image viewing software. The software allows searching of the image archive and display of a patient's images (in DICOM file format).

PACS are commercially available from multiple vendors and have mature support regimes. The implementation of PACS has been associated with workflow efficiencies and cost-saving [3–5]. A PACS primarily intended for a radiographic service can potentially be used to store and distribute non-radiographic images – for example, dermatology, gastroenterology, pathology and ophthalmology [6]. Teledermatology can leverage existing PACS hardware infrastructure, management processes and support staff thereby achieving economies of scale. Alternatively, an organisation can implement a PACS dedicated to dermatology.

Digital Imaging and Communication in Medicine (DICOM)

DICOM is a global information technology standard that facilitates biomedical image communication and workflow management (acquisition, storage, retrieval, transmission and display). As a standard, DICOM is a document that specifies a set of rules governing the formatting of images and the transmission of images between different biomedical imaging devices. It is implemented as a software application running on an imaging device (e.g. acquisition modality, storage archive or display workstation).

History

The American college of radiology (ACR) and the national electrical manufacturers association (NEMA) formed a joint committee in 1983 to develop a standard to [7]:

- Promote communication of digital image information, regardless of device manufacturer;
- Facilitate the development and expansion of PACS that can also interface with other systems of hospital information;
- Allow the creation of diagnostic information databases that can be interrogated by a wide variety of devices distributed geographically;

This standard was first published in 1983. Since then it has gone through a number of revisions. The current version is DICOM 3.0. The DICOM standards committee now releases yearly corrections, updates, retirements and supplements to the base standard in lieu of major version changes. At the time of writing, the DICOM standard had 16 parts in the base standard and 151 supplements.

DICOM Organizational Overview

Memberships of the DICOM standards committee include manufacturing companies, professional bodies, other standards-developing organizations and government agencies. The original DICOM standard was specific to radiography. However, there are now numerous medical specialities that produce biomedical images. For this reason, the Committee may form special interest groups or working groups to represent non-radiographic imaging groups. Working Group 19 (WG-19) (now defunct) was a special interest group formed to develop dermatology specifications for the DICOM standard.

DICOM File Format

A DICOM file comprises of two parts – the first is the DICOM header and the second is the pixel data of the image. The *header* contains metadata relating to the patient, study and image. Real-world objects such as patient, study and image are known in the DICOM standard as *information entities (IE)*. There are various attributes that can be used to describe an information entity. The standard logically groups and orders these attributes and also specifies which elements are compulsory and which are optional. Attributes that described a patient may include: the patient name, date of birth and a unique patient identifier. A study is described by: a description of the image and acquisition date and time. The image metadata include matrix size, photometric interpretation and bit depth. Each of these attributes is referenced by a unique attribute tag in the format (group, element). All patient data is in group 10 with the attribute tag for patient name being (0010,0010) and the attribute tag for the patient's date of birth is (0010,0030) whereas, group 28 defines the pixel structure of the image – for example the matrix size of the image is the number of rows (0028,0010) by the number of columns (0028,0011).

The second part of a DICOM image – *the pixel data* – can be in most common image formats, probably the most common being JPEG. The two parts are melded into a single file – often called a DICOM object. It is this file structure that makes the practice of teledermatology using DICOM particularly advantageous for two reasons. Firstly, there will be a standardized set of metadata elements for every teledermatology image and secondly there is no risk of separation of the image and the relevant patient demographics that can occur with other modalities of store-and-forward dermatology.

Biomedical images acquired with a digital camera are known collectively in DICOM as *visible light objects (VLO)*. A VLO is how a dermatology image is encapsulated as a DICOM object. *DICOM Supplement 15 Visible Light Image for Endoscopy, Microscopy and Photography* defines the required and optional metadata elements in a definition called the Visible Light *information object definition (IOD)*. Alternatively, visible light objects can also be encapsulated as DICOM objects using the *secondary capture (SC)* IOD. However, the use of VLO is considered best practice for dermatology. The SC IOD contains no modality or speciality specific metadata elements. The purpose of the SC IOD was to define a generic IOD that allowed images captured in a non-DICOM format to be converted to a DICOM format. In commercially available software applications, support for secondary capture is more widespread due to the generalizability of the secondary capture IOD to multiple medical specialities and applications.

Table 16.1 lists the compulsory attributes defined in the VLO IOD. There are various sources for the attributes. Patient demographics are normally entered by the user at acquisition, whereas image attributes may be automatically parsed from the pixel data of the image component. PACS requires *unique identifiers (UIDs)* for each image, series and studies. UIDs are software-assigned at acquisition.

Message Exchange

DICOM works via message exchange between communicating biomedical devices. Each message has a command or a request issued by the sending device and a response from the receiving device. The response normally contains a status as to whether the command was carried out successfully. There are two categories of messages. The first is composite messages which contain all information necessary to perform a certain operation. The second is a normalized message. Multiple normalized messages are needed to accomplish a single operation. DICOM messages are know in the standard

Table 16.1 Information Object Definition showing compulsory attributes for a Visible Light Object

Information entity (IE)	Attribute tag	Attribute name
Patient	0010,0010	Patient's name
	0010,0020	Patient ID
	0010,0030	Patient's DOB
	0010,0040	Patient's Gender
Study	0020,000D	Study Instance UID
Series	0008,0060	Modality = XC (external camera)
	0020,000E	Series Instance UID
	0020,0011	Series Number
Equipment	0008,0070	Manufacturer
Image	0020,0013	Instance Number
	0028,0002	Samples per pixel
	0028,0004	Photometric Interpretation
	0028,0010	Rows
	0028,0011	Columns
	0028,0100	Bits Allocated
	0028,0101	Bits Stored
	0028,0102	High Bit
	0028,0103	Pixel representation
	0040,0555	Acquisition Context Sequence
	0008,0008	Image Type
	0028,2110	Lossy Image Compression Flag
	0008,0016	SOP Class UID
	0008,0018	SOP Instance UID

as DICOM message service elements (DIMSE). Composite messages are prefixed with a "C", whereas normalized messages are prefixed with "N". An example of a composite DIMSE is C-STORE which – as the name implies – is used to invoke the storage of a DICOM object on a remote device such as an image archive. Further examples of composite DIMSE include: C-FIND used to initiate the query of stored DICOM objects, C-MOVE used to move a DICOM object from one device to another – say, from and image archive to a review station. Examples of normalized DIMSE operations include: N-SET used to the get the status of network printer and N-CREATE used to create a print job on a network printer.

Service Classes

DICOM has a service class definition for actions that can be undertaken on a DICOM object. The actions result in the communication of the DICOM object from one biomedical device to another. Actions may include storage of an image onto a PACS archive (DICOM storage service class), printing on a network printer (DICOM print management service class) or interrogating a PACS archive for a particular image so it can be displayed on a review station (DICOM query/retrieve service class). Each service class definition describes three components:

- The expected outcome of the action;
- The DIMSE needed to accomplish the action; and
- The DICOM objects that the action can be performed on.

There is a functional relationship between the service class and the DICOM object known as a *service object pair (SOP)* class. In simple terms, a SOP class is a combination of the DICOM object and the service class – for example, VL Image Store SOP Class or SC Image Store SOP Class. A PACS intending to store dermatology images must support a SOP class matching that of the acquisition device. This could be any or all of the following SOP classes: VL Image Store, VL Photographic Image or SC Image Store. A DICOM-compatible device will optionally support a SOP class. Supported SOP classes for a device are listed in a document called a DICOM conformance statement published by the device's vendor.

Acquisition

The initial challenge in using DICOM to facilitate teledermatology is converting a digital camera image – most often a JPEG image – into a DICOM object. Commercial, open-source or purpose-written software will need to be used to achieve this. One such commercial product is shown in Fig. 16.1. This is a multi-function application that creates a DICOM object from two inputs:

- Images are imported from the local hard-disk or a peripheral device;
- Patient demographics obtained from a user input via a fill-out form.

The demographics and other machine-assigned attributes will become the metadata elements of the DICOM header when they are melded with the pixel data to create a DICOM object.

Another challenge is whilst DICOM may elegantly address image encapsulation and transmission there are ancillary components to a store-and-forward

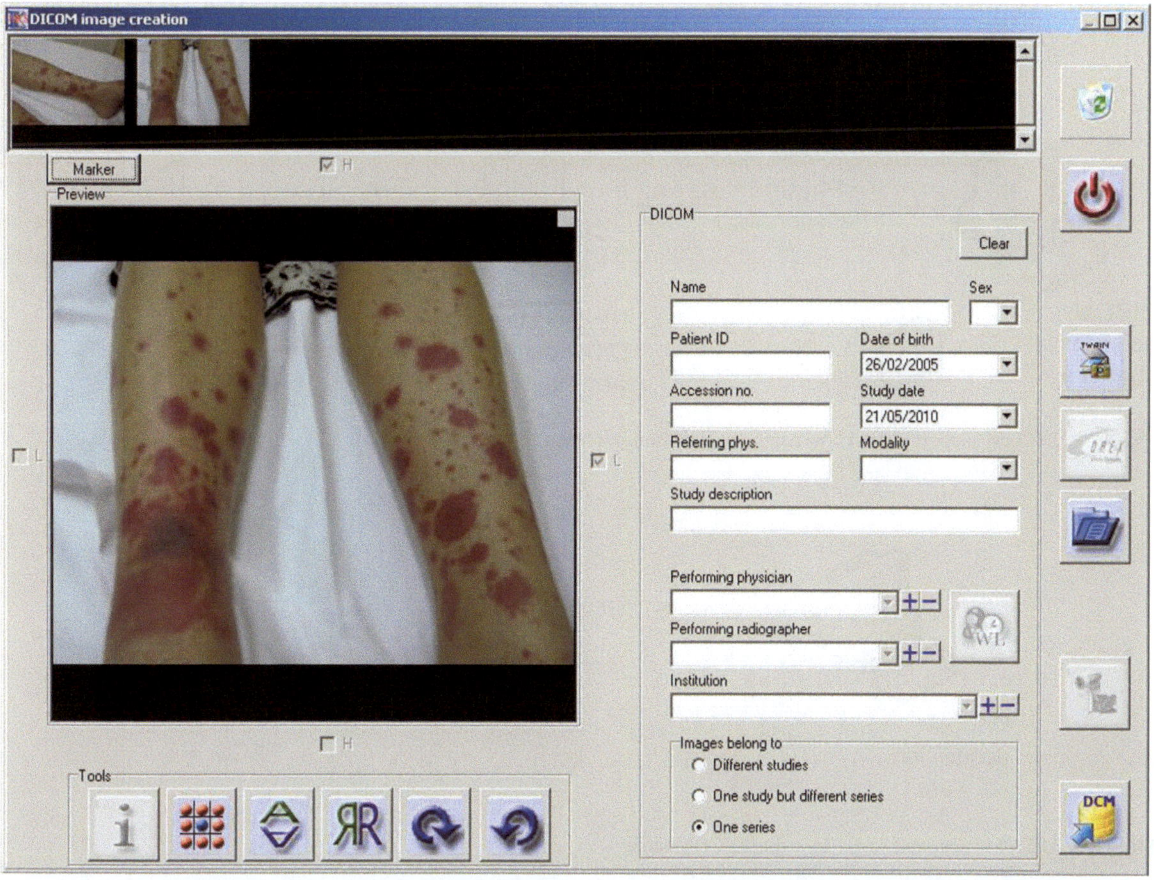

Fig. 16.1 Acquisition software that converts a digital camera image into a DICOM object

teledermatology consultation – for example, patient history and clinical notes. Opportunity exists to scan these documents and encapsulate into a DICOM objects using the methods described in *Supplement 104 DICOM Encapsulation of PDF Documents.* An encapsulated DICOM object is like a DICOM image object in that it contains two parts; the first is the header containing metadata. The second part of a DICOM image object is the pixel data. Whereas, the second part of an encapsulated DICOM object is the PDF document. Once created an encapsulated object, can be stored or transmitted similarly to image objects.

Transmission of DICOM Objects

Once a VL Object has been created for teledermatology it will need to be sent to the remote dermatologist for review. The Standard defines a number of mechanisms the referrer can achieve this:

- Transferring the images to CD (or other portable data medium) for physical transfer;
- Storing the images to a PACS archive, so they can later be accessed by the remote dermatologist working on a review station; or
- Sending the objects via email attachments.

Part 10 of the DICOM Standard – *Media Storage and File Format for Data Interchange* – describes how DICOM images can be written to removable media – for example, CD. The resultant CD can be physically sent to a remote dermatologist who will be able to view the images with DICOM viewing software (Fig. 16.2). The CD may also contain web-content allowing images to be viewed in a web-browser. Physically transportation may be necessary in situation where there is no network connectivity between the referral site and the dermatology site. Once at the destination, the DICOM images can be archived to PACS using functionality inherent in the review software.

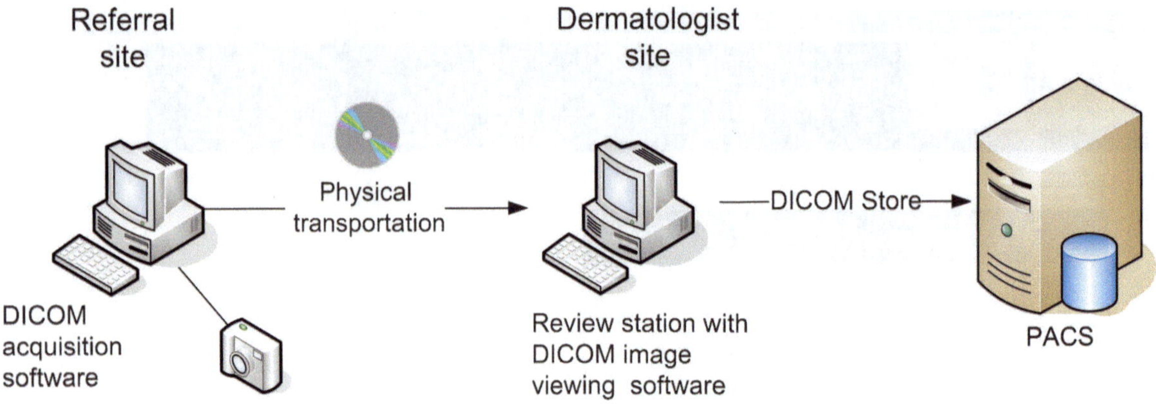

Fig. 16.2 DICOM supported workflow using physical transportation of removable media

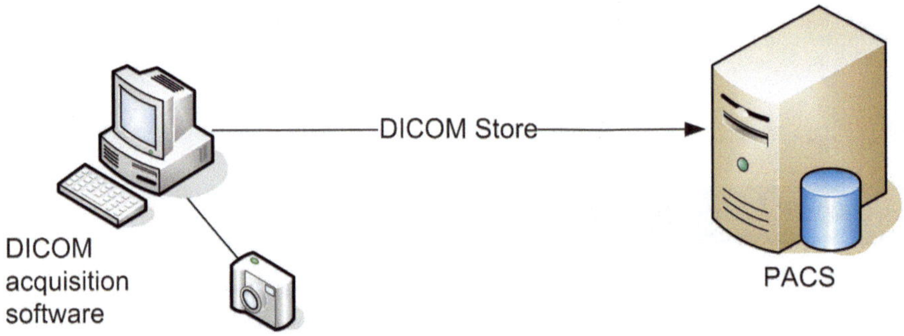

Fig. 16.3 DICOM supported workflow using DICOM store

Dermatology images in a valid DICOM file format can be archived directly from the acquisition modality to PACS given the two devices have network connectivity (Fig. 16.3). A TCP/IP network connection either over a *local area network (LAN)* or a *wide area network (WAN)* can be employed. Security concerns with transmission over a WAN which incorporates the public Internet can be addressed by *virtual private network (VPN)* connections between the communicating devices. The DICOM storage service class governs the exchange.

In addition to sending and receiving images via the TCP/IP protocol, DICOM images can be exchanged with standard email protocols – for example, *simple mail transport protocol (SMTP)*, *Internet message access protocol (IMAP)* and *post office protocol (POP)*. A *multipurpose internet mail extension (MIME)* type defines how non-text content – for example, images – can be encoded into an email message thus allowing them to be sent as email attachments. *Supplement 54 DICOM MIME Types* was published by the DICOM Committee in 2002 and defines a MIME type dedicated to encoding DICOM objects. DICOM email refers to the process of using standard email protocols as the transport mechanism for transmission of DICOM objects from the referral site to the remote dermatologist via DICOM MIME-encoded email. The message body or attached PDF files can be used to convey the patient history, clinical notes or the dermatologist report. DICOM email is the transport mechanism of choice when there is no persistent network connectivity between referrer and remote dermatologist. In addition, email encryption mechanism such as public key infrastructure (PKI) can be utilized to secure the privacy of communication.

DICOM email has been used extensively in Germany to support teleradiology services. [8, 9] The widespread adoption of DICOM email for teleradiology has led to the development of dedicated DICOM email software applications resulting in a high-level of automation and seamless integration with existing PACS infrastructure such as review stations and PACS archive. One example of automation is an auto-polling application that periodically checks an

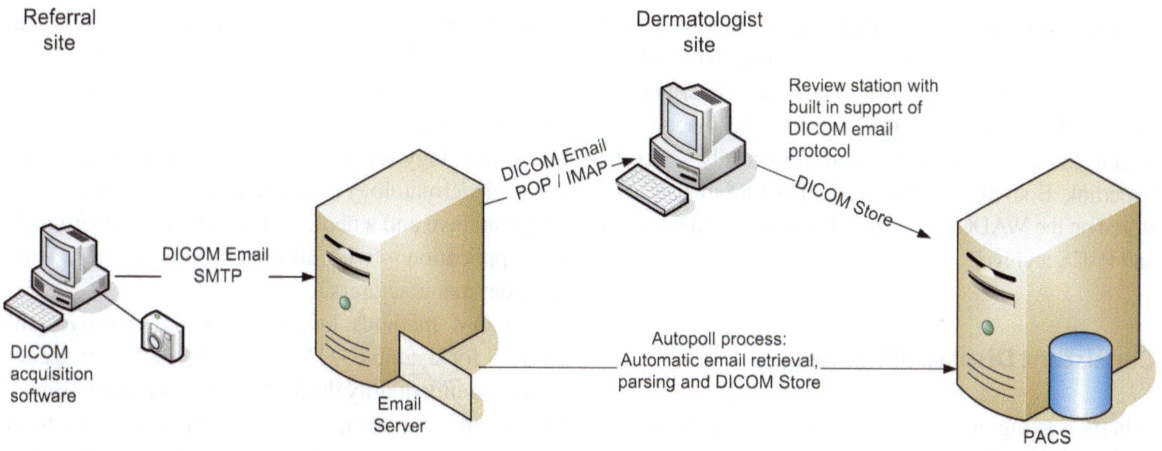

Fig. 16.4 DICOM supported workflow using DICOM email

organization's email server for an incoming email message containing attached DICOM images. The auto-polling application downloads the email and initiates a DICOM store of the attached images. Alternatively, the dermatologist can manually initiate the retrieval of the DICOM email as would happen with an ordinary email client (Fig. 16.4).

Dermatologist Review of Stored Images

The transmission protocols described in the previous section demonstrate how DICOM can be used at the referral site of a teledermatology consultation. As discussed, the referrer can archive images directly to a PACS from the acquisition station or alternatively images may have been archived by a DICOM email auto-poll process. Either way, the dermatologist will need to access images stored on the PACS archive. To achieve this, they use a review station with DICOM viewing software for the display of DICOM objects. In addition, the review station software will be able to search a PACS archive for images that meet certain criteria – for example, the patient name – and display images that meet that criterion. The ability to search and retrieve images is defined by the DICOM query/retrieve service class.

Web-Access to DICOM Objects (WADO)

As alternative to the query/retrieve, DICOM defines *web-access to DICOM objects (*WADO). WADO is Part 18 of the DICOM base standard. It provides mechanism for displaying DICOM objects from a web-browser using *hypertext transfer protocol (HTTP)* or *secured hypertext transfer protocol (HTTPS).* WADO methods are used in web-based review stations or EHR portals.

The use of WADO relies on the availability of web-enabled DICOM server which can perform the following functions:

- Transmit images to a web-client in response to the client's HTTP get request; and
- Interact with images stored on the PACS.

The HTTP get request can contain parameters the server must respond too. These parameters include: study, series or image UID, image format (DICOM, JPEG, JPEG2000, etc.) and matrix size to render the requested image. The DICOM committee recommend a WADO server also support methods that can be used to serve non-image components. [7] In teledermatology these methods can be used to convey patient history, case notes and the dermatologist's report. Non-image based content type include:

- Plain or rich text;
- Hypertext markup language (HTML) or extensible markup language (XML);
- Portable document format (PDF); or
- Clinical document architecture (CDA) as defined by HL7 [10]

Image-enabled web-portals – for example, an electronic medical record or a web-based teledermatology application – can integrate WADO methods in two ways. The first involves embedding images into the web-page – often called an inline image. Using this method the actual full resolution pixel data is displayed as part of the web-page content. The second method is embedding hyperlinks to stored images. The hyperlink may be textual description or thumbnail of the linked image. To display the image would require the user of the web-portal to manually select the hyperlink. Both methods require the DICOM images to be stored on the WADO server or an integrated WADO server and PACS archive.

Consistent Display of Images

Whether using a PC-based or a web-based review station, DICOM images are viewed on the display monitor of workstation. DICOM has developed a means to ensure consistency of display regardless of which monitor the images are viewed on – namely, the greyscale standard display function (GSDF). DICOM has defined a characteristic luminance response curve for ideal image display. The characteristic curve (i.e. GSDF) is based on Barten's model of human visual perception. [11] The luminance response of a display monitor is measured using an external photometer (sometimes referred to as a puck) and this information is fed into a software application. The software applies a correction to compensate for differences between the measured and the ideal characteristics. GSDF does not specify functions for display of color images. However, color monitors can be calibrated to the GSDF, thereby ensuring consistency of display.

Review stations often allow the user to manipulate images – for example, color or grey scale transformations (windowing), spatial transformations (flipping, rotating) or graphical transformations (annotations, text or overlays). The use soft copy presentations states allow these transformations to be stored and reproduced. DICOM defines a greyscale, color, or pseudocolor softcopy presentation state. The presentation state is stored as a separate DICOM object to the image. It is possible with some review stations to automatically display an image with the soft copy presentation applied whenever the study is reviewed.

Advantages and Disadvantages of Teledermatology PACS

A PACS predominantly used for radiographic images can be used to store dermatological images allowing the teledermatology service to leverage an organization's existing infrastructure, management processes and suport personnel. Using a standards-based approach to image management means devices from different manufacturers can be seamlessly coupled. Hence, a teledermatology service could be built from say, a dedicated teledermatology acquisition station, a radiographic image archive and a dedicated web-based teledermatology application – with all components possibly from different manufacturers.

DICOM methods leverage existing security standards – for example, HTTPS, VPN, PKI – to secure patient confidentiality during transmission and retrieval. One further advantage of DICOM is the methods defined to ensure consistency of display namely, greyscale standard display function and the softcopy presentation states.

The use of DICOM and PACS does have disadvantages over other modalities of store-and-forward teledermatology – for example, ordinary email and web-services. Requirements of DICOM-based services are much more complex than other service-delivery modalities. Further, ordinary email and web-services use ubiquitous components for acquisition, transmission and review of teledermatology images. DICOM will require dedicated software applications.

Conclusions

This chapter has described the use of DICOM methods for the acquisition, transmission, storage and review of dermatological images. To implement a teledermatology service based on the DICOM standard will require dermatological images (acquired with a digital camera) to be encapsulated and stored in the DICOM file format. A dedicated acquisition software application is required to convert a digital camera image to DICOM format. The DICOM file format combines the pixel data of the image with a defined set of metadata elements containing patient, study and image demographics. The metadata requirements are defined by DICOM's visible light photographic IOD. The DICOM file format prevents the separation of images and patient demographics that can occur with other modalities of teledermatology and provides consistent metadata for each dermatological consultation.

Acquisition of DICOM objects is done at the referral site and the resultant DICOM objects are transmitted to the remote dermatologist for review – via a LAN or a LAN. DICOM defines a number of transmission methods

– such as DICOM email, direct DICOM store or physical transportation of removable media. A dermatologist will review images on a review station that can display images in DICOM format. In addition to using a review station, images could also be reviewed with a web-based review station, EHR portal or a dedicated web-based teledermatology application (provided the web-application supports WADO methods). Teledermatology can be implemented with any combination of the transmission and retrieval methods described.

The potential of DICOM-based teledermatology remains largely untested. However, DICOM has been credited with the success of teleradiology. In addition to this precedent, the ATA's prediction of the likely impact of DICOM will have on practice of teledermatology adds further support to the consideration of DICOM-based teledermatology services.

Glossary of Terms

Clinical Document Architecture (CDA) CDA refers to the HL7-based exchange of clinical documents (e.g. discharge summary or a diagnostic report) between information system. The clinical document is encoded as an XML documents.

DICOM Message Service Element (DIMSE) DIMSE is a DICOM message or a command used by communication devices to invoke an action – for example, the DIMSE *C-STORE* is issued by one device to invoke the storage of a DICOM object on a remote device.

Digital Image Communication in Medicine (DICOM) DICOM is a global information technology standard. DICOM was developed conjointly by the American College of Radiologists (ACR) and the National Electrical Manufacturers Association (NEMA). The aim of DICOM is to facilitate the network transfer of medical images from one device to another regardless of device's manufacturer.

Greyscale Display Function (GSDF) DICOM defined method that facilitates the consistent display of images regardless of which monitor they are viewed on. GSDF relies on monitors being calibrated to characteristic curve.

Health Level 7 (HL7) Global standard used for the network transfer of health information from one information system to another. HL7 is predominantly concerned with the transfer of text based information.

Hypertext Transmission Protocol (HTTP) Hypertext Transfer Protocol governs the transfers of web pages from server to client (web browser).

Hypertext Transmission Protocol Secure (HTTPS) The encrypted transfer of web pages from server to client using a secure socket layer (SSL) or similar encryption technique.

Information Object Definition (IOD) A DICOM definition that list the metadata required in the header of a DICOM file – for example, the Visible Light IOD will list all the metadata elements in the header of a Visible Light image.

Internet Message Access Protocol (IMAP) IMAP is a protocol that governs how a email client accesses emails stored on a server. The IMAP protocol is used when the client wants to access email stored on a server without downloading or deleting the email from the server.

JPEG A standard digital image file format named after named after the Joint Photographic Experts Group who created the standard. A JPEG image results from a compression algorithm being applied to the pixel data of an image.

Multi-part Internet Mail Extension (MIME) MIME is a standard that defines structure and encoding in the body of an email. The MIME standards were developed to allow email to:
- Be formatted in ways other than plain text – for example, HTML;
- Be written in non-English character sets; and
- Contain attached files.

Post Office Protocol (POP) A protocol used by email software to retrieve email from a remote mail server and download it onto the user's local computer.

Public Key Infrastructure (PKI) PKI is a data encryption technique that uses public/private keys to encrypt/decrypt electronic information. PKI relies on a trusted third party or certification authority to issue public/private keys and verify their use. PKI can be used by email application to secure email communication.

Secondary Capture Object A generic DICOM defined object used for the DICOM encapsulation of images originally acquired in a non-DICOM format. The Secondary Capture IOD contains no modality or specialty specific metadata elements.

Service Object Pair (SOP) Class A combination of a DICOM service (action) and the DICOM object. In the SOP Class *Secondary Capture Image Storage* – the Secondary Capture is the object and the storage is the service.

Simple Mail Transfer Protocol (SMTP) SMTP is a protocol that governs the transfer of emails from email server to email server.

Unique Identifier (UID) A globally unique numbering system overseen by the ISO.

Virtual Private Network (VPN) VPN is a security mechanism used to encrypt the data transfer between two devices that communicate over a public network – for example, the Internet.

Visible Light Object A DICOM categorization for images acquired with a digital camera.

Web Access to DICOM Persistent Objects (WADO) Part of the DICOM base standard that defines mechanisms allowing the display of DICOM objects by a web-browser.

References

1. Krupinski E, Burdick A, Pak H, Bocachica J, Earles L, Edison K et al (2008) American telemedicine association's practice guidelines for teledermatology. Telemed J E Health 14(3):289–302
2. Queensland Government. Queensland Health (Clinical Records) Retention and Disposal Schedule: QDAN 546 v.3. http://www.archives.qld.gov.au/downloads/QDAN00546V3.pdf. Accessed June 2010
3. Mackinnon AD, Billington RA, Adam EJ, Dundas DD, Patel U (2008) Picture archiving and communication systems lead to sustained improvements in reporting times and productivity: results of a 5-year audit. Clin Radiol 63(7):796–804
4. Nitrosi A, Borasi G, Nicoli F, Modigliani G, Botti A, Bertolini M et al (2007) A filmless radiology department in a full digital regional hospital: quantitative evaluation of the increased quality and efficiency. J Digit Imaging 20(2):140–148
5. Canadian Association of Radiologists. PACS Position Paper. http://www.car.ca/Files/media_PACS.pdf. Accessed June 2010
6. Bergh B (2006) Enterprise imaging and multi-departmental PACS. Eur Radiol 16(12):2775–2791
7. National Electrical Manufacturers Association. DICOM Home Page. http://medical.nema.org/. Accessed June 2010
8. Weisser G, Engelmann U, Ruggiero S, Runa A, Schroter A, Baur S et al (2007) Teleradiology applications with DICOM-e-mail. Eur Radiol 17(5):1331–1340
9. Weisser G, Walz M, Ruggiero S, Kammerer M, Schroter A, Runa A et al (2006) Standardization of teleradiology using Dicom e-mail: recommendations of the German Radiology Society. Eur Radiol 16(3):753–758
10. HL7. CDA frequently asked questions. http://www.hl7.org/documentcenter/public/faq/cda.cfm. Accessed June 2010
11. Barten PGJ (1999) Contrast sensitivity of the human eye and its effects on image quality (Thesis [doctoral]). SPIE Optical Engineering Press, Technische Universiteit Eindhoven

Further Reading

The DICOM standard can be downloaded in PDF format from the DICOM home page http://medical.nema.org/. All base parts and supplements are in a separate document. Accessed June 2010

Oleg Pianykh has written a comprehensive text book on DICOM. Pianykh, Oleg S (2008) Digital Imaging and Communications in Medicine (DICOM) – a practical introduction and survival guide. Springer

The UK's National Health Service has produced a 'Beginner Guide to PACS'. It is available for download from Centre for Evidence-based purchasing web site. http://www.pasa.nhs.uk/PASAWeb/NHSprocurement/CEP/CEPproducts/DES+catalogue+-+Diagnostic+imaging.htm#PACS. Accessed June 2010

17 Photographic Imaging Essentials

Janelle Jakowenko, Matthew J. Smith, and Anthony C. Smith

Core Messages

- There are many different tools available to the clinician to capture clinical images, the clinicians must familiarize themselves with the particular photographic equipment available to them in order to be able to utilize it effectively.
- This guide will provide a basic foundation on how a digital camera works to capture an image, as well as fundamental theory and techniques required to take good clinical photographs.
- This guide is not exhaustive and it is essential to refer to the relevant user manual of the digital camera in use in order to get a full understanding of its controls and operation.
- Clinical photography is about accurate and scientific visual reproduction. This requires good even lighting, correct exposure, proper composition and scale.

J. Jakowenko (✉) • A.C. Smith
Centre for Online Health, School of Medicine, Queensland Children's Medical Research Institute, The University of Queensland, Royal Children's Hospital, Brisbane, QLD, Australia;
e-mail: janelle@nomadmedia.com.au; asmith@uq.edu.au

M.J. Smith
Queensland Ambulance Service, Queensland Government, Australia

Introduction

Photography by its very nature is part art and part science. It has been used for centuries in many different ways, capturing images of the tiniest fungi growing on a forest floor, to huge stars millions of kilometers away from Earth.

Photography in a clinical or forensic setting has a specific set of requirements that set it apart from most other forms of photography [1]. While one must keep in consideration the artful skills of composition and lighting, clinical photography is very much about recording a true and accurate picture of the subject in order to derive quantitative information. This means that the image captured needs to be as close as possible to what one would see with the naked eye. The aim of this chapter is to help clinicians achieve this goal while overcoming some of the hurdles that may be confronted in various clinical environments.

Digital Cameras

Digital cameras are now the mainstay of the photographic industry. They have several benefits over their film counterparts, many of which prove to be extremely beneficial to a clinician.

Firstly, they allow the ability to instantly review an image on screen right after it has been captured. This permits the photographer to see if the image taken is satisfactory and without errors. If it is not suitable, then it is simply a matter of retaking the

H.P. Soyer et al. (eds.), *Telemedicine in Dermatology*,
DOI 10.1007/978-3-642-20801-0_17, © Springer-Verlag Berlin Heidelberg 2012

Table 17.1 Advantages and disadvantages of SLR and compact cameras

	Advantages	Disadvantages
Digital SLR camera	Higher image quality, better performance in low light, fast shutter response	Bigger, heavier, more expensive. Macro ability requires a specific macro lens
Digital compact camera	Cheaper, compact, lighter, usually good macro ability	Poorer performance in low light, shutter lag delay

photo, perhaps altering a setting or changing the composition or lighting.

Unlike film, there is no need to wait for a film to be developed and printed – the computer is now the darkroom of digital photography. Once downloaded to a computer, images are widely available through the Internet, email and internal hospital databases.

Another advantage of the digital camera is the ability to effectively "change film" or their sensitivity to light at the flip of a dial. This allows the photographer to quickly adapt to different lighting conditions without having to fumble around changing film.

There are two main types of cameras, which are generally used for photography in the clinical setting. They are the *digital compact* camera and the *Digital SLR* (*Single lens reflex*) camera.

Both cameras have their advantages and disadvantages, which are summarized below in Table 17.1.

Technology is constantly advancing at an accelerated rate, and the gap between digital compact cameras and digital SLR cameras is being bridged by "hybrid" models that combine some of the benefits of an SLR with the compact size and features of a digital compact.

Cameras such as the Panasonic GF-1 and Olympus EP-1, which employ a format described as a "Micro Four Thirds" system, are two such examples. These cameras have a large image sensor, close to the size of most digital SLRs, which gives them the advantages of higher image quality than smaller sensor equipped compact cameras. However they differ in that they do not employ a lens reflex mirror and pentaprism design like that of an SLR, thereby reducing size and weight considerably.

They do however, like an SLR, possess a lens thread, which allows the photographer to attach different lenses for various applications.

Although both types of cameras have their differences, the basic premise of taking a photograph remains the same. One must ensure they have selected the right setting for the situation; they must compose the photograph, focus the lens and press the shutter release. This all sounds relatively easy, but in a clinical setting the aim is to obtain an *accurate* image. That is, an image that is as close as possible to natural in terms of lighting, color and perspective – as that viewed by the naked eye.

Equipment and Accessories

Tripod

Tripods can make a big difference to the quality of your image. It stabilizes the image, and makes the photographer think about composition. If you don't like the awkwardness of a tripod, consider a monopod or use a bench top or something stable to rest the camera on. Tripods can be essential with macro and specimen photography. A tripod will help ensure sharper images especially when capturing close up macro photography.

Flash

All consumer digital cameras have a built-in flash. Often this is too bright, not bright enough or non-adjustable. Many cameras will not have the possibility to use a second flash. The options will open up if the camera has a hot-shoe, or it's possible to attach a ring flash via the lens thread. A ring flash will throw light at the subject from all directions, thereby eliminating harsh dark shadows. A flash in a hot shoe has a rotating head, so it can be turned towards the ceiling or an adjacent wall to bounce light indirectly onto your subject, resulting in a much softer, smoother light with less shadows.

Dermoscope

The use of digital imaging benefits teledermoscopy, it enables forwarding of dermoscopic images for second opinion (Fig. 17.1). There are different ways of obtaining digital dermoscopic images: The compact digital camera, can be attached directly to a simple handheld

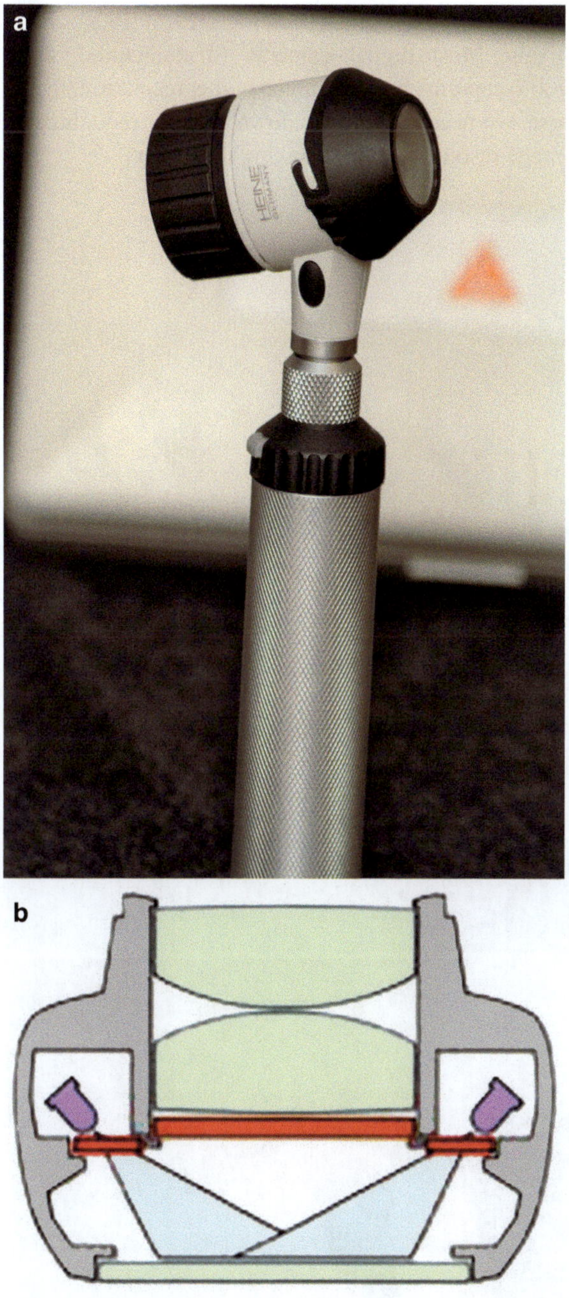

Fig. 17.1 Handheld Dermatoscopy. The LED light source of the dermatoscope is balanced to daylight and flash. A dermoscope view covers 25 mm of surface area and captures at a magnification between 8× and 20×. (**a**) The Heine Dermatoscope. (**b**) Cross-sectional diagram of a dermatoscope

dermatoscope (Fig. 17.2a) and does not require any additional setting changes (leave your camera on *Auto*!). This is a non-invasive (low cost) method for viewing structures just underneath the skins surface. There are also specially designed dermoscopy lenses that can be coupled to a digital camera (Fig. 17.2a, b). This method offers a better image quality than macro photography. Attachments for mobile devices such as the iPhone also perform a similar function (Fig. 17.2a, c) There are also digital skin photography systems available that use videodermoscopic imagery and integrated software. These more expensive systems provide digital dermoscopic images that can be used for teledermoscopy (Fig. 17.3).

How a Digital Camera Captures an Image

All digital cameras contain an image sensor, which is the digital equivalent of film. The image contains millions of tiny photo sensors, which when exposed to light; covert it to a tiny electrical charge, which in turn is converted into digital information by the cameras internal processor.

This information is converted into pixels, the building blocks of a digital photograph.

When the term *megapixels* is used in camera specifications, it is describing the total number of pixels able to be captured by the image sensor.

Compact digital cameras have a smaller image sensor than their digital SLR counterparts. This is due to the size restrictions and the relative expense of manufacturing a larger sensor. If an image were captured on a DSLR and a compact digital camera, both with 10 megapixel sensors, more noise artefacts would be visible on the image produced by the compact camera.

Digital noise artefact is simply a result of the individual photo sensors producing inaccurate and random information as the "gain" or ISO setting is increased on the camera. Larger photo sensors are simply able to capture more light in a given time than smaller photosites, so the ISO setting of a larger sensor does not need to be increased as much to obtain the same exposure as the equivalent compact digital camera with the smaller sensor and denser photo sensors.

Resolution

Image resolution is a three dimensional calculation, it takes into account the number of pixels on a horizontal plane, vertical plane and the bit depth of the pixel. The greater the number of pixels the higher the resolution.

The Internet uses low resolution images, in order to quickly generate web pages, whereas high quality 3D tomographic diagnostic imaging requires high resolution images. The output or viewing platform for most clinical images is a computer monitor. A standard 15″ monitor has a total viewing area of 1920×1080 pixels. Most digital cameras (manufactured since 2006) capture images of much higher resolution, therefore, we need to consider downsizing or reducing the image resolution prior to taking the photo.

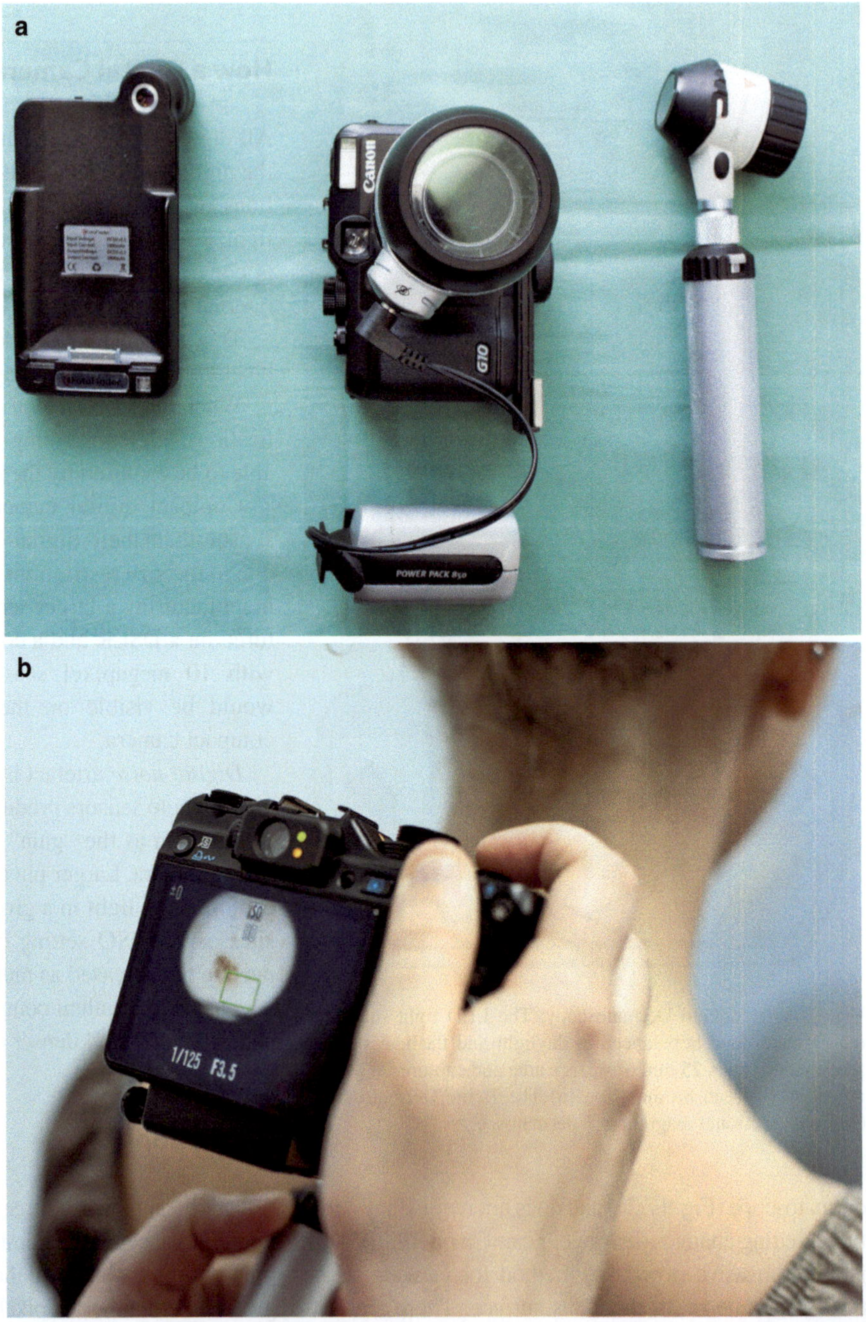

Fig. 17.2 (**a**) Options for obtaining digital dermoscopic images (from *left* to *right*): iPhone dermatoscope attachment, digital camera with dermatoscopic attachment and handheld dermoscope. (**b**) Using a digital camera with a dermatoscopic attachment. (**c**) Using an iPhone with a dermoscopic attachment

Fig. 17.2 (continued)

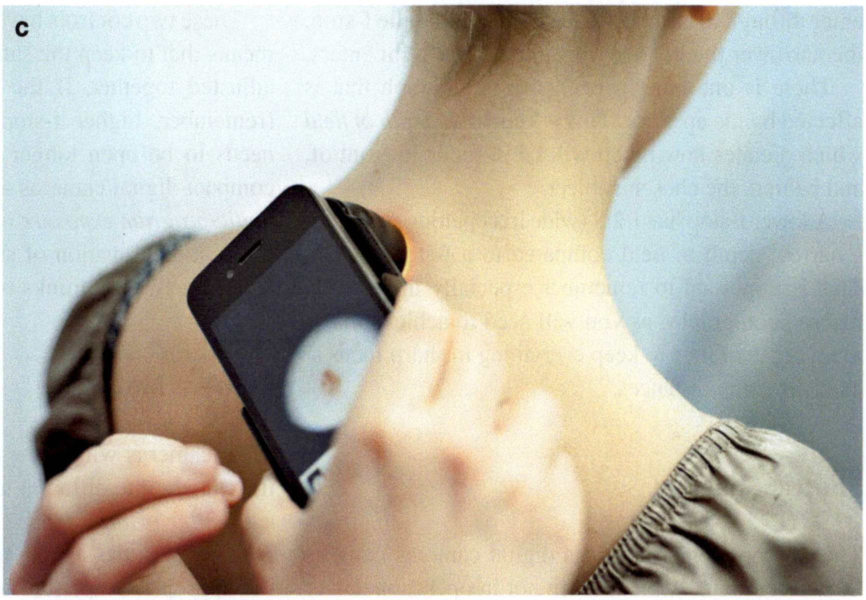

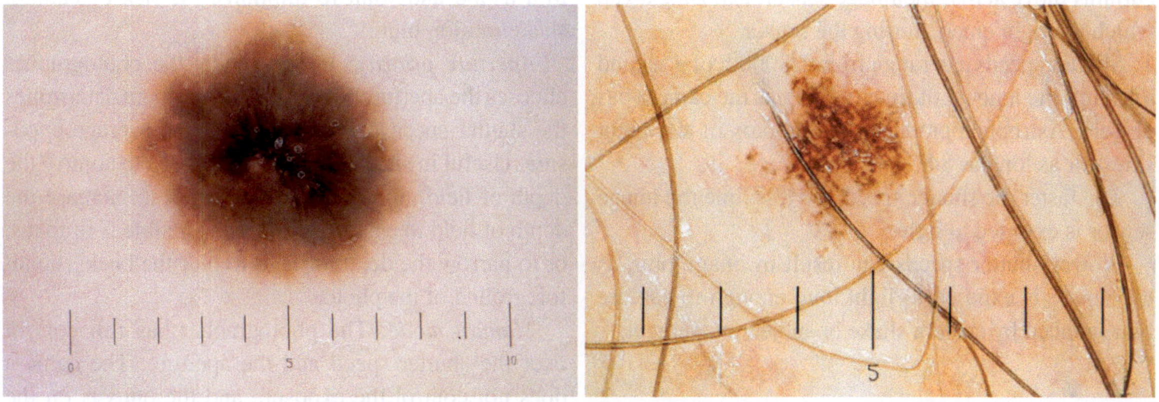

Fig. 17.3 Examples of high quality dermoscopic images including millimetre scale

Exposure: The Three Fundamental Parameters of Image Capture

There are three fundamental parameters, which control the exposure of a photograph. They are: *aperture*, *shutter speed* and *ISO*. Each parameter can be manipulated by the photographer to obtain a correct exposure. These three parameters are paramount to understanding how to take a properly exposed photograph.

Aperture

The aperture acts in a very similar way to the iris of the human eye, contracting and expanding to regulate the amount of light entering the opening. It is constructed of very thin material that contract and expand in a circular motion. They are usually located at the back of a cameras lens. The aperture is given a numerical value referred to as an *f stop*. The lower the f-stop, the wider the aperture and the more light is allowed to enter through the iris of the lens. The higher the f-stop, the narrower the iris opening and the less light enters.

There is one other aspect of a photograph that is affected by the aperture. This is known as *depth of field* which dictates how much will be in focus in front of, and behind, the chosen subject.

A lower f-stop like f/2.8 (wide iris opening) provides a narrow depth of field compared to a f-stop of f/16. This is important to remember especially in close up macro photography, as you will need to achieve maximum depth of field to keep everything in sharp focus at close focusing distances.

Shutter Speed

The shutter on most modern digital cameras consists of two "curtains" which, when not in operation, cover the image sensor and prevent light from reaching it. When the shutter release button is pressed, the shutter curtains move across the image sensor, exposing a gap which the light enters, hitting the sensor.

Shutter speeds can range from 1/8000th of a second to an infinite amount of time (as long as the camera has power). Astrophotographers take photos of the night skies for as long as 8 h.

The faster the shutter speed, the less time the image sensor is exposed to light.

Slower shutter speeds can result in image blur, as the sensor is exposed to light long enough to capture blur induced by camera shake or subject movement.

ISO

ISO refers to the sensitivity level of the sensor, or in the case of film, the sensitivity of the chemical layers embedded in the film. Not surprisingly, the resulting effects of adjusting the ISO in both digital and film photography are similar, the higher the sensitivity (increased ISO number) the increased granularity of the image.

Controlling the exposure of a photograph is a balancing act between the above three fundamental controls. The photographer must choose settings to match the circumstances.

When taking a photo the photographers must determine how much depth of field they require to select an appropriate aperture; how much ambient light is available and how likely there is to be subject movement or camera shake (to determine the importance of shutter speed).

These two controls have a direct relationship, which means that to keep the same exposure they need to be adjusted together. If the aperture (iris) is narrowed (remember, higher f-stop number) then the shutter needs to be open longer to allow more light in. On compact digital cameras and SLR cameras with *automatic/program exposure* modes, the camera works out the best combination of shutter speed and aperture to determine what it thinks is an accurate exposure.

Camera Modes

Most cameras will allow the photographer to change the camera into different modes.

Shutter priority mode: In this mode, the photographer chooses the shutter speed and the camera selects the appropriate aperture to achieve an average exposure. Useful in situations where you need to control the shutter speed. For example, when you have no access to a tripod and want to minimize the risk of camera shake/motion blur.

Aperture priority: In this mode, the photographer chooses the aperture (f-stop) and the camera determines the shutter speed needed to achieve an average exposure. Useful in situations where you need to control the depth of field more accurately – either to increase the depth of field to ensure as much as possible is in focus, or to narrow the depth of field to blur the background/foreground of the photo.

Manual mode: The photographer has full control over the shutter speed and the aperture. The camera does not control the exposure and the onus is on the photographer to select a combination, which will achieve an accurate exposure.

In most situations the automatic program mode offered by the camera will be sufficient for taking diagnostic photos, however it is useful to understand the other modes and when they may be required.

A camera employs a *metering system* to determine what constitutes an accurate exposure. This system takes average readings from selected areas of the image and attempts to achieve a good balance between exposing correctly for the darkest and lightest areas of an image. In short, the camera will try to exposure everything as an average tone.

This is why in one of the cameras program modes (anything other than full manual mode), if you were to take a photo of a pure white subject filling the frame, the image would come out with that subject looking slightly

Table 17.2 Various light sources and the corresponding color temperatures

Light source	Degrees Kelvin
Sunrise or sunset	2000
40 W tungsten lamp	2650
100 W tungsten lamp	2865
Fluorescent lamp	3400–4800
Early morning/late afternoon light	4300
Flash/bright daylight/moonlight	5500
Overcast sky	6000
Average summer shade	7100

grey. The camera has *underexposed* the image to try and achieve average grey tones. Conversely, taking a photo of a largely dark object filling the frame, and the camera will *overexpose* the photo in order to bring the dark tones of the subject up to average tones.

There is a control on most digital cameras to help control this behavior. It is called *Exposure compensation* or *EV compensation*. Using this control, the user can force the camera into under or over exposing the image from what it thinks is the correct exposure.

The EV compensation is measured in *stops* and can usually be set to adjust in 1/3 or 1/2 stop increments.

Thus when you are taking a photo of a subject that contains a lot of white/very light tones, you can apply positive (+) EV compensation to force to camera to increase the exposure and display those tones as they would look to the naked eye. The opposite applies to images containing a large ratio of dark tones.

Color: How Cameras Interpret Light

Light is emitted from various sources, each with its own hue that is measured in Degrees Kelvin (Table 17.2). The resulting image will be affected by the color of the light illuminating the scene. Digital cameras are equipped with a *white balance* adjustment that allows the camera to compensate for the color of the light source and thus avoiding unnatural coloring in the rendered image.

Digital cameras have white balance settings to correct for different conditions, such as daylight or fluorescent bulbs, overcast and flash. The automatic setting, that is normally very accurate, adjusts the white balance for any lighting condition. Some cameras will permit the white balance to be set manually by pointing the camera at a neutral white or grey surface and recording the reference for this image.

Light Sources

Below is a definition of various light sources, where they might be encounter and how to use, or avoid them. The aim when photographing clinical subjects is to create an environment with neutral white, diffuse and even light. Below are various situations where clinical photos might be taken, and some suggestions on how to approach the situation.

Daylight

Natural lighting can result in uniform and well-lit images, with high quality color reproduction. However, as light intensity and color vary widely depending on the time of day and weather conditions, such desirable results may not always be possible. This inconsistency also makes it difficult to achieve reproducible conditions, which will cause problems when photographing an individual's skin complaint over a prolonged period of time. Rooms that are only sunlit should be arranged in order to admit as much light as possible, while minimizing the amount of shadow. Note however that images should never be taken in direct sunlight, as this is extremely bright and will produce sharp shadows.

Shade

Shadow gives a blue cast, however the diffused light provides a good even light source.

Overcast

Gives a slightly blue cast, however the diffused light is good to use as an even light source.

Night (Moon-Light)

The moon is a direct reflection from the sun, so it is the same color temperature as daylight. Long exposures in full-moon situations will recreate the scene as if it was the middle of the day. However there are no practical situations where this is useful when patients are involved!

Flash

Most cameras contain a built-in flash that can be turned on or off, or set to automatic.

The auto flash function determines whether there is sufficient natural light illuminating the scene and fires the flash as necessary. However using the flash can create problems. As the flash points directly at the subject a strong shadow can be created, which is likely to cause problems when taking close-up images. A strong flash can result in an over-exposed image with a whitish glare, which can erase much of the detail. Increasing the distance between the camera and the subject can significantly reduce this overexposure. It is also possible to reduce the flash by reducing its intensity using a semi-transparent white plastic bag.

Fluorescence

Fluorescence angiography is useful in determining blood-flow from the optic nerve in the pupil. It is a specialist technique that requires a dedicated digital camera. Fluorescence has also been used to photograph skin patches of suspected leprosy.

Fluorescent

Fluorescent lighting is very difficult to reproduce and even repeat using the same light source. The color temperature of the tubes changes during their life span, and they also exist in many different color temperatures, some of which are daylight balanced. Most emit a green hue. Under fluorescent lighting conditions some cameras may produce images with horizontal or vertical bands, which is a result of the flickering tubes.

Tungsten/Incandescent (Including Sodium Vapor, Mercury Vapor)

Professional photographic studios used tungsten light sources for many years, however a special tungsten balanced film was used to correct for the yellow cast. It is still possible to use tungsten light sources but this will need to be corrected in your cameras white balance settings. Both sodium and mercury vapor lights are used in street lighting. Sodium gives a yellow cast whilemercury a green cast.

Halogen Lamps

Halogen lamps provide intense light, which is easy to direct. However some error in color reproduction may result. Generally, they are daylight balanced, but this can vary, and should be displayed on the packaging.

Fiber Optics

Daylight balanced fiber optic cables are often used in macro and microphotography, as they allow very good positioning of a small light source. They are expensive and used in specialized fields.

Reflected Ultraviolet

Ultraviolet (UV) photography is useful in dermatological applications such as the changes in skin pigmentation, however it is not possible to record UV on ordinary digital camera, so specialized equipment must be purchased.

Reflected Infrared

Infrared recording techniques are useful for penetrating the epidermal layers of the skin to examine blood-flow. This is useful in detecting cases of varicose veins, collateral circulation and other vascular diseases. Again the sensors in digital cameras all react quite differently to infrared reflection so specialized equipment must be purchased.

Radiological Images (X-Rays, MRI and CT)

These three imaging techniques go well beyond the visual spectrum and are not performed by clinical photographers. However they are useful to keep in mind, as similar to clinical photography there are standard series of images that must be captured in specific medical situations.

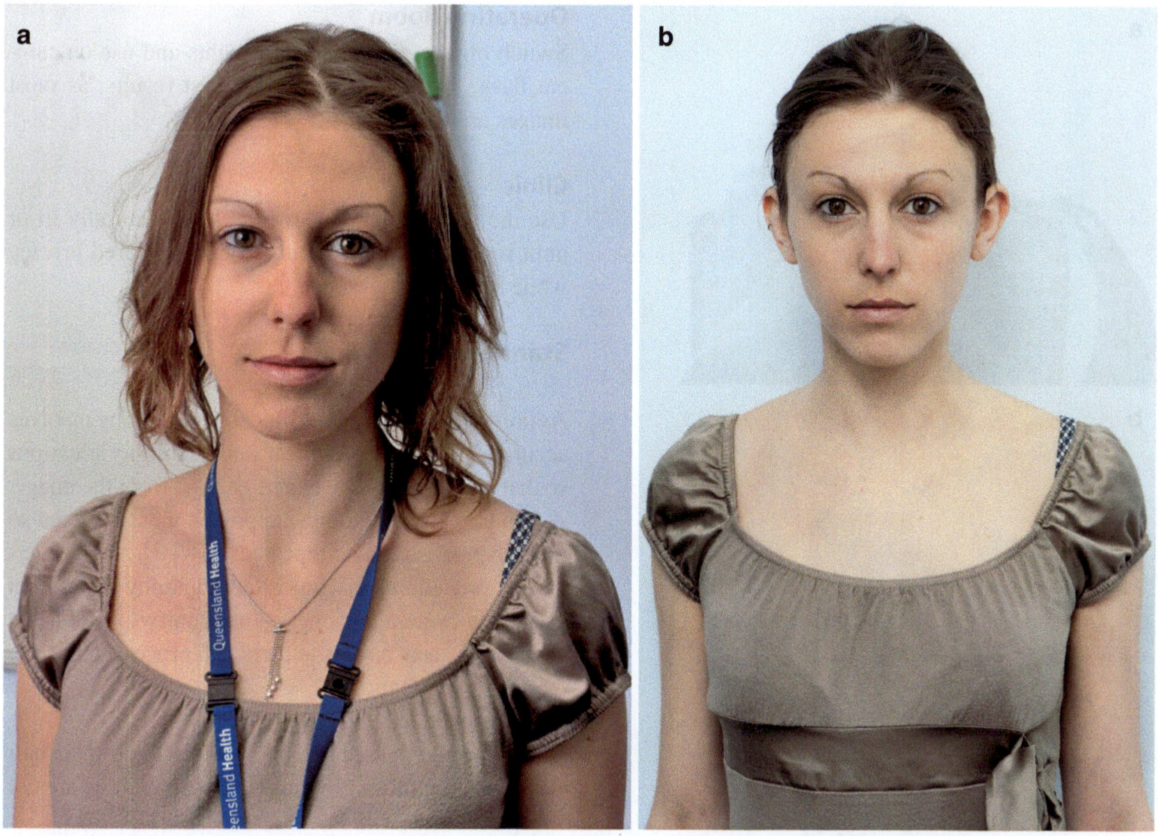

Fig. 17.4 The difference between backgrounds, composition and exposure. (**a**) Underexposed subject, not centered in frame, distracting background elements. (**b**) Good even lighting, subject centered in frame with a plain neutral background

Practical Guidelines: Background, Composition and Lighting

Background of a Photograph

The perfect background is a non-reflective and neutral grey (18%). Given that this is not always available; the next best option is a green or blue surgical drape or a white sheet. The neutral grey background is preferred, as the colors do not influence any of the colors in the image. If a drape or sheet is not available, a clean wall or the back of a door is appropriate (Fig. 17.4).

Lighting

Studio

The ideal environment for photographing patients is in a studio. The background should be neutral grey and non-reflective. The patient should stand approximately 1 m in front of the background. Two diffuse "softbox" light sources should be positioned 45° from the patient.

Naturally Lit Room

Well-lit rooms with natural lighting are very useful. The patient should not stand in direct sunlight as this causes excessive contrast and dark shadows. The "shaded" area of the room will offer even, diffuse lighting. If the light is strong enough there should be no need to use the built in flash.

Room Without Natural Lighting

Use the built in flash, or on camera flash. For best results diffuse the flash light source using a flash "sock" a white plastic bag or some opaque sticky/cello/durex tape (Fig. 17.5). This will slightly reduce the contrast created by the shadows.

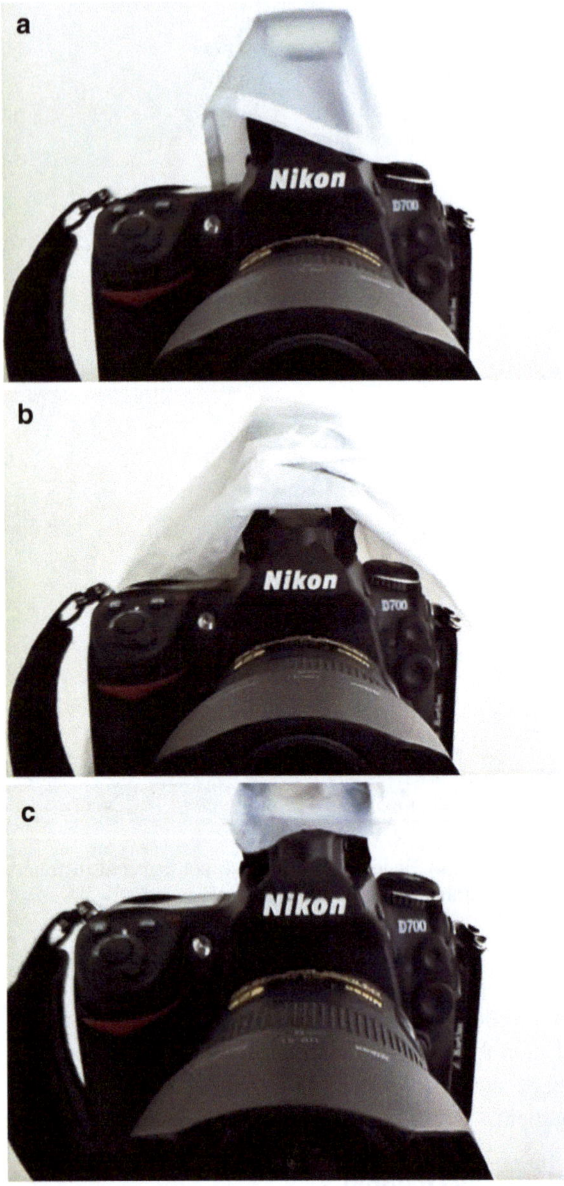

Fig. 17.5 "Point and shoot cameras often result in over exposure when using the flash for macro photography. Three methods to reduce this over exposure include: (**a**) a tissue, (**b**) a plastic bag and (**c**) sticky tape

Outside

Photograph the patient in a shaded area. The sun is a "pin-hole" light source, which means harsh distracting shadows will be cast on the patient if they are photographed in direct sunlight.

Operating Room

Switch off the operating room lights and use on camera flash. A ring flash provides best results, as most images are close-ups.

Clinic

Use the same principles as in either a naturally lit or unlit room. Make sure your patient is offered privacy while being photographed.

Standardization

As previously mentioned clinical photography involves accurately capturing clinical and scientific situations so that quantitative data can be derived from the image. A standard and methodical approach must be taken so that the process can be repeated.

The procedures in clinical photography should not vary from camera to camera – or country to country. It should be seen as a standardized process requiring thought and attention.

Steps include:

- Having the patient remove jewellery, tie their hair back and remove clothing that obstructs the area of interest.
- Clean the area, removing blood, fixing tape and other obstructions.
- Use a clinical background such as a drape or a plain wall.
- Have the camera settings ready and an idea of which patient series (to follow) you need to capture.
- When using a scale or color chart, make sure it is parallel to the frame of the image.
- *Always* use correct anatomical positions (Fig. 17.6).

Practical Scenarios

Photographing a Patient

Equipment required: Background, scale, optional use of a tripod and other accessories

1. Ask the patient if they consent to photography AND explicitly explain where the images will be used. This is called "*Informed Patient Consent.*" Have the patient sign a consent form, or if they are under 18, have a parent or guardian sign the form.
2. Know the desired output (Internet, study, publication etc.) and adjust your *camera settings* accordingly.

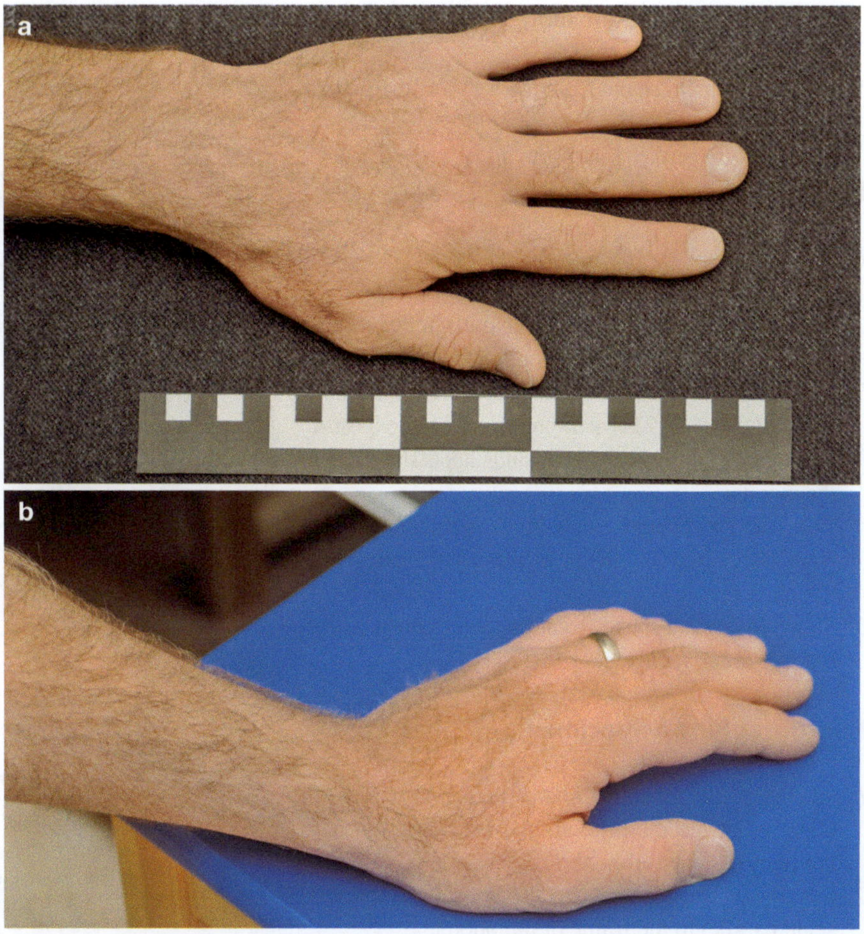

Fig. 17.6 Various anatomical aspects: (**a**) correct positioning; (**b**) incorrect positioning

3. Check the *environment*. Private room, plain background, consider lighting, have the patient remove clothes, jewellery, glasses and clean the area of interest if necessary.
4. *Photograph the patient sticker* or something that will later enable identification of the patient. This is very useful if numerous patients are photographed, or the memory card is not downloaded for some time.
5. *Photograph the patient* using a standard series and then additional pictures as desired.
6. *Download* to computer, rename files and *store* in a database.

While taking the photos consider these things:

- Overview
- Regional
- Regional with scale or markings
- Close-up

The four characteristics of an exceptional clinical photograph are:

- Correct perspective
- Use scales and color charts (aligned with the image frame)
- Even lighting
- Plain, preferably neutral background

Photographing an X-Ray

Equipment required: Light box and tripod

1. Clean the light box
2. Mount the camera on a tripod and align it with the centre of the image on the light box.
3. Set your camera to B&W.
4. Turn off room lights and block light coming in from doors and windows; the backlight from the light box is what needs to be recorded. Any excessive

light spilling out from the light box should be blocked by pieces of card.

5. To avoid camera shake from the long exposure, *use the self-timer setting.*

Photographing a Monitor

Equipment required: Monitor and tripod

1. Clean the monitor.
2. Mount the camera on a tripod and align it with the centre of the image on the monitor.
3. For Cathay Ray Tube (CRT) monitors *set you camera to "night" mode.* This will produce a long exposure that will avoid the horizontal bands appearing across the monitor.
4. Turn off room lights, and block light coming in from doors and windows, as these will reflect off the glass monitor.
5. To avoid camera shake from the long exposure, *use the self-timer setting.*

Photographing a Specimen

Equipment required: Background, scale and tripod

1. Clear a flat place on the ground (as normally they are photographed from above).
2. Lay down background and the specimen. Place a scale parallel to the frame of the photo.
3. If the room is not sufficiently lit use a tripod. Specimens are often reflective, so it is best to diffuse the flash.
4. *Photograph the patient name, or a description of the specimen.*
5. Take the photo.

Photography in the Operating Room

Equipment required: Camera with a flash

1. Clean the area of interest.
2. Ask for the operating lights to be momentarily switched off.
3. Take the photo as parallel to the subject as possible, this might require getting up on a stepladder or stool.

Dental Photography

Equipment required: Retractors, dental mirrors and an external light source (or ring flash)

1. Ask the patient if they consent to photography AND explicitly explain where the images will be used. This is called "*Informed Patient Consent.*" Have the patient sign a consent form, or if they are under 18, have a parent or guardian sign the form.
2. Warm the mirrors by placing them in warm water. This will stop the mirrors fogging when they are placed in the patient's mouth.
3. Organize the external light source and change the white balance settings on your camera accordingly.
4. *Photograph the patient sticker* or the patient holding a color chart with their name and date of birth underneath.
5. Have the patient lick their lips before inserting retractors or mirrors.
6. Aim to capture the image series below by photographing the reflection of the teeth on the mirrors.

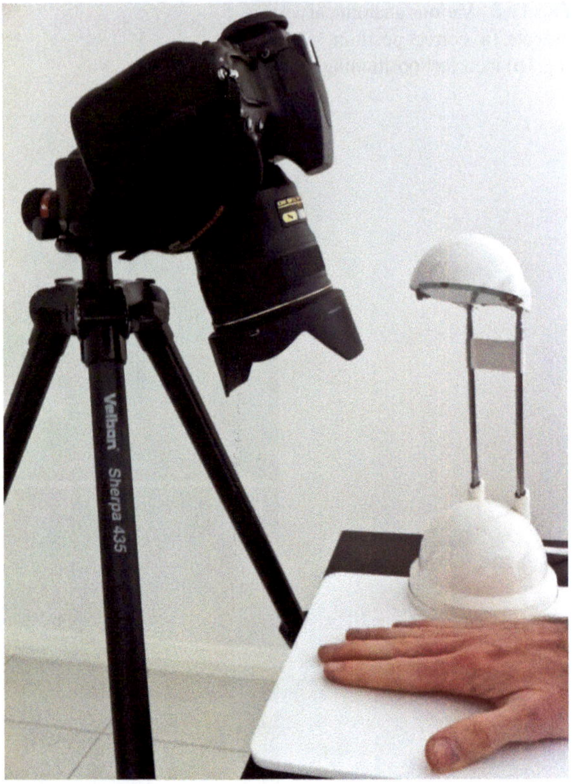

Fig. 17.7 This example shows a desk light being used as an additional light source; it is also good when two such lights can be used at 45° angle to the subject

Macro Photography

Equipment required: Background, scale and an appropriate light source (built-in flash, external light source or ring flash)

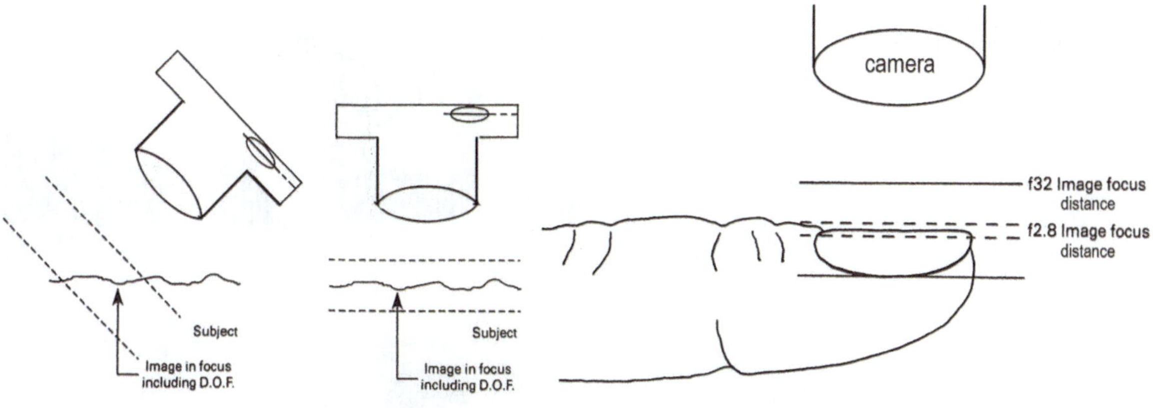

Fig. 17.8 The depth of field (*DOF*) is decreased by a smaller working distance, smaller *f* number (not often adjustable in consumer cameras) and by not being parallel to the subject (Vetter JP: Biomedical photography, Boston, 1992, Butterworth- Heinemann)

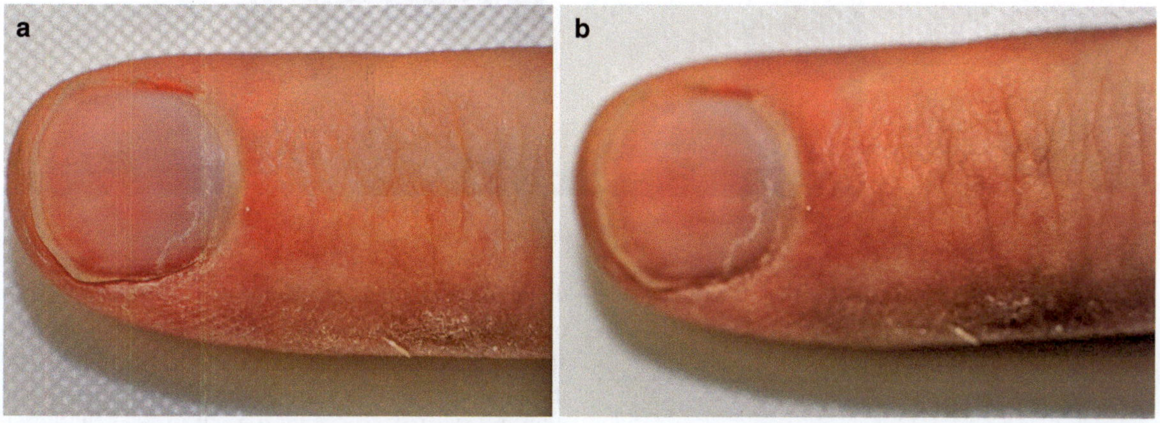

Fig. 17.9 Examples of in and out of focus macro photographs. The close up of the fingernail in (**a**) is in focus, whereas (**b**) shows the fabric back ground in focus

Close-up photography or macro photography is a useful technique to master, as it constitutes such a large part of dermatology photography. If a remote doctor is to be offered advice or a diagnosis from an image, the image needs to be sharp and the color and texture must be accurately reproduced. Professional macro and micro photographers use dedicated lenses and flashes, which are purpose-designed for photographing objects at 1:1 magnification. It is possible to achieve similar results with modern compact digital cameras, provided the macro functions are understood.

The many challenges associated with macro photography include the limited amount of sharpness in front and behind the main point of focus (Figs. 17.7–17.10). This is known as depth-of-field, which is very shallow at limited working distance. It is possible to get a sharper fingernail bed but the skin in front and the nail behind will become disappointingly soft. One option is to shoot from a further distance and crop the photo later. The overall subject is sharper, but the photo quality may not be as good because you have fewer pixels, resulting in a lower resolution, grainier image. The other option is to become better acquainted with the macro function and capabilities of your camera.

1. Ask the patient if they consent to photography AND explicitly explain where the images will be used. This is called "*Informed Patient Consent.*" Have the patient sign a consent form, or if they are under 18, have a parent or guardian sign the form.
2. Organize the external light source and change the white balance settings on your camera accordingly.
3. *Photograph the patient sticker* or something that will later identify the patient.
4. Change the camera settings to macro.

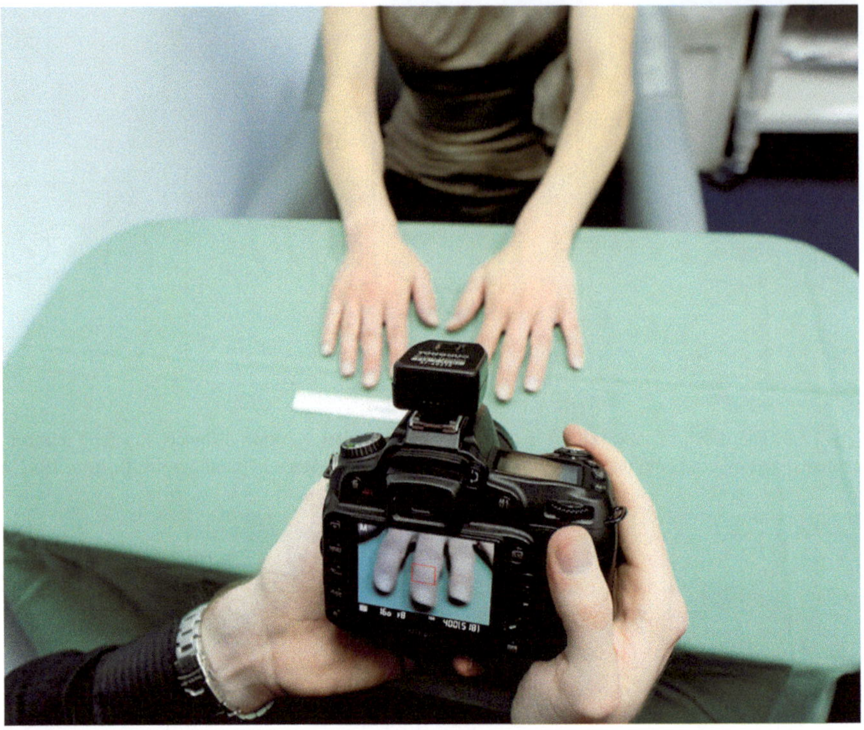

Fig. 17.10 Using the live view screen of a camera to get a large view of the in focus area

5. Take the image making sure that the focus and exposures are 100% accurate.

Informed Patient Consent

Obtaining informed consent should become part of the clinical photography routine and must be obtained prior to photography. An image or video should be treated as any part of the patients' medical record, in confidence and handled according to consent legislation. As well as consenting, the patient must acknowledge, in writing if their images to be used anywhere outside their own medical record. This extends to emails, publications, studies or the duplication of images for case discussion or referral.

Conclusion

High quality clinical photography is integral to a patients medical record, more so in dermatology than other medical specialities. High quality images (but not necessarily high resolution) can be used for diagnosis, treatment and to identify a lesions change over time. When capturing photographs in a clinical setting, the clinician must keep in mind the purpose of the photographs. They are being viewed objectively with the aim being to accurately illustrate and record the specific patient injuries, illnesses and abnormalities. The aim of the clinical photographer is to capture images containing quantitative information by making adjustments to the lighting, composition and exposure to ensure the image can be relied upon for its intended purpose.

Doing this requires an understanding of the camera and the clinical photographic principles as outlined in this chapter. By following these guidelines the clinician will have a better chance of creating high quality, standardized, accurate clinical photographs.

Reference

1. Jakowenko J 2009 Clinical photography. J Telemed Telecare. 15:7–22

Legal Issues 18

Leif Erik Nohr

Core Messages

- It is of vital importance to clarify legal issues and ensure that teledermatology services are performed within the relevant health care legislation.
- Information processing in telemedicine and e-health must ensure confidentiality, privacy and be secured by information security regimes.
- Teledermatology services must meet legal and ethical requirements with regard to responsible practice. Furthermore, hospitals and other institutions shall fulfill system responsibility duties.
- Patients' Rights become increasingly more important in health care. The patients' rights to consent must be respected both with regard to telemedicine examinations and treatment and processing of information.
- To realize the potential of cross-border teledermatology, special consideration must be given to legal issues, in particular concerning licensing, responsibility and information security.
- Legal clarification and certainty could be ensured through the development and use of guidelines and contracts.

L.E. Nohr
Norwegian Centre for Integrated Care and Telemedicine, University Hospital of North Norway
Tromsø, Norway
e-mail: leif.erik.nohr@telemed.no

Introduction

Health care is an area of strict and comprehensive legislation. Providing high-quality health care for the population is essential. Legislation is one way of securing quality and accessibility of care as well as the funding governments and citizens invest into health care.

Health care legislation is mainly based on and related to traditional means and methods of providing care. Obviously, new methods mean new legal challenges. Telemedicine and eHealth is still developing rapidly, and it is safe to say that legislation is often lagging behind. Still, telemedicine services must operate within existing legal frameworks, and it is important both to have knowledge about this framework and to know how to adapt services to it. Our purpose with this chapter is to give an introduction to legal issues that are commonly believed to be the most important in telemedicine and eHealth and through this create awareness and hopefully contribute to quality assurance of teledermatology services with regard to legal aspects.

There are few, if any, *specific* legal issues within the specialty of teledermatology. This chapter presents issues and aspects that will have relevance for telemedicine and eHealth services in general. Having said this, teledermatology is one of the most mature telemedicine services and many of the issues discussed here have come up through projects and services in the field of teledermatology.

H.P. Soyer et al. (eds.), *Telemedicine in Dermatology*,
DOI 10.1007/978-3-642-20801-0_18, © Springer-Verlag Berlin Heidelberg 2012

Privacy, Confidentiality and Information Security

Introduction

Health professionals depend on enough, good enough and relevant information from and about the patient in order to be able to assess the patient's condition, examine and treat the patient. The patient needs to be informed about his/her condition, the examinations, possible treatments and risks in order to be able to govern his/her own situation and disease. In addition, a potentially large number of other people and providers might, at different stages of the course of treatment, have legitimate need for information or be providers of information. These could be health care personnel from other hospitals, laboratories, pharmacies, etc.

Privacy

The right to privacy is considered a fundamental human right both under the United Nations Universal Declaration of Human Rights from 1948 and the European Convention on Human Rights from 1950. Article 8 of the latter reads:

1. Everyone has the right to respect for his private and family life, his home and his correspondence.
2. There shall be no interference by a public authority with the exercise of this right except such as is in accordance with the law and is necessary in a democratic society in the interests of national security, public safety or the economic well-being of the country, for the prevention of disorder or crime, for the protection of health or morals, or for the protection of the rights and freedoms of others.

Both the Declaration and the Convention codifies the general principle of privacy as a matter of respect for every individual's personal autonomy. This autonomy is built on an understanding that each person has a right to set her or his own limits to any infringements of her/his personal "sphere". This sphere does not just include a person's body and thoughts but extend beyond this to encompass a person's family, home and correspondence.

The term *information privacy* is relating to all kinds of information that identifies or relates to an individual. Under the Australian Privacy Act personal information is defined as

> ...information or an opinion (including information or an opinion forming part of a database), whether true or not, and whether recorded in a material form or not, about an individual whose identity is apparent, or can reasonably be ascertained, from the information or opinion [1].

A similar definition is given in Article 2 (a) of the European Data Protection Directive [2] which in turn is the basis of information privacy legislation in most European Countries.

In 2008, in a ruling based on the above mentioned Article 8 [3], the European Court of Human Rights ordered the Finnish government to pay a citizen damage for the state's failure to protect confidentiality. The ruling is important as it links data security directly to human rights.

Personal information shall only be processed based on consent or if there is a specific legal basis. An example of the latter is laws on keeping of medical records. Furthermore, only necessary and relevant information shall be stored and processed and only data relevant for the purpose of giving care can be stored.

Confidentiality

If information is considered a major commodity in health care, confidentiality might be seen as the currency that makes it possible to use and utilize this information in a medical treatment setting. A duty of confidentiality, ensured by law and professional ethics, is basically what the health care worker has to offer in exchange for vital and potentially sensitive information from the patient.

The duty of confidentiality is mentioned already in the Hippocratic Oath, an early codification of ethical duties of the medical practitioners:

> Whatever I see or hear in the lives of my patients, whether in connection with my professional practice or not, which ought not to be spoken of outside, I will keep secret, as considering all such things to be private. [4]

Under the Norwegian Health Personnel Act [5], article 21, the duty of confidentiality is codified like this:

> *§ 21 General rule relating to the duty of confidentiality*
> Health personnel shall prevent others from gaining access to or knowledge of information relating to people's health or medical condition or other personal information that they get to know in their capacity as health personnel.

The wording and details of the legal duty of confidentiality vary from country to country, but there are some basic characteristics that one will find in most legislation:

- A duty of confidentiality applies to health/medical information received by the professional in the capacity of a health care worker.
- The duty implies keeping information confidential from unauthorized persons.
  - The patient her-/himself is, with few exceptions, always authorized
  - Only colleagues and other health care personnel that are cooperating in the care process are authorized to information
  - Family and next of kin can only have information if the patient gives consent.

How to Keep Information Confidential

Legislation establishes the principles of confidentiality, not the means and methods on how to keep information safe from non-authorized persons. Preserving confidentiality is about keeping silent, keeping control over documents and other means of information as well as actively making sure that non-authorized persons are unable to gain access to the information.

Information Security

Information security is about managing risk related to processing of personal information. In one sense, information security is a trade-off between securing and protection of the information on one hand, and having in place sensible and usable systems for use of and access to the information on the other. Traditionally, the following aspects are included in the term information security:

- Confidentiality
  Ensuring that confidential information is kept from unauthorized access.
- Integrity
  Ensuring that information is not altered or removed in an unauthorized manner.
- Access
  Ensuring that information is accessible for those who are authorized to access it.
- Quality
  Includes ensuring that information is stored and processed in a way that does not reduce the information quality or damage the information.

To have in place an information security regime is a fundamental basis and prerequisite for processing patient information in telemedicine and eHealth settings. A hospital, a doctors office or any other enterprise or entity that handles personal health information must establish, use and maintain information security regimes on all levels. These should be updated regularly and in this process, *risk assessment* is an important tool.

Information security relates to several dimensions – including legal, organizational and technological. The legal is about the legal requirements to information security, the organizational about the need to establish information security as a routine in the different organizations as well as establishing an organization that place responsibilities and duties. The technical, which is especially relevant in teledermatology, is about having technology in place that makes it possible to process information securely, both in terms of protecting it and keeping it confidential and in terms of making it usable and accessible.

Responsibility and Liability

Professional Responsibility

Another important legal duty for all health care personnel is to do their work in a responsible way. To act in accordance with professional, legal and ethical principles, standards and regulations on good practice. Duties of responsibility shall ensure high quality health care for the patients and keep the patients safe from harm. The health care provider who fails to meet these requirements might be held liable for her/his wrongdoing and be met with formal reprimands, loose of license or even criminal prosecution.

The duty to act responsibly is expressed differently under different legislations, but the core principle is that health care personnel shall do their work in accordance with a standard of good practice. This is a so-called legal standard and as such the detailed content and framework of the duty will be decided based on an assessment of the situation at hand and the education, practice and skills of the health care professional.

In English law, a reasonable standard of care is often assessed using the so-called *Bolam test*, based on a jury direction statement from a case in 1957 [6]. According to this test, a doctor will not be guilty of malpractice if he acts:

> (...) in accordance with a practice accepted as proper by a responsible body of medical men skilled in that particular art (...)

In a given case, it will be necessary, through witnesses and other evidence, to establish the more detailed content of this standard, based on factors like education, skills, knowledge, equipment, etc. of the medical professional and the situation at hand.[1]

Under Norwegian law, the duty to act responsibly is codified under the Health Personnel Act (see note 5) Article 4:

> Health personnel shall conduct their work in accordance with the requirements to professional responsibility and diligent care that can be expected based on their qualifications, the nature of their work and the situation in general.

In relation to teledermatology (and telemedicine in general) a core question is whether or not examining or treating the patient using telemedicine is considered responsible and in accordance with legal and ethical codes of good and professional conduct. The answer to this question must be found in national laws, regulations and professional guidelines.

One quite common approach is to consider face-to-face contact to be the responsible way of meeting the patient and tele-solutions to always be secondary to this. This view can for instance be found in the Ethical Guidelines in Telemedicine adopted by the Finnish Medical Association [7]. These guidelines are based on guidelines and recommendations by the World Medical Association [8]. The guidelines states that:

> Preferably, all patients seeking medical advice should see a doctor in a face to face consultation, and telemedicine should be restricted to situations where a doctor can not be physically present within acceptable time. The major application of telemedicine is the situation in which the treating doctor seeks another doctor's opinion or advice, at the request of or with the permission of the patient.

The Norwegian Health Authorities have taken a more pragmatic approach with regard to telemedicine and responsibility. In the regulation, the fact that medical decisions are based on information about the patient and her/his condition is emphasized and with regard to the use of telemedicine a very important principle is formulated: The important factor in assessing if a medical – or telemedical – practice is performed responsibly is whether or not the health professional have received sufficient and relevant information not *how* the information is received.

This approach is pragmatic in the sense that it does not rule out any types or means of information sharing. A doctor might get information from and about the patient by a face-to-face consultation, via videoconferencing or via email.

Taking an approach where the telemedicine service is considered secondary based on an assessment where this solution – more or less at the outset – is inferior to face-to-face consultations, implies reducing the telemedicine service to be used for second opinion and advisory situations.

As more and more telemedicine and e-health solutions and services are being developed, tested, implemented and used, users gain more knowledge and experience. Together with a growing number of evidence based studies this contributes to the development of telemedicine also with regards to assessing how services apply to codes of conduct and legal responsibility requirements.

Teledermatology services are probably of the most mature within the realm of telemedicine and many hospitals have used different teledermatology solutions as routine services for years. Based on this knowledge there should be no reason to classify teledermatology services as secondary to traditional face-to-face services, at least not at the outset and not through legal constraints. The legal standard should be the same for teledermatology and for traditional dermatology practices and the assessment of whether or not the standard is met should be based on the service and situation at hand, research, experience and the competence of the participating health professionals.

Acknowledging that teledermatology can be provided in accordance with legal and professional standards also means that a doctor can *take* responsibility in a given teledermatology consultation. This is especially important for services where the remote doctor is a specialist and the patient is referred via videoconferencing or store-and-forward solutions. In these situations/consultations it is vital for the nature of the service that a specialist can be regarded as the responsible party in the sense that she or he is the one making the decision(s) with regard to the patient's condition. The consequence of this is that the doctor or nurse at the patient's end of the consultation have only a limited responsibility and is not the overall responsible physician. As mentioned this in turn means that the

[1]It should be said that this test has been discussed and also opposed to by many. One example is discussions about its relevance and importance under Australian law, see for example Kirby M (1995) Patients' rights – why the Australian Courts have rejected Bolam. J Med Ethics 21(1):5–8.

specialist should be able to have the consultation remunerated as a traditional consultation.

The doctor that is responsible for the consultation can also be held liable for malpractice or wrongdoings.

System Responsibility

On a more overall level, the professional duty of responsibility must be assessed in connection with the institution's duty to organize the workplace and the environment for health care provision in a safe and professional manner. This is often referred to as system responsibility. A health care institution or employer has a duty to have in place physical, technical and organizational "regime" that makes it possible for the health care worker to provide the best possible care. This includes aspects like equipment, staff, information security regimes, guidance, education and training, routines, etc.

In telemedicine it is especially important that for instance video conferencing equipment is accessible, usable and of good quality and that information security regimes are in place and documented. These are issues that fall within the area of system responsibility.

Liability

Liability is of course closely connected to responsibility. If a person or an institution is to be held liable, she or it must be responsible. In assessing liability, a court or a supervising authority will assess if a person have acted in a responsible manner, meeting legal and professional requirements for the actions in question. And in the same way an institution's systems and organizations will be assessed and evaluated according to legal and other standards.

We know of no examples of court decisions or decisions by supervising authorities where telemedicine practices have been tested.

Patients' Rights and Consent

Introduction

Over the last decades, there has been a worldwide trend toward recognizing patients as having specific and fundamental rights as patients. The content and legal protection of these rights vary, but we see that more and more countries secure patients' rights through law. Finland was the first country in the world to pass a Patients' Rights act in 1992. Even without a specific Act on patients' rights, such rights are often recognized and can be enforced under many jurisdictions.

On a general basis, patients' rights can be categorized in three:

- The right to treatment
- Rights as a patient
- Procedural rights

With the exception of consent (see below) we will not go into detail on the many and important aspects of these rights. Here, and for our purpose, it is important to be aware of the existence of patients' rights and respect the value of these. Services and practices in teledermatology must appreciate such rights and through design, guidelines and organizations take patients' rights into consideration. Among other things, this means giving the patient information and allowing the patient to participate in examinations and treatment to the extent possible. It means respecting the patients' right to confidentiality and it means respecting the patient's right to consent.

Consent from the patient is a basic and fundamental condition for any examination or treatment. Without it, examining or treating the patient will violate her or his personal autonomy and right to be in command over her or his own body. For some procedures, action without valid consent would easily constitute a serious criminal offence.

In telemedicine and eHealth, consent issues must also be considered and respected with regard to processing of patient information, being it for record keeping or more general information and treatment purposes.

Consent Requirements

Use of the term "valid consent" shows that there are requirements that need to be met before anyone can do anything based on consent.

Competence

The consenting person must be *competent* before giving consent. Competence is related both to age and capacity. The age of consent usually follows the age of majority. In addition, some legislation also recognizes that children under the age of majority can give consent on their own in matters concerning their own health. Under Australian legislation, the competence to consent follows the age of legal competence (18 years) in principle, but there exist provisions, cases and principles that recognize that children under this age can be considered competent [9]. When a child is not competent to consent, her or his parents or guardians gives consent on behalf of the child.

An otherwise formally competent person might not be actually competent to give consent because she or he is temporarily or permanently incapable to consent. This can be due to medical conditions, intoxication or degrees of dementia because of old age. In such circumstances, health care personnel might be referred to not starting treatment or examination and to wait for the patient's condition to improve. The important exception is of course emergency situations where the principle of necessity and the goal of saving lives or reducing damage and injuries gives basis for medical action. In the case of age-dementia, a person should have a guardian appointed to take care of her or his interests also in health matters.

Informed Consent

Consent shall be based on thorough information. In health care, all health care workers have an obligation to give patients relevant and thorough information about the patient's condition, examinations, procedures and treatment. This information must be adapted to the individual patient and the health care professional have a duty to make sure that the patient understands the information as well as the implications of giving or not giving consent. In medical care, a point is often made about informing the patient of possible risks of a given procedure.

Withdrawal

Consent is a unilateral legal action. In this sense it is different from contractual situations. The consenting party can at any time, and without reason, *withdraw* her or his consent. A patient should also be informed that she or he has this possibility, as well as possible consequences of such withdrawal.

Consent in Practice

In most daily practices, consent issues are relatively uncomplicated. The doctor who sees a patient at her office can presume that the patient is giving consent to at least common and routine examinations and treatment.

In *telemedicine*, the question has been asked whether or not it is necessary to ask for specific consent from the patient before engaging in a telemedicine consultation. The answer is probably yes. As long as telemedicine is relatively uncommon and not routine practice, the patient should be informed about the procedures, the risks and the benefits and asked to consent before a telemedicine consultation takes place.

Cross Border Teledermatology

There is undoubtedly a huge potential in telemedicine for providing services across country borders. This has been realized since the first days of modern telemedicine, but to this day this is still a largely unexploited potential. There have been a number of projects and pilot studies on cross border telemedicine, but with the exception of teleradiology, very few have developed into routine services.

There are of course a multitude of explanations to why telemedicine have not utilized this potential despite arguments and proofs that cross border solutions can provide expert health care globally. National legislations is probably one of the more important barriers.

The legal barriers and challenges in telemedicine become even stronger and more manifest in cross border care.

Licensing/Authorization

In all countries health care personnel must be licensed in order to practice lawfully. Health care personnel from another country must obtain a national license before she or he can practice. In some cases, for instance within the EU/EEA region, obtain a license is almost a formality [10], whereas applicants from outside Europe might need to provide more documentation or even take additional exams or tests.

In telemedicine, the situation is, or might be, different in the sense that the doctor provides services from the country or state where she is licensed, to patients (or other doctors/health care personnel) in another country. The question then is whether or not the doctor needs to be licensed in the other country as well.

It is difficult to give a definitive answer to this question, depending on the service provided and the legal requirements in the respective countries. In the absence of specific legislation or guidelines on this issue with regard to telemedicine, the general rule will probably apply: A doctor that wants to practice telemedicine in another country should be licensed in this country. This is at least the best advice in order to be on the safe side.

A similar approach is recommended in the Core Standards for Telemedicine Operations, adopted by the American Telemedicine Association (ATA) [11]. Their Administrative Standards for Health Professionals states:

1. Health professionals providing telehealth services shall be fully licensed and registered with their respective regulatory/licensing bodies and with respect to the site where the patient is located, administrative, legislative, and regulatory requirements.
2. Health professionals providing telehealth services shall be aware of credentialing requirements at the site where the consultant is located and the site where the patient is located, in compliance with and when required by regulatory and accrediting agencies.

(...)

The American Academy of Dermatology makes the following statement in their Position Statement on telemedicine:

> Licensing
> Interactive telemedicine requires the equivalent of direct patient contact.
> In the U.S., teledermatology using interactive technologies is restricted to jurisdictions where the provider is licensed.

Services where health professionals merely give general advice or where consultations are between health professionals in different countries will not require licensing in the receiving state. In these cases, the sole responsibility lies with the doctor who asks for and receives advice.

It is in any case advisable to investigate and clarify these issues with the relevant national authorities before engaging in a cross-border teledermatology service.

Responsibility and Liability

The above mentioned aspects of responsibility and liability must be addressed also in a cross-border setting. In services that involves direct patient contact, it is of vital importance that the patients' rights are respected and that the tele-doctor take on and accept professional responsibilities towards the patients.

Information Security

To the extent it is relevant to transfer patient information across national borders, information security must be ensured. National legislation in this area might differ from state to state with regard to aspects like patient consent, encryption standards, formats, etc.

Within the EU area, the Directive on processing of personal data (see [5]), establish a regime where personal data can be transferred between member states. The condition is that the states have adopted the Directive and adapted their national legislation accordingly.

Guidelines and Contracts

Guidelines

In this chapter a number of references have been made to guidelines on telemedicine and teledermatology. To some extent, making and using guidelines prove to be a solution to overcome legal barriers. Guidelines can be the instrument or measure that provides clarity and security for patients, providers, organizations and authorities. Guidelines are more dynamic and less bureaucratic than formal laws and regulations. It is important, however, if such guidelines shall have any impact, that they are within the national legislative frameworks. Where national laws prohibit a given telemedicine practice, a guideline cannot legitimate it.

Loane and Wootton [12] gives the following definition of a guideline:

1. A statement or other indication of policy or procedure by which to determine a course of action;
2. Guidance relative to setting standards or determining a course of action;
3. A rule or principle that provides guidance to appropriate behavior.

The authors also points out the fact that "(...) *there is little reference in the literature to guidelines for telemedicine.*" And we might add: One have to look even more to find guidelines on *legal aspects* of telemedicine. Having said that, also other guidelines, general or on other topics, might have relevance for legal aspects of teledermatology. And one might find useful guidance and advice in guidelines on other specialties.

As of today, most guidelines seems to be about more technology specific issues. As telemedicine becomes more routine and integrated in everyday services and common technology, one might expect to see more guidelines dealing with more general and underlying issues, for example regulatory aspects.

The American Academy of Dermatology (AAD) [13] has a so-called position statement on telemedicine that serves as guidelines. The Statement addresses some legal issues. Both the World Medical Association (WMA) and The Standing Committee of European Doctors (CPME) have addressed telemedicine aspects in a number of documents that can be found on their websites [14, 15].

Guidelines are issued by different bodies, and as Loane and Wootton points out, there are no consensus as to who should be responsible for formulating and issuing these. Health care professionals should obviously be involved in creating clinical and probably also technical guidelines. It is therefore natural that medical associations are responsible for most guidelines in existence today. It is less obvious who should take responsibility for guidelines on legal aspects of telemedicine. Such guidelines are on a more general level and must, as mentioned, be rooted in national laws and regulations. The ideal "parents" to such guidelines would probably be health authorities in close cooperation with medical associations.

The quality of guidelines will vary and there are no definitive standards as to how they should be made or what they should contain. Loane and Wootton are referring to an article by Hayward et al. [16] that gives some advice on assessing guidelines:

1. Are the recommendations valid?
2. Were all important options and outcomes considered?
3. Was en explicit and sensible process used to identify, select and combine the evidence?
4. Was an explicit and sensible process used to consider the relative value of different outcomes?
5. Are the guidelines likely to account for important recent developments?
6. Have the guidelines been subject to peer review and testing?

Another challenge regarding guidelines is related to their use – their penetration or impact in the telemedicine world. It is difficult to know to what extent a guideline is actually being used. Involving relevant stakeholders in the creation of guidelines is probably a key factor to make sure that they have some impact.

Contracts

A contract is an obvious choice as a tool for establishing a legal framework for a telemedicine service. Contracts can be dynamic and will address the exact issues relevant for a given service. The parties can also regulate payment and dispute issues in a contract.

The same main rule applies for contracts as for guidelines: Contractual provisions must be within the national legal framework. A contract or a contractual clause that contradicts laws will be considered invalid.

In the R-bay project [17], the partners developed a set of draft contracts for the provision of (tele)radiology services across national borders. The contracts tried to include and relate to different national legislations as well as professional guidelines in the field. The draft contract templates are published in the final report that can be found on the project website.

Conclusion

This chapter has probably showed how difficult it is to present and discuss legal aspects of teledermatology in general terms. We hope, however, that we have been able to give an overview of some of the aspects believed to be most important and to have contributed to some clarifications. It is essential for the success of a teledermatology service that it is provided within the legal frameworks. This is a vital condition to ensure quality of service for patients and other stakeholders. When planning a teledermatology service, in projects or as routine implementation, legal aspects should be included from day one. This is the best way to prevent laws and regulations from being barriers.

References

1. Privacy Regulations (2006) http://www.comlaw.gov.au/comlaw/Legislation/LegislativeInstrument1.nsf/0/1CEB84A1FB10217ACA25724100162984?OpenDocument. Accessed 27 June 2010
2. Directive 95/46/EC of the European Parliament and of the Council of 24 October 1995 on the protection of individuals with regard to the processing of personal data and on the free movement of such data
3. I v Finland, Judgement, Strasbourg (17 July 2008) http://www.cl.cam.ac.uk/~rja14/Papers/echr-finland.pdf. Accessed 29 June 2010

4. http://www.nlm.nih.gov/hmd/greek/greek_oath.html. Accessed 30 October 2009
5. Lov om helsepersonell m.v. av 2. juli 1999 nr 64 (Act of 2 July 1999 No. 64 relating to Health Personnel etc. Unofficial translation: http://www.regjeringen.no/en/dep/hod/documents/lover_regler/reglement/2002/act-of-2-july-1999-no-64-relating-to-hea.html?id=107079. Accessed 30 October 2009)
6. Bolam v Frieren Hospital Management Committee (1957) 1 WLR 582
7. http://www.laakariliitto.fi/e/ethics/telemed.html. Accessed 21 January 2010
8. http://www.wma.net/en/10home/index.html. Accessed 21 January 2010
9. Bowles K (2010) Age of consent to medical treatment. http://www.findlaw.com.au/article/10022.htm. Accessed 10 May 2010
10. Council Directive 93/16/EEC of 5 April 1993 to facilitate the free movement of doctors and the mutual recognition of their diplomas, certificates and other evidence of formal qualifications (2010) http://eur-lex.europa.eu/smartapi/cgi/sga_doc?smartapi!celexapi!prod!CELEXnumdoc&lg=en&numdoc=31993L0016&model=guichett. Accessed 27 May 2010
11. www.americantelemed.org. Accessed 20 June 2010
12. Loane M, Wootton R (2002) A review of guidelines and standards for telemedicine. J Telemed Telecare 8:63–71
13. http://www.aad.org/Forms/Policies/ps.aspx. Accessed 20 June 2010
14. http://cpme.be/. Accessed 21 June 2010
15. http://www.wma.net/. Accessed 21 June 2010
16. Hayward RSA, Wilson MC, Tunis SR, Bass EB, Guyatt G (1995) How to use a clinical practice guideline. JAMA 274:570–574
17. www.r-bay.org. Accessed 20 June 2010

Health Economics

19

Mark E. Bensink, Paul A. Scuffham, and Anthony C. Smith

Core Messages

- Economics is about making choices when resources are limited.
- Health economics applies economic theory to the specialized area of health care and provides, amongst other things, a set of tools to weigh the cost and consequences of alternative courses of action.
- This focus on cost and consequences is critical, health economics does not focus solely on cost, instead it is the impact an investment has on patient outcomes compared to the alternative/s.
- Understanding the difference between the tools that are available in the health economics tool box and using them appropriately to answer a specifically and carefully developed research question is a critical first step.
- The overall aim of investigating the cost and consequences of alternatives is to provide evidence to decision makers that investment in a particular alternative is a good one.
- Providing evidence of the value of investment in a teledermatology alternative is essential information to justify and foster the uptake of new and innovative ways to provide dermatological services.

M.E. Bensink (✉)
Centre for Online Health, Level 3, Foundation Building, Royal Children's Hospital, The University of Queensland, Brisbane, QLD, Australia

Centre for Applied Health Economics, School of Medicine, Griffith University, Brisbane, QLD, Australia

Research and Economic Assessment in Cancer and Healthcare (REACH) group, Fred Hutchinson Cancer Research Center, Seattle, Washington, USA
e-mail: mbensink@fhcrc.org

P.A. Scuffham
Centre for Applied Health Economics, School of Medicine, Griffith University, Brisbane, QLD, Australia

A.C. Smith
Centre for Online Health, School of Medicine, The University of Queensland, Queensland Children's Medical Research Institute The University of Queensland, Royal Children's Hospital, Brisbane, QLD, Australia

Introduction

It's choice, not chance that determines your destiny
(Jean Nidetch)

Economics is all about choice. Why? Because of the raison d'être for economics, scarcity. Scarcity exists when the resources available are insufficient to cover every course of action or intervention we may want, or need, to implement. As a result choices must be made.

Health economics then is the application of economic principles, founded on the concepts of choice and scarcity, to the health care context. It has emerged as a distinct discipline within economics because of the unique characteristics of the health care market, one of the main ones being uncertainty [1].

In the health care environment where resources are scarce and choices need to be made between the interventions that are and are not funded, health economic evaluation provides a set of analytic tools for the "comparative analysis of alternative courses

H.P. Soyer et al. (eds.), *Telemedicine in Dermatology*,
DOI 10.1007/978-3-642-20801-0_19, © Springer-Verlag Berlin Heidelberg 2012

of action in terms of both their costs and consequences" [2]. This process of weighing costs and consequences is basic rational behavior and something the vast majority of individuals do every day. For example, in deciding which groceries to buy the individual weighs their needs and the related cost of alternatives before making a decision on what they purchase.

When the decisions that are being made involve much larger sums of money and the consequences involve the health and well-being of patients, these decisions should be made in a systematic, transparent and justifiable way. This is the role economic evaluation can play in health care.

What does this mean for teledermatology? Faced with a new alternative for the provision of dermatological care to a patient group that involves the application of a telecommunications technology (i.e. a teledermatology intervention), economic evaluation provides the means to transparently and systematically evaluate both the cost and consequences of this new alternative when compared to the existing form of dermatological care. The overall aim of economic evaluation is to provide evidence to decision makers that the decision to investment in the new alternative is a good one [3].

The aim of this chapter is to provide the reader with an overview of economic evaluation in health care and its application to teledermatology. Examples from the general dermatological literature as well as specific teledermatology examples and other analyses are used to place this overview within context and hopefully, to foster and encourage the much needed application of economic evaluation to teledermatology studies.

The Six Steps of Economic Evaluation

The White Rabbit put on his spectacles. 'Where shall I begin, please your Majesty?' he asked. 'Begin at the beginning,' the King said gravely, 'and go on till you come to the end: then stop.' (Lewis Carroll, Alice in Wonderland)

Although there are different analytic techniques within the tool box of economic evaluation, there are six common steps to be completed in any evaluation (Table 19.1).

Table 19.1 Summary of the steps required to complete and economic evaluation

Step	
1	Formulation of the research question to be answered
2	Selection of an appropriate economic evaluation method
3	Definition and measurement of the resources used/consumed and assignment of costs
4	Definition and measurement of consequences
5	Incremental analysis and dealing with uncertainty
6	Presentation and interpretation of results

Box 19.1 What Questions Do We Want Answers to: Technical and Allocative Efficiency

Efficiency in economics revolves around the maximization of health outcomes using the available resources [4]. When we are interested in choosing different combinations of resources to maximize the health benefit obtained for a given investment, we are asking a question about technical efficiency. And when we are interested in the mixture of health care programs to maximize the health of society, we are asking a question about allocative efficiency. In effect, these efficiency measures are at the micro (specific) and macro (general) levels in scope (Fig. 19.1). Economic evaluation using measures of clinical effectiveness or health outcomes, such as quality-adjusted life years (QALYs) provides answers at the technical efficiency level.

1 – Formulation of the Research Question: The PICO-EE Structure

As noted in the introduction, the overall aim of economic evaluation is to provide evidence to decision makers (see Box 19.1).

With the notion of providing evidence to decision makers at different levels in mind, the evidence-based medicine PICO structure (**P**atient, **I**ntervention, **C**omparator, **O**utcome) [5] is an ideal means of focusing a research question. However, when completing an economic evaluation, some additional components are required namely, specification of the economic perspective of the evaluation and the economic decision maker or decision-making context of the evaluation (Fig. 19.2).

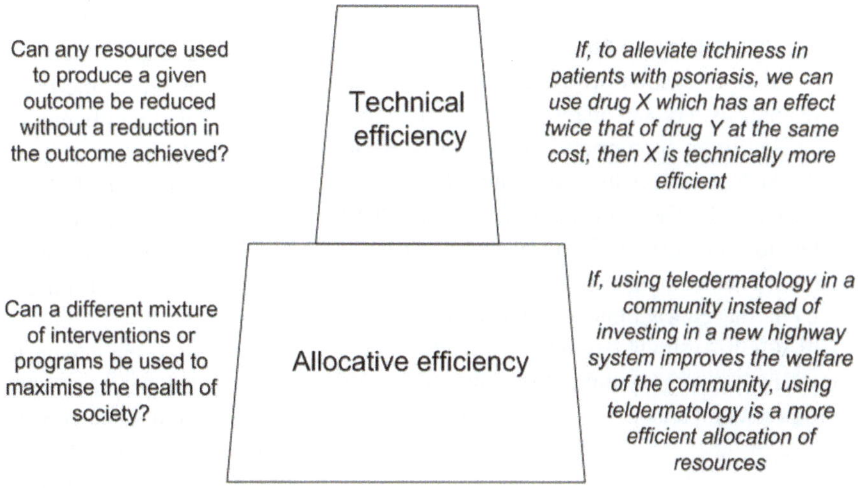

Fig. 19.1 Summary of the efficiency hierarchy in health economics

P	Population or problem
I	Intervention
C	Comparator
O	Outcome

E	Economic perspective
E	Economic decision maker

Fig. 19.2 Summary of the six elements of a focused economic evaluation research question, the PICO-EE structure expanded from Centre for Evidence Based Medicine PICO structure available at http://www.cebm.net/index.aspx?o=1036

As for the more general PICO structure, it is important to realize that the PICO-EE structure provides a set of components to formulate a focused research question. Each component does not necessarily need to be included in the order given. If we take the PICO-EE structure and apply it to a study from the literature, for example the evaluation completed by Pitt et al. [6], "a cost-utility analysis of pimecrolimus vs. topical corticosteroids and emollients for the treatment of mild and moderate atopic eczema" the place of each of the six elements of a focused economic evaluation research question becomes clear (Table 19.2).

Although this produces a rather long research question, requiring a careful balance between brevity and precision, the key components of the evaluation,

Table 19.2 Example of a focus economic evaluation research question using the PICO-EE structure

Structural component	Related research question component
E – Economic perspective	From the perspective of the provider of public health services in the UK
E – Economic decision maker	Should the NHS support
I – Intervention	The use of pimecrolimus as a first or second line treatment
P – Population	For patients with mild and moderate atopic eczema
O – Outcome	As a more cost-effective alternative
C – Comparator	Than topical corticosteroid (TCS) treatment alone

including the comparator (see Box 19.2) are captured in a single comprehensive statement.

The added components of perspective and decision maker are essential and need to be defined from the outset as they have important implications for the evaluation itself.

The implementation of a new alternative will affect different stakeholders in different ways. The concept of perspective is used to specify the scope of the evaluation. As for the Pitt et al. study, this can be limited to the funder of health services, in this case the NHS. The perspective may be limited to an institutional, third party, patient or governmental perspective or it may incorporate a more comprehensive and exhaustive societal perspective.

The choice of perspective will have important implications for data collection as well as the type of question that can be answered. For example, asking whether the NHS should fund a given intervention but

Box 19.2 Selecting a Comparator

Economic evaluation always involves comparative analysis. For any analysis to be meaningful, selection of an appropriate comparator is essential. The National Institute for Clinical Excellence (NICE) in the UK stipulate the use of the "best alternative practice" as the most appropriate comparator in an economic evaluation [7]. In contrast, the Pharmaceutical Benefits Advisory Committee (PBAC) in Australia require "the practice that is used by the largest number of patients" as the required comparator.

Box 19.3 The Economists View of Cost: Opportunity Cost

Although many see economics as being focused only on money, economists view the cost of alternative decisions as encompassing more than dollars. If one health care intervention is invested in over another, there will of course be differences in the costs involved. However, the opportunity cost of this decision is best measured by the health benefits that could have been achieved had the next best alternative intervention been funded [9].

For example, in choosing to spend $1 million on a new telemedicine service for robotic surgery instead of a teledermatology outreach service for children in rural communities, the opportunity cost is the outcomes that would have been gained from the teledermatology outreach service. In choosing A we lose the opportunity of doing B.

taking the perspective of a single GP practice will not provide the right information. In addition, it may or may not be important to take into account the perspective of patients and their families.

Although a number of different perspectives can be taken in an economic evaluation, a societal perspective provides the most comprehensive one indicative of the true opportunity cost to society as a whole [8] (see Box 19.3). From a societal perspective, *all* of the costs involved must be accounted for, as should *all* of the consequences. This includes direct costs (those where an actual transaction occurs e.g. the cost of a surgical procedure or the cost of patient travel to attend an appointment) and indirect costs or productivity costs (i.e. the cost of time off from work for patients and family members involved in disease treatment and care) as well as the value of leisure time lost and the value of life lost. In addition, form a societal perspective, long-term costs, savings and outcomes should also be included. The inclusion of these costs can often be constrained by the availability of reliable data.

At times, the perspective will match with the decision maker (e.g. the Pitt et al. example). At other times the two will need to be specified as separate and distinct components. For example, the decision maker may be the health department as the funder of a particular intervention, yet we may still want to consider a more holistic societal perspective to include patient and family direct and indirect costs.

The opportunity cost is the health benefits forgone when resources are used in a particular way

2 – Selection of an Appropriate Economic Evaluation Method

Given that economic evaluation involves the costs and consequences of alternatives, there are three types of evaluation that can be used namely cost-effectiveness analysis (CEA), cost-utility analysis (CUA) and cost-benefit analysis (CBA).

The primary difference between the different economic evaluation methods is that each form of analysis answers different questions as each expresses the consequences of alternatives using different metrics

Cost-effectiveness analysis (CEA) measures consequences in terms of natural units or intermediate outcomes. An evaluation may compare the cost of two alternative means of reducing patient weight or reducing patient depression scores. The metric used reflects the focus of the research question. For example, a CEA could be used to answer a question about the most cost-effective alternative for reducing blood pressure with the metric used being the incremental cost per millimeter of mercury reduction in blood pressure ($/mmHg) or the most cost-effective alternative for reduce patient weight with the metric being the incremental cost per kg of body weight lost ($/kg).

Cost-utility analysis (CUA) measures consequences in terms of quality adjusted life years (QALYs). Of note, some journals and texts do not distinguish CUA as a distinct economic evaluation method, instead it is considered a specific form of cost-effectiveness analysis that uses QALYs as the measure of consequence.

The composite QALY indicator combines quality and quantity of life into a single index [10]. The underlying concept of QALYs is utility or preferences for different health states. The greater the preference for a given health state, the greater the utility. Utility is expressed on a numerical scale from 0, the health state "Dead" to 1, the health state "Perfect health" [11] or "best imaginable health"[35]. With information on preferences for different health states (their utility) and information on the duration of time spent in that health state, in terms of years, the number of QALYs can be calculated.

Cost-benefit analysis (CBA) measures both costs and consequences in monetary terms. This allows a calculation of net monetary benefit to be made (the overall monetary balance of choosing one intervention over another). When the benefits of an intervention outweigh the costs (i.e. when the net monetary benefit is positive) funding of the intervention is economically justified. If on the other hand the benefits are outweighed by the cost (i.e. when the net monetary benefit is negative) funding of the intervention is not economically justified.

Cost-minimization analysis (CMA) is sometimes included as a forth economic evaluation method. However, this form of analysis assumes, or identifies, that the consequences of the alternative under evaluation are the same. For this reason it is often referred to as a method of partial economic evaluation [2] (see Box 19.4).

As previously noted, the fundamental difference between the different forms of economic evaluation is that each form of analysis answers different questions as each expresses the consequences of alternatives using different metrics.

The use of intermediate outcomes in CEA limits the decision making context to the set of interventions whose consequences can be measured in terms of the selected intermediate outcome. For example, an evaluation that uses depression scores as the metric for quantification of consequences will only provide information for decisions about interventions focused on depression. It will obviously not allow extension of that decision to other health intervention such as immunization or promotion of breast feeding.

Box 19.4 A Note on Cost-Minimization Analysis

It has been argued that CEA is the analytic tool of choice rather than CMA which is often inappropriately employed [12]. Ideally, the assumption of equivalent consequences of alternatives should be confirmed with well designed and conducted randomized controlled trials and meta-analysis, the level of evidence required for pharmacoeconomic evaluation [13]. Even if this data is available, the focus of any evaluation should be on the estimation of the incremental cost, the incremental effect and quantification of the uncertainty surrounding the resulting incremental cost-effectiveness ratio [12] (or net monetary benefit if CBA is used).

Despite this, CMA is often used in telehealth with the assumption that the tele-intervention is equivalent to a face-to-face usual care alternative. In some situations this may seem a reasonable assumption in others the assumption may be less reasonable. Whatever the case, the results of these evaluations must be considered with caution. Although an intervention may be less costly, without careful evaluation of the consequences, important implications may be overlooked possibly to the detriment of patients.

In addition, intermediate measures of effectiveness, rather than final outcome variables such as QALYs, may have no link to the preferences of patients. For example, from a clinical perspective it may seem appropriate to complete an evaluation of two treatment options for the management of osteoporosis with the outcome measured in terms of the reduction in loss of bone mass. The issue is the relationship between bone mass and the perceived benefit of patients. Reduced loss of bone mass may have follow-on effects that are perceived by the patient; however, the direct relationship is unclear if the evaluation is limited to bone density as the measure of effect.

Certain treatments may also have a number of effects not necessarily in the same direction. It may be intuitive to use the cost per point reduction in subjectively rated skin irritation in a CEA of two Eczema treatment options. However, one option may provide improved skin irritation scores on the one hand yet also have gastrointestinal side effects on the other. The multidimensional facets of effectiveness are not usually accounted for when intermediate outcomes are used.

In contrast, the use of QALYs as the metric in CUA addresses many of the issues that using intermediate outcomes presents to CEA.

CUA allows the cost and consequence of diverse health care interventions to be compared using a common metric, the cost per QALY. This allows decision making to extend beyond a single clinical context. The cost-effectiveness of a teledermatology intervention could be compared to the cost-effectiveness of a childhood immunization program with the consequences of both alternatives measured in terms of the quality and quantity of life gained. The use of QALYs as the effect metric also addresses the issues of individual preferences and multidimensionality. By their very nature QALYs, whether obtained directly using Standard Gamble or Time Trade-Off methods, or indirectly using multiattribute health status scoring systems, the preferences of individual's is incorporated (see Box 19.4). In addition, the use of QALYs attempts to estimate a more holistic, multidimensional view of health care effects to provide a final outcome measure incorporating quality and quantity of life.

The dollar per QALY measure is currently the preferred metric for cost-effectiveness analysis in health and medicine [14]

Yet QALYs are not perfect [11, 15] and the dollar per QALY metric is not perfect either. Improvements in quality of life that are not health related are not measured by QALYs. Such improvements might include a more comfortable or convenient treatment option, improvements that may be perceived as valuable to patients. These types of benefits can never be measured correctly with either CEA or CUA. Instead, measures of patients' willingness-to-pay for these benefits need to be incorporated into the evaluation, something that can only be done using CBA.

Despite the challenges associated with quantification of quality and quantity of life as a monetary value, the distillation of consequences to the dollar metric in CBA has some major advantages. The first one is that CBA allows comparisons of very divergent interventions. For example, a health care intervention to reduce the incidence of cancer and the construction of a new freeway to prevent road accidents can be compared using CBA. Again, CBA provides answers to different questions and at a different level of decision making.

Another advantage provided by CBA is the direct link with the normative economic theory known as welfare economics [16] providing it with a sound theoretical, although not uncriticised [17], foundation. The third advantage is the calculation of net monetary benefit. This final metric makes the decision making criterion explicitly clear, fund interventions that have a positive net monetary benefit, don't fund those interventions that have a negative net monetary benefit. Whilst CEA and CUA both provide information on the additional cost per unit of outcome (e.g. the cost per millimeter of mercury reduction in blood pressure or the cost per additional QALY) they do not enable a conclusion on the overall value of investment. For CEA and CUA this last step is separated from the analysis and made the responsibility of the decision maker (although willingness-to-pay thresholds for a QALY are often used as a guide for decision making with CUA, but more on this latter). CBA on the other hand incorporates this component of the analysis in the evaluation itself (see Box 19.5).

The advantages allowed by expressing consequences such as improved quality of life and prolonged life into a dollar value, also presents the greatest drawback of CBA. As such it is not often used as an evaluation technique for health care interventions.

Although these methods have been presented as distinct forms of analysis they are not necessarily mutually exclusive. For example, if the scope of questions ranges from a clinician wanting to know the most cost-effective means of reducing skin irritation in patients with eczema and the health department want to know how this translates into a cost per QALY for decisions regarding funding of a specific therapy, both CEA and CUA can be employed.

Although the selection of which method to use will depend on the question being asked, it is important to realize that these methods may be employed in parallel.

3 – Definition and Measurement of the Resources Used and Assignment of Costs

Although the collection of information on costs seems to be an obvious component in an economic evaluation,

Box 19.5 Clinical Trial or Decision Analytic Model?

With an understanding of the different methods of economic evaluation, it is also important to distinguish between the two different techniques that can be used to complete an economic evaluation of any type, namely as part of a clinical trial or as a decision analytic model.

Clinical trials are the gold standard for establishing the efficacy and effectiveness of new medical therapies or health care interventions [18]. During the past 20 years clinical trials have also become a potential source of information for economic evaluation with the collection of data on health service use and patient related costs as part of the trial [19]. Information provided by economic evaluations conducted alongside clinical trials provide valuable information, yet there are also limitations. The length of follow-up selected, the treatment comparators used and the patient populations studied, result in trial results that do not answer all treatment adoption questions.

Decision analytic modeling addresses these issues by providing a systematic approach to decision making under uncertainty [20]. When applied to the process of economic evaluation, decision analytic modeling allows the definition of a possible set of consequences that flow from a set of alternative options being evaluated (e.g. usual care or teledermatology) using mathematical relationships [21]. The probability of each consequence (e.g. symptom alleviation or no alleviation) is entered into the model along with the corresponding cost ($, €, £) and outcome (mmHg, kg, QALY, $, €, £). For each option evaluated, the expected cost and the expected outcome of each consequence is weighted by the probability of that consequence to provide quantification of the incremental cost per unit of outcome (CEA or CUA).

Why does decision modeling provide answers that clinical trials cannot?

1. Synthesis – Decision modeling is designed around the use of all relevant evidence so results from multiple clinical trials (ideally in the form of a meta-analysis), rather than a single trial, can be brought to bear on the decision problem under evaluation.
2. Comparators – To identify the cost-effectiveness or net monetary benefit of a given intervention, all alternative options that could feasibly be used in practice need to be included, something not feasible, affordable or necessarily ethical in clinical trials.
3. Time horizon – Ideally, the study period needs to be of sufficient length to capture all of the costs and all of the benefits of an intervention, for some interventions this is effectively a life-time horizon.
4. Uncertainty – Surrounding the evidence available to answer a given decision there is always a level of uncertainty. As such decision makers need to know the probability that a given decision is the correct one whilst accounting for the uncertainties in each of the model parameters, this is the role of decision modeling probabilistic sensitivity analysis (although more recent advances in clinical trial economic evaluations include acceptability curves that provide just this type of information). In addition, quantification of this uncertainty can be used to inform on the value and design of additional research (something a clinical trial cannot do).

Ultimately, it is clear that there is a place for both techniques in economic evaluation. Clinical trials inform decision models, decision models provide information to inform decisions and at the same time provide information on what new studies may be conducted and their value in terms of reducing uncertainty around the decision question being asked.

In the end, the choice of technique comes down to the availability, or lack of, evidence and the overall aim of the evaluation. Where the evidence supporting the effectiveness of the intervention or program is well documented, decision analytic modeling may be the technique of choice. Where the evidence is sparse or non-existent, a clinical trial may be indicated as a step in the process of providing information to inform future decision making. On the other hand, when the evidence is sparse, a value of information decision model may provide just the information required to justify the completion of a clinical trial or decision analytic modeling may also be used early in and investigation to demonstrate, within the constraints of the currently available evidence, that a new alternative is a potentially cost-effective approach to a given problem or issue.

this process is actually completed in two steps. Obtaining information directly from health service budgets is not necessarily the first or most appropriate source of information. Likewise, collecting expenses information directly from patients may also be fraught with complications.

The first step is to define what resources need to be accounted for and how best to measure their use. The second step is to identify a per unit value for these resources from which to calculate a cost.

Differentiating these steps is important. The price paid for a resource is not necessarily indicative of its cost. Many hospitals or health care organizations have bulk purchase plans for certain items, if these prices are used in an evaluation the cost will be underestimated. As the underlying aim of any evaluation is to inform decision making, the information used in an evaluation must be indicative of the true cost rather than the price paid. There are some exceptions: where the market price is very close to the marginal cost (e.g. telecommunications) and where the agency is a non-profit organization where the price is thought to equal cost (e.g. government agencies or schedules such as the *Medical Benefits Schedule* item numbers [22] for health services in Australia or the *British National Formulary* [23] for drugs in the UK can be used to value health care resources and services) (see Box 19.6).

Another important component in measuring costs is the annuitization of equipment related expenses. This process allows an initial outlay for equipment to be converted into an annual cost for owning that capital item. Yearly maintenance costs can be included in the calculation as can a salvage price (the asset may be salvageable at the end of the period of use and sold for example, as part of an ongoing upgrade mechanism). The time period which the annuitized cost is spread across is dependent on the useful life of the piece of equipment (usually between 3 and 10 years depending on the item and the upgrade time frame). A discount rate is applied to account for costs occurring at different times (see Box 19.7).

The selection of discount rate can be arbitrary. Some governments specify discount rates when evaluating public investment projects and/or for capital investments. The Australian government for example, set discount rates for high, medium and low risk project proposals at 12%, 10% and 8% respectively in 2007 [29]. With information on the discount rate and time frames, the equivalent annual cost (EAC) of equipment can be calculated, for ease of computation, in two steps:

1. The selected discount rate (*r*) and the time period (*t*) are converted into an annuity factor (A) (19.1).

$$A = \frac{1}{r} \times \left(1 - \left[\frac{1}{(1+r)^t}\right]\right) \tag{19.1}$$

2. The annuity factor is then combined with the initial asset price (*Ap*), the discount rate (*r*), the time period (*t*), the annual maintenance cost (*M*) and the salvage price (*S*) (19.2) (see Box 19.8).

$$EAC = \left(\left[A_p - \frac{S}{(1+r)^t}\right] \times \frac{1}{A}\right) + M \tag{19.2}$$

Cost-effectiveness in health care is not necessarily synonymous with the cheapest option instead it is the cost per unit of outcome that should drive decisions.

4 – Definition and Measurement of Consequences

The metric of consequences is defined implicitly with the specific economic evaluation method selected. When CEA is selected the definition and measurement of consequences must focus on the appropriate natural unit to be measured and the measurement method to be used. The working group on core measures of the burden of skin diseases identified 11 skin-specific quality of life measures that pertain to Adults [34] including the skindex [35] and the Dermatology Life Quality Index (DLQI) [36]. Although the point has already been made, it is essential to remember that the use of these types of tools for economic evaluation provides limited answers to questions of cost-effectiveness. These scales were developed as measures of skin disease related, rather than preference-based, quality of life instruments and do not provide utility scores for the calculation of QALYs. Whilst the cost per point reduction in the Skindex instrument may provide useful information within a given context, it will not provide information for questions of productive efficiency.

For the calculation of QALYs in a CUA, utility scores can be obtained using direct or indirect methods.

Direct elicitation of preferences to derive utilities can be achieved using Standard Gamble (SG), Time Trade-

Box 19.6 Classification of Costs

Direct costs are those that accompany the occurrence of a transaction. For example, in the Pitt et al. cost-utility analysis of pimecrolimus direct health costs included the cost of drugs and health care personnel (in other circumstances the cost of hospitalization might be included as a direct health cost). Travel costs incurred by patients to attend outpatient visits are another form of direct, although non-health related, cost.

In the Pitt et al. example, pimecrolimus treatment was valued at £62.35/100 g and low-potency topical corticosteroids at £2.47/100 g as per the *British National Formulary* [23]. The quantity of either of these drugs was based on the weight required for a specific body part for each monthly treatment, for example the face required 30 g with a resulting cost of £18.71 for pimecrolimus treatment and £0.74 for topical corticosteroids. As you can see, information on the volume of the resources and a valuation of its price, where used in tandem to calculate the cost used in the analysis.

Costing other items in this way can be more of a challenge. For patient transport such as road travel, the approach taken in some evaluations has been to measure the distance travelled by the patient and to multiply this by the tax refund allowed for business use of a personal vehicle, in the 2008/9 financial year in Australia the rate was $0.74/km for a medium sized car [24]. The aim of this is to avoid confounding variations in petrol prices, car sizes and associated fuel consumption whilst still providing a reasonable valuation of patient travel in the analysis. Identifying the cost of air travel is also a challenge. One approach is to use the lowest available air fare identified using available online information (e.g. WebJet.com.au, Cheapflights.com, skyscanner.net).

Indirect costs are those that traditionally do not involve a direct transaction, for example unpaid care provided by family members or decreased productivity when at work. There are a number of approaches for calculating these costs including the human capital approach, friction cost approach and US Panel approach for paid time.

Unpaid time such as time spent performing informal care activities, leisure time or time for those not in the work force, is rarely included in economic evaluations due to challenges of measurement and valuation. There are approaches that attempt to do this (e.g. the replacement cost of informal care and valuing the impact of caring on carer's quality of life) however detailed information on the time spent in these situations is required. In general, an attempt should be made to account for these indirect costs for inclusion, at the very least, in sensitivity analysis.

Costs can be further classified as fixed or variable. Differentiating costs in this way is important so decision makers have a clear indication of the costs involved in maintaining the base requirements of a service and those that will change depending on the level of use of the service.

Fixed costs are those that do not vary with the level of activity. This may include equipment costs, installation costs or basic infrastructure costs (office space or buildings). *Variable costs* on the other hand are those that vary with the level of activity. This may include staff costs (the more activity in a service, the more staff that will be required), telecommunications costs (e.g. telephone lines, Internet accounts) or travel costs.

Sunk costs are those that occur as one-off costs (e.g. telephone line installation). If the analysis involves the use of an existing service where the required telecommunications infrastructure is already in place, sunk costs can be ignored. Usually however, installation costs are an important component to include in an analysis so the decision maker is aware of costs to include in the implementation of a new service, one-off or otherwise.

Off (TTO), or discrete-choice experiment methods. These methods can be used with members of the general population or with patients with a particular disease or condition and results used in modeling-based evaluations. They can also be used directly with patients during a study. At times however, the completion of these methods is impractical. In this situation, indirect methods should be used.

Indirect methods for estimating utilities alongside trial-based studies include instruments to measure health states which patients can complete directly during a study (e.g. EQ-5D, HUI, AQoL) [37–39].

Box 19.7 Accounting for Time Preferences: Discounting Future Costs and Outcomes

It is human nature to value things gained, or lost, now more than things gained or lost in the future. The use of credit cards displays the phenomena of positive time preference perfectly. Many individuals prefer to have the enjoyment provided by an item purchased now and delay the cost of that purchase until latter, despite the fact that it will cost more in the end when done this way dependent on the interest rate attached to the card. Another example is smoking cigarettes, smokers value the pleasure of smoking now more than the health losses resulting from smoking in the future [25].

Discounting is the process of making current costs and benefits worth more than those occurring in the future to account for time preferences. Although the discounting of health effects has raised some debate in the past [26], it is now common practice to report both discounted and undiscounted results in analyses so decision makers can see the results of the analysis in terms of absolute costs and effects, regardless of when they occur, and the same results accounting for time preferences [27].

A discount rate of 3.5%, for both costs and effects, is recommended by NICE in the UK. A discount rate of 5% is recommended in Australia [28]. The impact on results of different discount rates should be included as part of the sensitivity analyses completed. With the discount rate selected (*r*), a calculation of the present value (*PV*) of a future cost (or effect) incurred in (t) years time (i.e. the future value [*FV*]), can be made. The formula for calculating *PV* is shown in Eq. 19.3 with an example presented in Table 19.3.

$$PV = \frac{FV}{(1+r)^t} \qquad (19.3)$$

Table 19.3 Discounting a future cost of $1,000 and effect of 1 QALY occurring in 5 years time, to see its present value using different discount rates

Future value	Discount rate (%)	Present value
Cost ($)		
1,000	0	1,000.00
1,000	3.5	841.97
1,000	5.0	783.53
1,000	10.0	620.92
Effect (QALYs)		
1	0	1.00
1	3.5	0.84
1	5.0	0.78
1	10.0	0.62

Box 19.8 The Cost of a Teledermatology Project a Worked Example Part 1: Annutization

Chan et al. [30] investigated the use of videoconferencing for remote specialist diagnosis and treatment planning for elderly patients with dermatological conditions from two hospitals in China. In this study, patients were first seen by a resident medical officer. If specialist opinion was required, consenting patients were assessed by a dermatologist using videoconferencing. On the same-day a face-to-face consultation with the same dermatologist was conducted to compare the diagnoses and management plans.

The cost of providing the teledermatology service to patients and the cost of providing usual care to patients, including travel costs, were calculated. Of note, only direct costs were included in this analysis presumably due to the fact that patients were institutionalized elderly patients, no account of lost *leisure* time for either option, teledermatology consultation or usual care was incorporated into the analysis. Table 19.4 presents a summary of the annuitization of the videoconferencing system cost from the Chan et al. [30] as an example of this process.

Table 19.4 Annutization of equipment used in a published evaluation of a teledermatology service in Hong Kong [30]

Step	Calculations	Inputs
1. Calculating the annuity factor	$A = \frac{1}{r} \times \left(1 - \left[\frac{1}{(1+r)^t}\right]\right)$ $A = \frac{1}{0.08} \times \left(1 - \left[\frac{1}{(1+0.08)^5}\right]\right)$ $A = 3.99$	Discount rate = 8% Time period = 5 years
2. Calculation of EAC	$EAC = \left(\left[A_p - \frac{S}{(1+r)^t}\right]\right) \times \frac{1}{A} + M$ $EAC = \left([67{,}500] \times \frac{1}{3.99}\right) + 7{,}200$ $EAC = 24{,}106$	Asset price (A_p) = 67,500 Annual maintenance cost (M) = 7,200[a] Salvage price (S) = 0

[a]In the original publication it is unclear what the annual on-site maintenance cost of HK$7,200 actually covered, for this example, it has been assigned solely to the videoconferencing system for demonstration purposes

Box 19.8 The Cost of a Teledermatology Project a Worked Example Part 2: Measuring, Valuation and Costing

Table 19.5 uses annuitized costs for all equipment to show the mix of fixed and variable costs for both the teledermatology service and usual care alternatives compared in the Chan et al. study.

Whilst the Chan et al. study provides an interesting example for this analysis of cost, their conclusion that teledermatology is cost-effective (stating that it cost HK$57.7 to see each patient via teledermatology and HK$322.8 to send them for usual care resulting in a saving of HK$265.1 per patient) highlights some of the misunderstandings about economic evaluation prevelant in the telehealth literature.

It is true that the lower cost intervention can be said to be the most cost-effective when the alternatives under evaluation have been shown to be identical in terms of their outcomes however, assertions on the equivalence of treatment options require specifically designed and well powered randomized controlled trials [31, 32]. It is inappropriate to conduct a cost-minimization analysis on the basis of an observed lack of significance in the effect differences between treatments alone [12]. Whilst the authors of the Chan et al. study considered diagnostic and management accuracy as part of the study, the equivalence of the two modalities, in terms of patient outcomes, was not specifically tested. Instead the recommendation is that "the analytic focus should be on the estimation of the joint density of cost and effect differences, the quantification of uncertainty surrounding the incremental cost-effectiveness ratio and the presentation of such data as cost-effectiveness acceptability curves" [12].

Table 19.5 Summary of costs included in an investigation of teledermatology for elderly patients reported in Hong Kong dollars (HK$) with no base year specified [30]

Cost	Teledermatology[b]	Usual care[e]
Fixed costs[a]		
Videoconferencing system	24,106	–
Television	949	–
Cordeless headphone system	113	–
Document camera	1,252	–
PCMCIA network card	301	–
Sub total	*26,721*	*0*
Sunk costs[c]		
ISDN line instillation	1485	–
Variable costs		
ISDN line rental	12.960	–
ISDN call charges	9,240	–
Consultation time for 74 patients at HK$57.7/patient for teledermatology HK$42.8/patient for usual care[d]	4,270	3,167
Transportation cost for 74 patients at HK$230/patient	–	17,020
Escort cost for 74 patients at HK$50/transport	–	3,700
Sub total	*13,523*	*23,887*
Total cost	**41,729**	**23,887**
Average variable cost per patient	183	323

ISDN integrated services digital network, *PCMCIA* Personal Computer Memory Card International Association

[a]In the original publication equipment costs do not appear to have been annuitized, annuitization has be completed in this summary using the published asset cost, maintenance cost and a discount rate of 8% over 5 years

[b]In the original analysis a set-up cost per site of HK$89,426 was presented; however, the cost of all of the equipment and the ISDN installation as published was HK$77,941 with the source of this discrepancy being unclear, the equipment costs as reported in the original publication have been used here

[c]Included as a one-off installation cost and therefore not annuatized

[d]The difference in per patient consultation is reportedly to account for the reduced level of diagnostic accuracy (74.3% versus 100%) of teledermatology

[e]The original publication included a third option, having the dermatologist travel to the remote hospital to provide consultation however, in the interest of space this has been excluded here

Box 19.8 The Cost of a Teledermatology Project a Worked Example Part 3: A Note on Assumptions, Budget Impact and Sensitivity Analysis

In the example from Chan et al. of costing a teledermatology project, it is important to recognize that a number of key assumptions have been made. These assumptions may have important ramifications for the analysis, the information it provides to decision makers and the generalizability of results to other contexts.

Firstly, Chan et al. assumed that the physical space required to conduct teleconsultations at both the referring and specialist ends was available at no cost. This may or may not be a reasonable assumption depending on the context. Secondly, they also assumed that the staff required to complete consultation at both ends, are available and have the time to complete teleconsultations. When telehealth replaces face-to-face consultations this may be a reasonable; however, when telehealth is an additional service, rather than a direct substitute, teleconsultations will add an additional load to the service requiring more staff.

These points will impact on the overall results as well as impacting the different stakeholders involved in different ways. A budget impact analysis allows for identification of cost-shifting from one stakeholder to another as well as an estimate of the impact of implementation on budgets at the national, regional or local level. [33] Undertaking a budget impact analysis can make these components clear. Sensitivity analyses (to be covered in more detail in section six of this chapter) can then follow to explore the impact on results overall, and for different stakeholders, of different assumptions and scenarios (e.g. patient transport covered by patients, the elder care institution or the referring hospital).

Algorithms (e.g. SF-6D) [40] have also been developed to convert scores from health-related quality of life instruments into utilities (e.g. SF-36, SF-12) [41, 42]. The key point with indirect methods is these instruments have scoring algorithms derived from the preferences of representative samples of the general population. That is, the utility weights are based on the valuations from the preferences of tax payers and consumers – these being the main players in any healthcare system.

All of these methods attempt to provide an indication of the utility of a patient at a given time point

Box 19.9 Calculating QALYs: The Area Under the Curve and the Complex Numbers Methods
A simple method for calculating QALYs from utility scores is called the area under the curve method. A patient with a utility of 0.6 at baseline, 0.8 at 6 month follow-up, 0.9 at 1 year follow-up and 1.0 at 2 year follow-up, will have an accumulated 1.725 QALYs. The proportion of a QALY for each time period is calculated as the average utility multiplied by the proportion of time relative to 1 year (Table 19.6).

Table 19.6 Calculating QALYs as a function of utility score at the beginning and end of each observation

Time period	Calculation(Average utility × proportion of 1 year)		QALYs
Baseline to 6 months	((0.6+0.8) × 0.5) × 0.5	=	0.35
6–12 months	((0.8+0.9) × 0.5) × 0.5	=	0.425
12–24 months	((0.9+1.0) × 0.5) × 1.0	=	0.95
Total		=	*1.725*

which, when collected over a number of time points, these can be used to calculate QALYs (see Box 19.9).

5 - Incremental Analysis and Dealing with Uncertainty

With research question in hand and having decided on the economic evaluation methods to be used along with the costs and effects to be measured, the next step is to complete an incremental analysis.

Incremental analysis in health economic evaluation involves calculation of the difference in cost, and outcomes, when one or more alternatives are compared to another [43]. For example, Moreno-Ramirez et al. [44] compared the difference between the cost and effect of a store-and-forward teledermatology system for skin cancer patients to the cost and effect of conventional skin cancer care. The cost of the teledermatology system ($Cost_{Tele}$) and the cost of the conventional care alternative ($Cost_{Conventional}$) were calculated and used to provide an estimate of the incremental cost (IC) (19.4).

$$Incremental\,cost = Cost_{Tele} - Cost_{Conventional} \quad (19.4)$$

For the Moreno-Ramirez et al. study, the incremental cost of the teledermatology system was −€49.59 (i.e. when teledermatology was compared to conventional care, the per patient cost was on average €50 less for patients in the teledermatology group).

Similarly, the difference between the effect of the teledermatology intervention ($Effect_{Tele}$) and the conventional care alternative ($Effect_{Conventional}$) was calculated to provide an estimate of the incremental effect (IE) (19.5).

$$Incremental\ effect = Effect_{Tele} - Effect_{Conventional} \quad (19.5)$$

For the Moreno-Ramirez et al. study, the effect was measured in terms of waiting intervals from time of first visit to the local doctor and subsequent follow-up in a skin cancer clinic. In this study the incremental effect was –76.31 days (i.e. when teledermatology was compared to conventional care, the patient waiting time was on average 76 days less for patients in the teledermatology group) (see Box 19.10).

When CEA and CUA are used, the final step in an incremental analysis is to produce an incremental cost-effectiveness ratio (ICER). This is a comparison of the difference in cost (IC) and the difference in effect (IE) (19.6).

$$ICER = \frac{IC}{IE} = \frac{Cost_{Tele} - Cost_{Conventional}}{Effect_{Tele} - Effect_{Conventional}} \quad (19.6)$$

This produces the final metric of the analysis, the cost per unit of outcome. For the Heinen-Krammerer et al. [47] study of etanercept in patients with moderate-to-severe plaque-type psoriasis compared to non-systemic topical therapy, the ICER for patients with severe disease was €18,154/QALY (i.e. etanercept therapy provided more benefit at a cost of €18,154 for each additional QALY).

Of course, this description of incremental analysis provides only a point estimate of the final ICER. In any evaluation there will be a level of uncertainty in the estimates of both incremental cost and incremental effect and correspondingly in the final ICER. It is important to quantify this uncertainty.

For clinical studies, the mean and 95% confidence interval (CI) provide information on the average patient response along with an indication of the uncertainty in this value. The same applies to ICER and NMB estimates. For ICERs completed alongside clinical trials this can be done using both parametric and non-parametric approaches.

Box 19.10 Statistical Methods for Incremental Analysis of Clinical Trial Data

When decision analytic modeling is used, incremental analysis is an inherent part of the analytic process. When individual patient data is collected as part of a clinical trial, statistical techniques need to be implemented. It is important to remember that it is the mean difference in cost that is the important metric for incremental analysis. Whilst the simplest of statistical technique is the *t*-test, cost data is typically non-normally distributed with highly skewed distributions. The temptation may be to analyze geometric mean or median or to use non-parametric techniques such as the Mann–Whitney *U* test or to perform some transformation. None of these approaches is appropriate as they do not quantify the arithmetic mean of the raw cost, the important summary statistic from both a social and budgetary perspective [45, 46].

In addition, more than treatment allocation may explain differences in cost between patients. Multivariable linear regression may be used however, again the distributional properties of the data are often limiting. Non-parametric bootstrapping in one option as well as generalized linear models (GLMs). GLMs can be used to address the specific distributional properties of the data as well as incorporating another additional feature of cost data that can be challenging, substantial zeros.

Given the challenging distributional properties of cost data obtained during clinical trials, it has been recommended that both simple univariate and multivariable analysis be used along with the presentation of different multivariable models so the uncertainty of results using different analytic techniques can be compared [19]. The same advice applies to effect data.

For both cost and effect data, incremental analysis involves reporting of the mean difference in cost and the mean difference in effect along with measures of variability, precision and an indication if the observed differences are likely to have occurred by chance.

Box 19.11 Uncertainty in Modeling Based Evaluations: Probabilistic Sensitivity Analysis

When decision analytic modeling is used a different technique is required for the construction of a 95% CI. The uncertainties surrounding each parameter are entered into the model (usually expressed as a distribution with mean x and standard error y). Monte Carlo simulations use repeated random sampling to construct a 95% CI accounting for the uncertainties, usually in each and every parameter, in the model. This probabilistic sensitivity analysis allows each and every variable in the model to vary simultaneously. Although computationally intensive, specialist software packages are available for this (e.g. TreeAge Pro) [50].

Fieller's parametric method assumes cost and effect pairs are bivariate normal and uses Student's *t*-distribution with $(n-1)$ degrees of freedom to construct a confidence interval for the ratio of two means [48]. Alternatively, non-parametric bootstrapping uses re-sampling with replacement from the given distribution from which to calculate a 95% CI. Again, as for the analysis of incremental cost and effect, results using different methods should be presented to allow readers to assess variability due to analytic technique [49].

After accounting for the uncertainty in the incremental cost, incremental effect and the final ICER or NMB using statistical methods, there remain additional uncertainties unrelated to sampling variation. This is the role of sensitivity analysis (see Box 19.11).

A one-way sensitivity analysis is used to evaluate the relative impact of the variables included in the analysis. Systematic variation of each variable across a plausible range of values, whilst holding all other variables constant, reveals the relative influence of each variable [51]. For example, the plausible cost of telecommunications may vary by 10% of the baseline value used in the analysis. Re-running the analysis with the telecommunications cost reduced by 10% and increased by 10% will reveal the impact of this variation in telecommunications cost on the overall result. Completing multiple one-way analyses with a fixed variation (i.e. ±50%) will reveal which variables have the greatest to the least impact on the overall result. Alternatively, best and worst case values can be

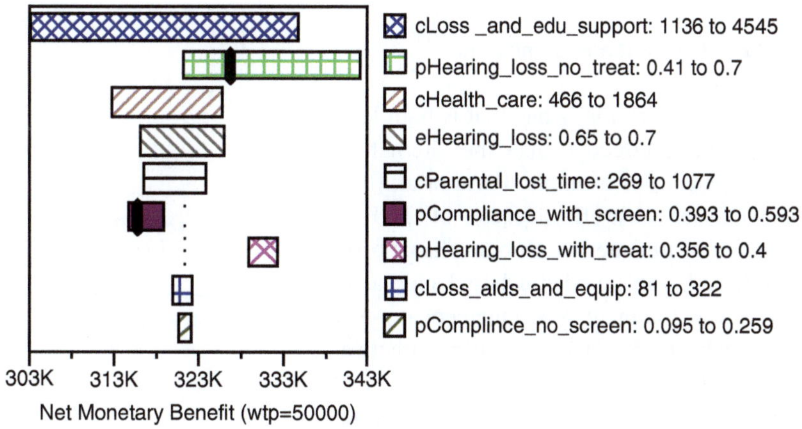

Fig. 19.3 An example of a sensitivity analysis tornado diagram from a hypothetical hearing loss study using modeling-based CEA

used. Another alternative form of multiple one-way sensitivity analysis is to complete a threshold sensitivity analysis. Instead of varying each parameter by a fixed amount, each parameter is varied to the extent where it changes the overall result of the evaluation. Threshold sensitivity analysis shows how much a particular variable needs to change for example, to result in the intervention under evaluation being no longer cost-effective.

Regardless, it is important to justify the form of sensitivity analysis selected as well as the choice of parameters included and, for sensitivity analyses other than threshold, the range over which these parameters are varied [52].

The results of sensitivity analyses are best presented in a table and/or diagrammatically, for example as a tornado diagram (Fig. 19.3).

Table 19.7 Summary results of a hypothetical teledermatology study using modeling-based CEA

Mean values	Option A – Standard care	Option B – Teledermatology
Undiscounted		
Cost	213,600	211,900
Incremental cost		–1,700
QALYs	10.312	10.414
Incremental QALYS		0.102
Cost/QALY	20,714	20,353
Incremental cost/ QALY		–16,667/**Dominant**
Discounted		
Cost	196,800	195,200
Incremental cost		–1,500
QALYs	9.498	9.591
Incremental QALYS		0.093
Cost/QALY	20,718	20,357
Incremental cost/ QALY		–16,129/**Dominant**

6 – Presentation and Interpretation of Results

With the incremental analysis complete a table should be used to report the results. The components to report from modeling based and trial based analyses will differ.

For modeling based evaluations, the mean cost and mean effect in each group, the difference in cost and effects and the calculated incremental cost-effectiveness ratio should be reported with both discounted and undiscounted results presented (Table 19.7).

The choice of threshold levels presented will be dependent on the context of the evaluation and the decision maker targeted. Although neither NICE or the Australian pharmaceuticals benefits advisory committee (PBAC) set $/QALY thresholds, the mean cost per QALY value for PBAC decisions between 1994 and 2004 was $A46,400 with an increase of $10,000/ QALY reducing the probability of listing by 0.06 [53]. The UK NICE guidelines are explicit – interventions with an ICER less than £20,000 should be accepted as cost-effective, those with an ICER between £20,000 and £30,000 need greater supporting evidence to be accepted as cost-effective and those with an ICER

Box 19.12 Dominant and Dominated Interventions

A dominant intervention is one that is both less costly and more effective than the alternative being compared. For example, Portu et al. [55] investigated the cost-effectiveness of TNF-α blockers for the treatment of chronic plaque psoriasis in Italy. Using a modeling based approach, infliximab was dominant over etanercept at week 24 and weeks 48–50 making it more effective and less costly.

This ideal situation makes decision making clear cut, fund dominant alternatives.

Dominated alternatives present the opposite scenario. In this situation the new alternative is more costly and less effective than the standard care alternative. Again, decision making is clear, do not fund dominated alternatives.

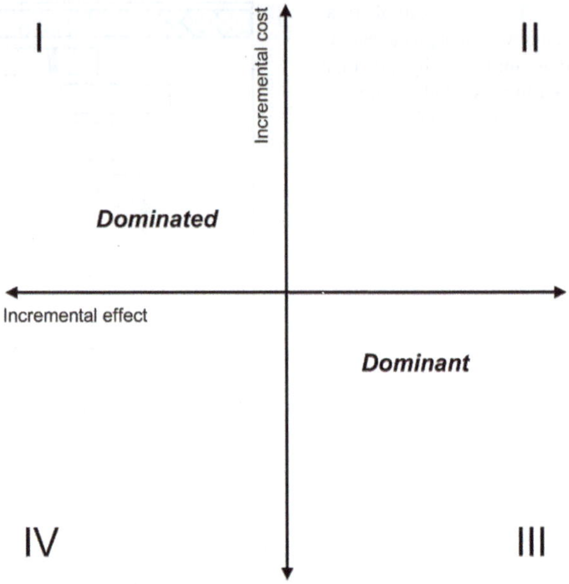

Fig. 19.4 The cost-effectiveness plane

Table 19.8 Summary results of a hypothetical teledermatology trial based CEA

Parameters	Intervention	Control
Undiscounted		
Cost (2007 AUD)	2,984	2,648
Incremental cost (95% CI, *p*-value)		336 (895 to −126, 0.19)
Effect (QALYs)	0.62	0.49
Incremental effect (95% CI, *p*-value)		0.13 (0.11–0.15, 0.03)
Incremental cost/QALY		2,585
Fieller's 95% CI		1,958–3,312
Bootstrapping 95% CI		1,268–5,159
Discounted		
Cost (2007 AUD)	2,763	2,415
Incremental cost (95% CI, *p*-value)		258 (763 to −118, 0.18)
Effect (QALYs)	0.61	0.47
Incremental effect (95% CI, *p*-value)		0.14 (0.10– 0.14, 0.03)
Incremental cost/QALY		1,843
Fieller's 95% CI		1,226– 3,211
Bootstrapping 95% CI		1,184– 4,986

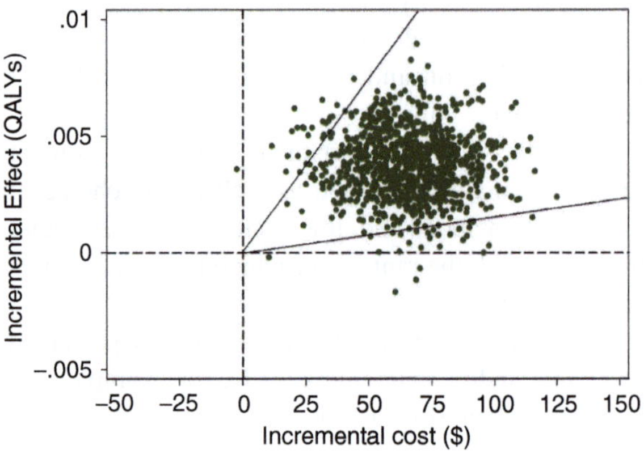

Fig. 19.5 The joint distribution of incremental cost and effect for a hypothetical teledermatology clinical trial using 1,000 bootstrap replicates with 95% confidence internal marked for reference

greater that £30,000 need a strong compelling case for acceptance as cost-effective. In contrast, the World Health Organisation (WHO) define the threshold as three times the gross domestic product of a given country [54] (see Box 19.12).

For trial based evaluations, more information on the uncertainty of results is required as well as the results using different analytic techniques (Table 19.8).

The cost-effectiveness plane [56] can be used to present the results of both a trial based study and a modeling-based study. The cost-effectiveness plane is made up of four quadrants with incremental effect on the *x*-axis and incremental cost on the *y*-axis (Fig. 19.4).

With each of the four quadrants labeled from I to IV working from the top left in a clockwise direction, the

Table 19.9 Summary of the distribution of incremental cost and effect points on the cost-effectiveness plane for a hypothetical teledermatology CEA

WTP Threshold	Quadrant	$20,000/QALY	$30,000/QALY	$50,000/QALY
I – More costly and more effective	Less than threshold	18%	22%	25%
	Greater than threshold	8%	4%	1%
II – More costly and less effective	Dominated	1%	1%	1%
III – Less costly and less effective	Less than threshold	0%	0%	0%
	Greater than threshold	0%	0%	0%
IV – Less costly and more effective	Dominant	73%	73%	73%

cost-effectiveness plane helps to understand the results of the incremental analysis. Interventions that are both less costly and more effective, those that are dominant, fall in quadrant III. Interventions that are dominated fall into quadrant I. Decision making in these situation is more clear cut – fund those interventions that fall into quadrant III and reject those that fall into quadrant I. Interventions with a cost-effectiveness ratio in quadrant II and IV require a valuation of the threshold level at which the additional cost, or saving in quadrant IV, is acceptable. Generally, interventions that are less costly but also less effective are not funded. Interventions that are more costly and more effective and are below the given threshold, are accepted and those above are rejected.

For a trial based study, bootstrap replicates are used (Fig. 19.5). For a modeling-based study, the results from Monte Carlo simulations are generally used.

Despite the intuitive understanding inherent in the cost-effectiveness plane, the issue of uncertainty remains. This can be readily seen in the distribution of points on the cost-effectiveness plane. The uncertainty in the outcome can be quantified by accounting for the number of points above and below the threshold level selected. This can be presented in a table and graphically as a cost-effectiveness acceptability curve. A table would present the percentage of points in each quadrant across the different threshold levels selected (Table 19.9). A cost-effectiveness acceptability curve provides similar information with the probability that the intervention is cost-effective plotted against the different threshold levels (Fig. 19.6).

In presenting the results of the study an answer to the original research questions should be provided. The focus should be on transparency with results provided in aggregated and disaggregated forms [52], hence the use of comprehensive tables as outlined in this chapter.

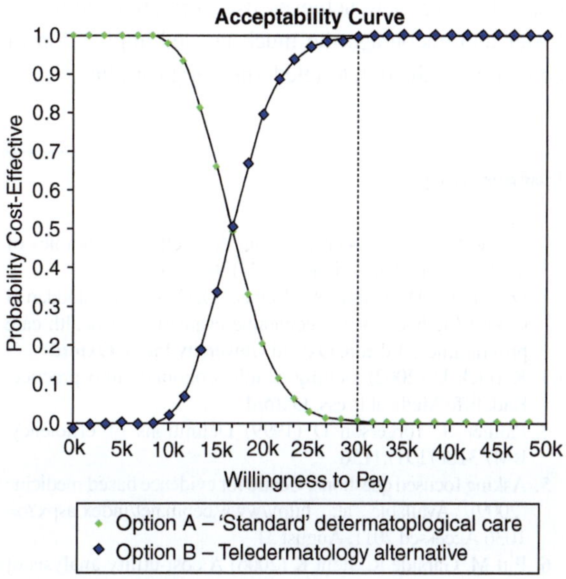

Fig. 19.6 Cost-effectiveness acceptability curves for a hypothetical teledermatology CEA

Conclusion

Economic evaluation in health care is concerned with answering decision making questions in a systematic, transparent and justifiable way. The overall aim is to provide evidence to decision makers on whether investing in a new alternative is a good decision or not. Economic evaluation provides the tools to compare the cost and outcomes of alternatives against a reference treatment or intervention within a given context.

The prescriptive steps used as a framework for presenting economic evaluation in this chapter provide a seemingly simple formula. It is important however to state that there are many decisions to be made along this path and many different facets in any analysis to be considered. Although this chapter has attempted to be as comprehensive as possible there are always additional issues and challenges in every evaluation. Despite the obvious conflict of interest in the statement, it nonetheless must be said that collaboration with a health economist early and consistently throughout an economic evaluation is highly recommended.

As every health system works within budgetary constraints and the issue of expanding health care expenditure becomes an even more critical problem, providing decision makers with information on the cost and effect of a teledermatology alternative will be essential. We hope this overview achieves its overarching aim - to foster and encourage the much needed application of economic evaluation to teledermatology studies.

References

1. Arrow K (1963) Uncertainty and the welfare economics of medical care. Am Econ Rev 53(5):941–73
2. Drummond M, Sculpher M, Torrance G, O'Brien B, Stoddart G (2005) Methods for the economic evaluation of health care programmes, 3rd edn. Oxford University Press, Oxford
3. Kernick D (2002) Getting health economics into practice. Radcliffe Medical Press, Oxford
4. Palmer S, Torgerson D (1999) Definitions of efficiency. BMJ 318(7191):1136
5. Asking focused questions: Centre for evidence based medicine (2009) Available at: http://www.cebm.net/index.aspx?o=1036 Accessed 2011, August 31
6. Pitt M, Garside R, Stein K (2006) A cost-utility analysis of pimecrolimus vs. topical corticosteroids and emollients for the treatment of mild and moderate atopic eczema. Br J Dermatol 154(6):1137–46
7. National Institute for Clinical Excellence (NICE) (2004) Guide to the methods of technology appraisal. London: NICE
8. Byford S, Raftery J (1998) Perspectives in economic evaluation. BMJ 316(7143):1529–30
9. Palmer S, Raftery J (1999) Opportunity cost. BMJ 318:1551–2
10. Patrick D, Erickson P (1993) Health status and health policy. Oxford Univeristy Press, New York
11. Nord E (1999) Cost-value analysis in health care: making sense out of QALYs. Cambridge University Press, Cambridge
12. Briggs A, O'Brien B (2001) The death of cost-minimization analysis? Health Econ 10(2):179–84
13. Vogenberg RE (2001) Introduction to applied pharmacoeconomics. McGraw-Hill, New York
14. Kind P, Lafata J, Matuszewski K, Raisch D (2009) The use of QALYs in clinical and patient decision-making: issues and prospects. Value Health 12(suppl 1):S27–30
15. Duru G, Auray J, Beresniak A, Lamure M, Paine A, Nicoloyannis N (2002) Limitations of the methods used for calculating quality adjusted life year values. Pharmacoeconomics 20:463–73
16. Boadway R, Bruce N (1984) Welfare economics. Basil Blackwell Publisher Ltd., Oxford
17. Little I (2002) A critique of welfare economics. Oxford University Press, Oxford
18. Sibbald B (1998) Understanding controlled trials: why are randomised controlled trials important? BMJ 316(7126):201
19. Glick H, Doshi J, Sonnad S, Polsky D (2007) Economic evaluation in clinical trials. Oxford University Press, Oxford
20. Raiffa C (1968) Decision analysis: introductory lectures on choices under uncertainty. Addison-Wesley, Reading
21. Briggs A, Claxton K, Sculpher M (2006) Decision modelling for health economic evaluation. Oxford University Press, Oxford
22. Australian Government Department of Health and Ageing: MBS Online. Commonwealth of Australia. Available from: http://www.health.gov.au/internet/mbsonline/publishing.nsf/Content/Medicare-Benefits-Schedule-MBS-1. accessed 31 August, 2011
23. British Medical Association & Royal Pharmaceutical Society of Great Britain (2005) British National Formulary, No. 49. Pharmaceutical Press, Oxfordshire
24. Australian Taxation Office. Claiming a deduction for car expenses using the cents per kilometre method. Australian Government. Available from: http://www.ato.gov.au/individuals/content.asp?doc=/content/33874.htm&pc=001/002/013/008/004&mnu=1220&mfp=001/002&st=&cy=1. accessed 31 August, 2011
25. Cairns J (1994) Valuing future benefits. Health Econ 3:221–9
26. Torgerson D (1999) Discounting. BMJ 319(7214):914–5
27. Smith D, Gravelle H (2001) The practice of discounting in economic evaluations of healthcare interventions. Int J Technol Assess Health Care 17(2):236–43
28. Australian Government Department of Health and Ageing (2008) Guidelines for preparing submissions to the Pharmaceutical Benefits Advisory Committee (Version 4.3). Canberra: Commonwealth of Australia
29. Australian Government Department of Finance and Deregulation (2007) The Australian government property ownership framework. Canberra
30. Chan H, Woo J, Chan W, Hjelm M (2001) Teledermatology in Hong Kong: a cost-effective method to provide service to the elderly patients living in institutions. Int J Dermatol 39(10):774–8
31. Borman P, Chatfield M, Damjanov I, Jackson P (2009) Design and analysis of method equivalence studies. Anal Chem 81(24):9849–57
32. Pater C (2004) Equivalence and noninferiority trials – are they viable alternatives for registration of new drugs? Curr Control Trials Cardiovasc Med 5(1):8
33. Mauskopf J, Sullivan S, Annemans L, Caro J, Mullins C, Nuijten M et al (2007) "Principles of good practice for budget impact analysis" report of the ISPOR task force on good research practices-budget impact analysis. Value Health 10(5):336–47
34. Chen S (2007) Dermatology quality of life instruments: sorting out the quagmire. J Invest Dermatol 127:2695–6

35. Chren M, Lasek R, Quinn L, Covinsky K (1997) Convergent and discriminant validity of a generic and a disease-specific instrument to measure quality of life in patients with skin disease. J Invest Dermatol 108:103–7
36. Finlay A, Khan GCED (1994) Dermatology Life Quality Index (DLQI): a simple practical measure for routine clinical use. Clin Exp Dermatol 19:210–6
37. Gusi N, Olivares P, Rajendram R (2010) The EQ-5D health related quality of life questionnaire. In: Preedy V, Watosn R (eds) Handbook of disease burdens and quality of life measures. Springer, New York, pp 87–99
38. Horsman J, Furlong W, Feeny D, Torrance G (2003) The health utilities index (HUI®): concepts, measurement properties and applications. Health Qaul Life Outcomes 1:54
39. Richardson J, Day N, Peacock S, Iezzi A (2004) Measurement of the quality of life for economic evaluation and the Assessment of Quality of Life (AQoL) Mark 2 Instrument. Aust Econ Rev 37(1):62–88
40. Brazier J, Roberts J (2004) The estimation of a preference-based measure of health from the SF-12. Med Care 42(9):851–59
41. Brazier J, Harper R, Jones N, O'Cathain A, Thomas K, Usherwood T et al (1992) Validating the SF-36 health survey questionnaire: new outcome measure for primary care. BMJ 305(6846):160–4
42. Ware J, Kosinski M, Keller S (1996) A 12-Item Short-Form Health Survey: construction of scales and preliminary tests of reliability and validity. Med Care 34(3):220–33
43. Schulman K, Seils D (2003) Clinical economics. In: Max M, Lynn J, eds. Interactive textbook on clinical symptom research. Bethesda: National Institutes of Health
44. Moreno-Ramirea D, Ferrandiz L, Ruiz-de-Casas A, Nieto-Garcia A, Moreno-Alvarez P, Galdeano R et al (2009) Economic evaluation of a store-and-forward teledermatology system for skin cancer patients. J Telemed Telecare 15:40–5
45. Thompson S, Barber J (2000) How should cost data in pragmatic randomised controlled trials be analysed? BMJ 320:1197–20
46. Ramsey S, Willke R, Briggs A, Brown R, Buxton M, Chawla A et al (2005) Best practices for economic evaluation alongside clinical trials: an ISPOR RCT-CEA task force report. Value Health 8:521–33
47. Heinen-Kammerer T, Daniel D, Stratmann L, Rychlik R, Boehncke W (2007) Cost-effectiveness of psoriasis therapy with etanercept in Germany. J Dtsch Dermatol Ges 5(9): 762–8
48. Jiang G, Wu J, Williams G (2000) Fieller's interval and the bootstrap-fieller interval for the incremental costeffectiveness ratio. Health Serv Outcome Res Methods 1(3–4): 291–303
49. Glick H, Doshi J, Sonnad S, Polsky D (2007) Economic evaluation in clinical trials. Oxford University Press, Oxford
50. TreeAge Software Inc. TreeAge Pro. Available from: http://www.treeage.com/products/overviewHealth.html. accessed March 27, 2009
51. Briggs A (1999) Handling uncertainty in economic evaluation. BMJ 319(7202):120
52. Drummond M (1996) Guidelines for authors and per reviewers of economic submissions to the BMJ. BMJ 313:275–83
53. Harris A, Hill S, Chin G, Li J, Walkom E (2008) The role of value for money in public insurance coverage decisions for drugs in Australia: a retrospective analysis 1994–2004. Med Decis Making 28:713–22
54. Tan-Torres Edejer T, Haltussen R, Adam T, Hutubesay R, Acharya A, Evans D et al (eds) (2003) Making choice in health: WHO guide to cost-effectiveness analysis. WHO, Geneva
55. De Portu S, Del Giglio M, Altomare G, Arcangeli F, Berardesca E, Pinton P, Lotti T et al (2010) Cost-effectiveness analysis of TNF-α blockers for the treatment of chronic plaque psoriasis in the perspective of the Italian health-care system. Dermatol Ther 23(1):S7–S13
56. Black W (1990) The CE plane. Med Decis Making 10(3): 212–4

Quality Assurance and Risk Management

20

Barbara Hofer, Christian Scheibböck, and Michael Binder

Core Messages

- Benchmarked guidelines, standards and quality management procedures for practicing teleconsultation have to be developed and adopted on a large scale.
- Successful teleconsultation services should be further transformed into a system of reliable and certified products and applications.
- Baseline, generic guidelines help ensure quality management across a broad range of different telemedicine services.
- In order to reduce and avoid human, technical and logistic errors and pitfalls, *checklists* have to be integrated into the practice of telemedicine.
- An appropriate illumination is important to obtain usable and diagnosable images.
- Filters can be useful to prepare the image or to emphasize relevant image areas.
- Because of potential loss of information, lossless image compression should be preferred rather than lossy compression.

B. Hofer (✉) • C. Scheibböck • M. Binder
Department of Dermatology, Division of General Dermatology, Medical University of Vienna,
Vienna, Austria
e-mail: barbara.hofer@meduniwien.ac.at;
christian.scheibboeck@meduniwien.ac.at;
michael.binder@meduniwien.ac.at

How Can the Teleconsultation Process Be Quality Proved?

Introduction

Without a doubt, the potential benefits of telemedicine are considered to be far-reaching and vast. "In the future, consulting and asking for a second opinion is likely be the gold standard of medical care…" [1] (Fig. 20.1).

If the above mentioned proposition shall become reality, there still remains substantial work to be done by professionals in the field of telemedicine. Even after a couple of decades of reports on successful (pilot-) projects, the majority of telemedicine services are yet to be implemented into greater (mainstream) health care systems. A considerable number of obstacles hinder and delay the implementation of telemedicine services on such a much greater scale. For example:

- Missing IT-standards and issues on interoperability
- Legal responsibilities, different regulations even within EU member states
- Remuneration for telemedicine services (provider and receiver)

H.P. Soyer et al. (eds.), *Telemedicine in Dermatology*,
DOI 10.1007/978-3-642-20801-0_20, © Springer-Verlag Berlin Heidelberg 2012

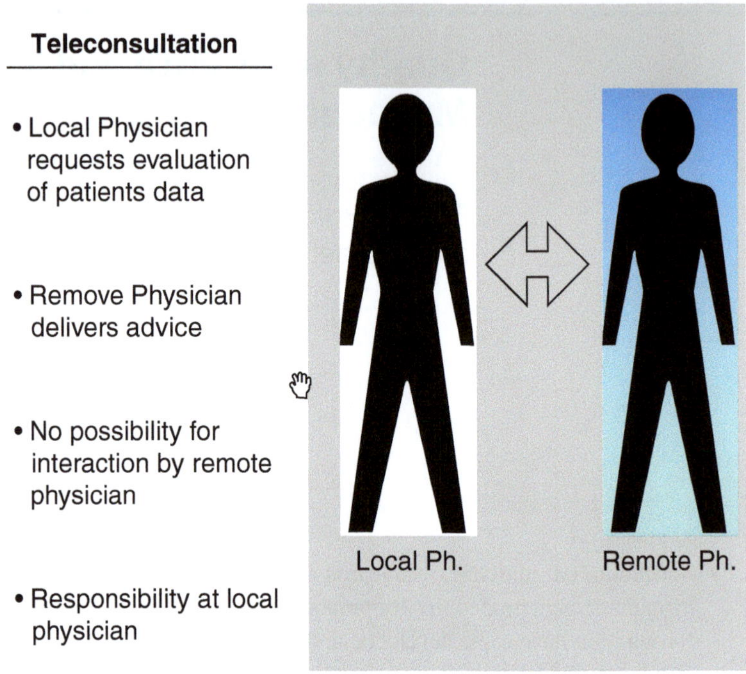

Fig. 20.1 Key facts: Teleconsultation between local and remote physician

Generic Guidelines for Teleconsultation Services

Eventually telemedicine should be considered as a potential alternative method of delivering health care. In that context that people are entitled to the same quality of care as provided through the conventional delivery of health care. Subsequently physicians and health care organizations are obliged to the same duty in the provision of health care irrespective of the systems they use to deliver health care [2, 3]. In Austria, like in the majority of countries worldwide, the legal duty of qualified care is the same for conventional medicine and for clinicians practicing telemedicine.

Although teleconsultation is nowadays used in a broad range of medical settings ranging from those "visual medical specialties" such as radiology, pathology, and dermatology, to other fields including gynecology, neurology and psychiatry – benchmarked guidelines, standards and quality management procedures for practicing teleconsultation have yet to be developed and adopted on a large scale.

Even though pilot projects can help identify and characterize crucial issues associated with successful telemedicine services overall, telemedicine systems developed, produced and implemented during (pilot) research projects have limited areas of application – therefore they cannot be easily integrated into a larger health care system and further developed to reach marketability without additional funding. In addition, differing proprietary systems in health care organizations (medical center, doctor's office etc.) can produce amongst others immense problems with interoperability and integration of different, *most of the times not-certified* telemedicine systems. This further complicates the process of developing teleconsultation services/systems/products to marketability. Hence there is considerable need to transform single successful (pilot) teleconsultation services into *a system of reliable and certified products and applications.*

Whereas standards and guidelines in the field of teleradiology are already developed and implemented to a much broader extent, the other fields of teleconsultation show a considerable lack of generally adopted *generic* standards, guidelines, policies and procedures.

Even though over the past years a great number of guidelines and reports by various organizations in the broad field of telemedicine and eHealth were developed, they are covering in the majority of cases specific questions for specialized topics and applications. A selection of a few examples for guidelines follows (not a comprehensive list):

- Practice Guidelines for Videoconferencing-Based Telemental Health. American Telemedicine Association (ATA). October 2009 [4].

- Practice Guidelines for Teledermatology. American Telemedicine Association (ATA). December 2007 [5].
- Core Standards for Telemedicine Operations. American Telemedicine Association (ATA). November 2007 [6].
- Telehealth Practice Recommendations for Diabetic Retinopathy. American Telemedicine Association (ATA). May 2004 [7].

Without a doubt, these are important steps in the right direction. But in our opinion, one of the limits to the widespread implementation of teleconsultation services (applications), products and systems is the above mentioned more or less considerable *lack of generic guidelines.* Pitfalls in the use of many differing sources for guidelines are the dangers of having redundant information sources in the best case, but contradicting guidelines in the worst case.

This chapter aims at presenting baseline, generic recommendations that help ensure quality management applicable across a broad range of different telemedicine services and varying geographic regions/areas. The recommendations in this chapter reflect the scientific evidence and state of knowledge at the current time.

General, Generic Guidelines for Teleconsultation Between Physicians

This chapter offers general, generic guidelines for teleconsultation between physicians, especially but not limited to those fields of teleconsultation where specific guidelines have yet to be implemented. These generic guidelines can be seen as framework to guide in the implementation of quality management principles.

(a) Definition of Inclusion/Exclusion Criteria
  - Definition of what happens in case of computer/network glitches
  - Backup communication, e.g. ISDN

(b) Define line of communication
  - A priori analysis
  - Planned mode of data transmission
  - Type of data transmitted

(c) Define system requirements
  - Computer hardware
  - Imaging hardware
  - Data compression/data format (e.g. DICOM)
  - Backup
  - Reliability of transmission line

(d) Reliability analysis
  - Contingency plan after system crash
  - Analysis of data integrity
  - Data modification after transmission
  - Uniqueness of data
  - Firewall efficacy

(e) Teaching and quality assurance
  - Defined training schedule for medical and non-medical personnel
  - Defined concept for quality assurance, e.g. test for cameras, screens

Responsibility Local Physician

- Have all necessary data at hand
- Identification of patient and patients data
- Archiving of transmitted and received data
- Compliance of local laws

Responsibility Remote Physician

- Check reliability of transmitted material (missing data, bad quality, obviously wrong data
- Archive received data
- Acknowledgement of data (sent and received)
- Documentation [8].

Towards a Quality Management of Teleconsultation Services

Alongside the development and implementation of adopted generic standards and procedures, quality management procedures and practices have to be developed and put into place [9].

Teleconsultation in the sense of consulting with one (or more) remote physician(s) by a locally present physician about a specific patient's medical case applying information and telecommunication technologies needs to be quality proved in the same or similar way as traditional medical consultations between two or more health care professionals. Based on our own experience, successfully organizing the quality management of teleconsultation services and applications is another key factor for implementing those systems on a larger scale.

Quality Management Systems (QMS)

There are different approaches to quality management (amongst others ISO 9000, TQM, Six Sigma), but in general a quality management system (QMS) describes the organizational structure, methods, processes, procedures and resources needed to implement quality management. To put it in other words, a certification to a certain quality management system's standard attests that formalized processes, methods, procedures etc. are being applied during the process of development and production of services or products.

Table 20.1 Exemplary ISO standards concerning telemedicine services

ISO/TR 16056–1:2004
Health informatics – interoperability of telehealth systems and networks – part 1: introductions and definitions [10]
ISO/TR 16056–2:2004
Health informatics – interoperability of telehealth systems and networks – part 2: real-time systems [11]
ISO/IEEE 11073–20601:2010
Health informatics – personal health device communication – part 20601: application profile – optimized exchange protocol [12]
ISO/IEEE 11073–10417:2010
Health informatics – personal health device communication – part 10417: device specialization – glucose meter [13]
ISO/IEEE 11073–10407:2010
Health informatics – personal health device communication – part 10407: device specialization – blood pressure monitor [14]
ISO/IEEE 11073–10404:2010
Health informatics – personal health device communication – part 10404: Device specialization – pulse oximeter [15]

For a (health care-)organization developing, using and offering telemedicine services, applications and products the International Organization for Standardization's ISO 9000 standards might be a useful quality management system.

Whereas *ISO 9000:2005* provides information about the fundamentals used in quality management systems, the *ISO 9001:2008* series addresses the principles and processes surrounding the design, development and delivery of a general product or service. Organizations can participate in a continuing certification process to ISO 9001:2005 to demonstrate their compliance with the standard, which includes a requirement for continual (i.e. planned) improvement of the QMS.

EN ISO 13485: 2003/AC:2007 describes required processes, procedures and resources needed during the development and manufacture of medical devices (Table 20.1).

Teleconsultation Workflow

In this chapter we introduce the general teleconsultation workflow as well as a comparison between the standard versus teleconsultation workflow.

General Teleconsultation Workflow

The general teleconsultation workflow – that is, the processes starting from the need for an expert/s opinion by the referring doctor until the delivery of the expected expert opinion can be outlined as follows (Fig. 20.2).

Comparison Standard Versus Teleconsultation Workflow

A comparison between the standard versus the teleconsultation workflow shows as the main difference the absence of personal, face-to-face contact between the patient and a medical expert without compromising on the standards of good medical care (Fig. 20.3).

Possible Errors in Consultations and Pitfalls

Various human, technical and logistic errors in telemedical consultations have to be avoided when practicing telemedicine. Practitioners in the various fields of telemedicine have to be aware of those pitfalls and take appropriate countermeasures (Table 20.2).

In order to reduce and avoid the above mentioned human, technical and logistic errors and pitfalls *checklists* have to be integrated in the practice of telemedicine. They are an excellent tool for error management and performance improvement. With the assistance of checklists mistakes can be avoided and overall outcomes can be improved.

Like any other medical procedure each telemedical procedure carries with it a probability of diagnostic and/or therapeutic risk. This chapter draws an outline of some of the fundamentals that are essential in developing and advancing successful risk management procedures in telemedical practice.

The essence of medical risk management in general and of telemedical risk management in particular is to provide safe diagnostic and therapeutic procedures for the patient. In that context medical risk management plays a crucial part in the development and advancement of continuing quality management initiatives. As already mentioned earlier in this chapter the authors consider checklists in (tele-)medicine as the key part in improving and guaranteeing medical care of highest standards.

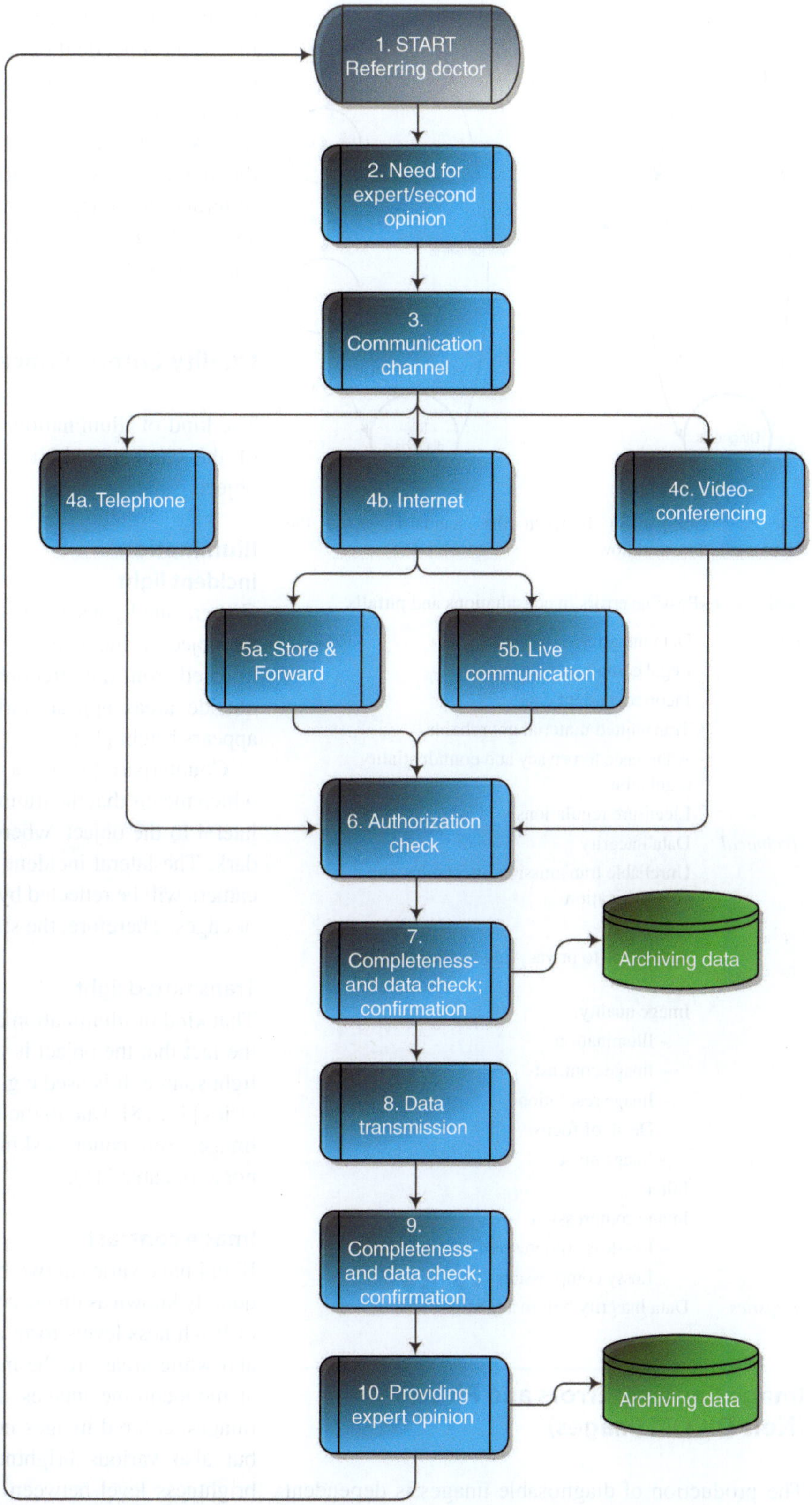

Fig. 20.2 General teleconsultation workflow

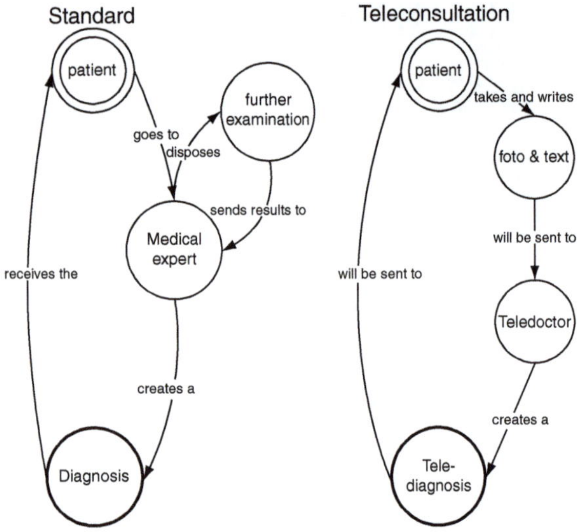

Fig. 20.3 Comparison between the standard versus the teleconsultation workflow

Table 20.2 Possible errors in consultations and pitfalls

Human	Data integrity
	Legal compliance
	Incorrect patient data
	Transmitted material not reliable
	Adherence to privacy and confidentiality regulation
	Licensure regulations
Technical	Data integrity
	Unreliable transmission line, no backup communication
	Firewall
	Adherence to privacy and confidentiality regulation
	Image quality:
	– Illumination
	– Image contrast
	– Image resolution
	– Depth of focus
	– Image noise
	Filter
	Image compression
	– Lossless compression
	– Lossy compression
logistics	Data integrity before and after transmission

Image Capture: Errors and Pitfalls (Non-DICOM Images)

The production of diagnosable images is dependent on camera quality and the skills/technique used by the photographer. The production of diagnosable images is dependent on camera quality and the skills/technique used by the photographer. It is apparent that different persons produce different image qualities. Also the camera constitutes a critical factor to the image quality. Furthermore, quality criterions like illumination, image contrast and image resolution should absolutely receive attention to produce optimal qualities [16].

Quality Criteria Concerning Image Quality

The kind of illumination results from the positioning of the camera and the illumination relative to the object.

Illumination

Incident light

Camera and light source are located at the same side as the object. If the object is at bright field, it will be illuminated from the direction of the camera. Therefore, outside areas appear dark whereas the object field appears bright [17].

Counterpart to the bright field is the dark field, which means that the illumination has a very low angle lateral to the object, whereby the object field appears dark. The lateral incident light in the direction of the camera will be reflected by the structures at the surface or edges. Therefore, the structures appear bright [17].

Transmitted light

That kind of illumination differs from incident light in the fact that the object is located between camera and light source. It is used e.g. for the measuring of geometries [17, 18]. Due to the fact that dermatologists take images from patient's skin, this kind of illumination is not applicable [16].

Image contrast

If an image varies in two brightness levels, it is consequently known as image contrast. More than two levels of brightness levels form a brightness gradient. Black and white areas are the maximum contrast difference at monochrome images. In contrast to monochrome images, colored images not only have various colors, but also various brightness levels. The higher the brightness level between two neighbored colors, the sharper the image will be perceived [19].

Image resolution

The technical ability of a camera to render fine structures is called image resolution. However, this ability can be influenced by several parameters:

- Quality of the lens
- Optimal focusing
- Aperture
- Shutter speed (risk of blurred images)
- Sensor
- Noise behavior of the sensors

Detail reproduction and image quality are determined by the weakest of these five parameters. Whereas in the past years the limiting factor concerning image quality was the number of pixels, nowadays the phenomenon of the optical diffraction can affect the image quality. The best imaging quality is in the centre of the image, whereby the image quality decreases steadily towards the image border. Therefore, it is decisive for detail reproduction to use a professional lens of high quality [20].

Depth of focus

Depth of focus is not primarily a quality factor of the lens, but rather a basic data attribute of the camera lens [18].

A substantial indicator for good image quality and an optimal depth of focus is the appropriate handling of cameras. During image taking, it is important that the camera is placed in an adequate distance to the photo motive. At a minimum distance of 10 cm with a physical focal distance of 5 mm, good cameras are able to take sharp images [16].

Image noise

Image noise describes the signal components in an image which are caused by thermally noise of the camera components or by transmission interferences. It can mainly occur as fluctuations in brightness which are detectable in dark image areas or as color stains. Higher sensitivity settings at the camera affect that the signal as well as image interferences and therefore image noise becomes intensified.

As in mentioned in Chap. 17, (see also 0) image processing can possibly suppress image noise. Such image processing methods mostly maintain edges and high contrasts, but single colored areas will become smoothed. Sometimes it can happen that the camera misrecognizes image details below a certain contrast as image noise. This means that these misrecognized areas will also become smoothed. Therefore it can entail a loss of structures [20–22].

Filter

To use noisy images there exists the opportunity to use image processing programs which include different image processing methods and algorithms. The elimination of the image noise effects that the image will be smoothed. Certainly, the higher the filter settings, the more details can be lost [23]. A further field of application for filters could be the image preparation. Sometimes it is helpful to intensify or extract the attributes of interest.

There are a large number of filters which can be used as single filter or cumulatively [24, 25]:

- Linear filter
- Median filter (non-linear filter)
- Sharpness filter
- Blur filter

Image Compression

Image compression describes the reorganization and reduction of image data volume. However, there are two kinds of compression algorithms. Lossless compression algorithms maintain the full image information and lossy algorithms accept a certain percentage of information loss. The higher the image compression, the higher is the information loss. According to this, there exist a variety of image formats to save images [26].

The quality of the compression algorithm can be characterized by two factors [26]:

- Compression factor – describes the relation between original size to the size of the compressed image.
- Compression method – lossless or lossy compression algorithms

Lossless compression

The relevance of lossless compression is justified by the fact that all pixels in every bit are identical to original data, after decompression. There exist various algorithms for lossy compression where the amount of image data can be reduced about factor 10–100. However in contrast to lossy compression, lossless compression is more difficult [26–28].

At lossless compression, redundancies will be recognized and summarized. Therefore, no information at all gets lost. More simply, repeating bit strings will be created once in a dictionary and then get only represented by a number.

The more same colored or similar patterned areas are available, the higher compression factors are possible. Color gradients can be decisive as well.

Rotation, mirroring and trimming of images are also image processing methods without loss of information [16].

Commonly used lossless algorithms among others are [29]:

- JPEG 2000 [28, 30]
- Run length encoding [28, 31]
- Lempel-Ziv-Welch algorithm (LZW) [28, 32]
- Huffman-coding [28, 33]

Lossy compression

By contrast to lossless algorithms, at lossy algorithms, high compression is of primary importance. Changes will be done on a scale that is still acceptable for the human eye, because these changes are hardly visible [16].

A typical compression algorithm for lossy compression is JPEG (Joint Photographic Expert Group), a well-known file format. JPEG uses the discrete cosine transform (DCT) to achieve a very high compression efficiency [34]. However, JPEG compression has visual problems. These are especially blocking (is caused by the partitioning of the image into small blocks) and ringing (is caused by the disadvantageous performance of the DCT at hard color transitions.

The compression of images to about 1.5–2 bit/pixel is visually lossless. 0.7–1 bit/pixel have good compression results, whereby at lower than 0.3 bit/pixel the JPEG is unusable (artefacts get out of hand) [29].

To sum up, the quality criterions concerning image quality an appropriate illumination is of utmost importance to obtain usable and diagnosable images. In addition filters can be useful to prepare the image or to emphasize relevant image areas. Because of potential loss of information, lossless image compression should be preferred rather than lossy compression.

References

1. Burg G et al (2005) Teledermatology: just cool or a real tool? Dermatology 210(2):169–173
2. Stanberry B (2000) Telemedicine: barriers and opportunities in the 21st century. J Intern Med 247(6):615–628
3. Wootton N (1998) Telemedicine in the National Health Service. J R Soc Med 91(12):614–621
4. Practice guidelines for videoconferencing-based telemental health. American Telemedicine Association (ATA), October 2009. Available from: http://www.americantelemed.org/files/public/standards/PracticeGuidelinesforVideoconferencing-Based TelementalHealth.pdf
5. Practice guidelines for teledermatology. American Telemedicine Association (ATA), December 2007. Available from: http://www.americantelemed.org/files/public/standards/Telederm_guidelines_v10final_withCOVER.pdf
6. Core standards for telemedicine operations. American Telemedicine Association (ATA), November 2007. Available from: http://www.americantelemed.org/files/public/standards/CoreStandards_withCOVER.pdf
7. Telehealth practice recommendations for diabetic retinopathy. American Telemedicine Association (ATA), May 2004. Available from: http://www.americantelemed.org/files/public/standards/DiabeticRetinopathy_withCOVER.pdf
8. Duftschmid G et al (2005) Guidelines for the planning and implementation of telemedical applications. Wien Kl Wochenschrift 117(19–20):673–683
9. Nerlich M et al (2002) Teleconsultation practice guidelines: report from G8 global health applications subproject 4. Telemed J E Health 8(4):411–418
10. ISO (2004) I.S.O., Interoperability of telehealth systems and networks – part 1: introductions and definitions. ISO/TR 16056–1: 2004. Available from: http://www.iso.org/iso/catalogue_detail?csnumber=37351
11. ISO (2004) I.S.O., Interoperability of telehealth systems and networks – part 2: real-time systems. ISO/TR 16056–2: 2004. Available from: http://www.iso.org/iso/catalogue_detail?csnumber=37352
12. ISO/IEEE 11073–20601:2010 Health informatics – personal health device communication – part 20601: application profile – optimized exchange protocol. Available from: http://www.iso.org/iso/iso_catalogue/catalogue_tc/catalogue_detail.htm?csnumber=54331
13. ISO/IEEE 11073–10417:2010 Health informatics – personal health device communication – part 10417: device specialization – glucose meter. Available from: http://www.iso.org/iso/iso_catalogue/catalogue_tc/catalogue_detail.htm?csnumber=54574
14. ISO/IEEE 11073–10407:2010 Health informatics – personal health device communication – part 10407: device specialization – blood pressure monitor. Available from: http://www.iso.org/iso/iso_catalogue/catalogue_tc/catalogue_detail.htm?csnumber=54573
15. ISO/IEEE 11073–10407:2010 Health informatics – personal health device communication – part 10404: device specialization – blood pressure monitor. Available from: http://www.iso.org/iso/iso_catalogue/catalogue_tc/catalogue_detail.htm?csnumber=54573
16. Scheibböck C (2008) Telemedizin in der dermatologie im rahmen einer klinischen studie - evaluation der verwendbarkeit der bilddaten mittels quantitativer bildanalyse. In: Department of dermatology. Technical University of Vienna, Vienna, p 96
17. Neumann B (2004) Bildverarbeitung für einsteiger: programmbeispiele mit mathcad. Springer, Berlin
18. Weissler GA (2007) Einführung in die industrielle bildverarbeitung. Franzis, Poing
19. Wikipedia, Kontrast. 2010

20. Wüller D (2007) Auflösung. Available from: http://6mpixel.org/?page_id=68
21. Huang HK (2004) PACS and imaging informatics: basic principles and applications, 2nd edn. Wiley-IEEE, Hoboken, N.J
22. Lehmann TM (2005) Digitale bildverarbeitung für routineanwendungen: evaluierung und integration am beispiel der medizin. DUV, Wiesbaden
23. Mainz A (2010) Bildrauschen. Available from: www.digitalfoto-tipps.de/content/view/13/32/1/1/
24. Erhardt A (2008) Einführung in die digitale bildverarbeitung: grundlagen, systeme und anwendungen. Springer, Wiesbaden
25. King JA (2002) Digitale Fotoretusche und-bearbeitung für Dummies.: Fotos reparieren und schöner machen, mitp-Verlag, Bonn
26. Barthel KU (2003) Lossless image compression, in it – information technology, p 9. FHTW Berlin. Available from: http://www.f4.htw-berlin.de/~barthel/paper/barthel_it.pdf; FHTW Berlin
27. Deever AT, Hemami SS (2003) Lossless image compression with projection-based and adaptive reversible integer wavelet transforms. IEEE Trans Image Process 12(5): 489–499
28. Dankmeier W (2006) Grundkurs codierung, 3rd edn. Vieweg+Teubner Verlag, New York
29. Salomon D (2007) Data compression: the complete reference, Band 10, 4th edn. Springer, London
30. Taubman DS, Marcellin MW (2002) JPEG2000: image compression fundamentals, standards, and practice, Band 1. Springer, Boston, Mass
31. Acharya T, Tsai PS (2004) JPEG2000 standard for image compression : concepts, algorithms and VLSI architectures, John Wiley & Sons, Hoboken, N.J
32. Slawsli D (2006) Digitale Bilder professionell bearbeiten. SmartBooks Publishing AG, Kilchberg
33. Blieberger J, Burgstaller B, Schildt G-H (2001) Informatik: grundlagen, 4th edn. Springer, Vennia
34. Pennebaker WB, Mitchell JL (2004) JPEG : still image data compression standard, Kluwer, Boston, Mass

Index

H.P. Soyer et al. (eds.), *Telemedicine in Dermatology*,
DOI 10.1007/978-3-642-20801-0, © Springer-Verlag Berlin Heidelberg 2012

MIX
Papier aus verantwortungsvollen Quellen
Paper from responsible sources
FSC® C105338

If you have any concerns about our products,
you can contact us on
ProductSafety@springernature.com

In case Publisher is established outside the EU,
the EU authorized representative is:
Springer Nature Customer Service Center GmbH
Europaplatz 3, 69115 Heidelberg, Germany

Printed by Libri Plureos GmbH
in Hamburg, Germany